ADVANCES IN MEDICAL ONCOLOGY, RESEARCH AND EDUCATION

Volume IV

BIOLOGICAL BASIS FOR CANCER DIAGNOSIS

ADVANCES IN MEDICAL ONCOLOGY, RESEARCH AND EDUCATION

Proceedings of the 12th International Cancer Congress,
Buenos Aires, 1978

General Editors: A. CANONICO, O. ESTEVEZ, R. CHACON and S. BARG, Buenos Aires

Volumes and Editors:

   I - CARCINOGENESIS. *Editor:* G. P. Margison

  II - CANCER CONTROL. *Editors:* A. Smith and C. Alvarez

 III - EPIDEMIOLOGY. *Editor:* Jillian M. Birch

 IV - BIOLOGICAL BASIS FOR CANCER DIAGNOSIS. *Editor:* Margaret Fox

  V - BASIS FOR CANCER THERAPY 1. *Editor:* B. W. Fox

 VI - BASIS FOR CANCER THERAPY 2. *Editor:* M. Moore

 VII - LEUKEMIA AND NON-HODGKIN LYMPHOMA. *Editor:* D. G. Crowther

VIII - GYNECOLOGICAL CANCER. *Editor:* N. Thatcher

 IX - DIGESTIVE CANCER. *Editor:* N. Thatcher

  X - CLINICAL CANCER - PRINCIPAL ŞITES 1. *Editor:* S. Kumar

 XI - CLINICAL CANCER - PRINCIPAL SITES 2. *Editor:* P. M. Wilkinson

 XII - ABSTRACTS

(Each volume is available separately.)

Pergamon Journals of Related Interest

ADVANCES IN ENZYME REGULATION
COMPUTERIZED TOMOGRAPHY
EUROPEAN JOURNAL OF CANCER
INTERNATIONAL JOURNAL OF RADIATION ONCOLOGY, BIOLOGY, PHYSICS
LEUKEMIA RESEARCH

ADVANCES IN MEDICAL ONCOLOGY, RESEARCH AND EDUCATION

Proceedings of the 12th International Cancer Congress,
Buenos Aires, 1978

Volume IV
BIOLOGICAL BASIS FOR CANCER DIAGNOSIS

Editor:

MARGARET FOX

Department of Experimental Chemotherapy
Paterson Laboratories
Christie Hospital and Holt Radium Institute
Manchester

PERGAMON PRESS

OXFORD · NEW YORK · TORONTO · SYDNEY · PARIS · FRANKFURT

U.K.	Pergamon Press Ltd., Headington Hill Hall, Oxford OX3 0BW, England
U.S.A.	Pergamon Press Inc., Maxwell House, Fairview Park, Elmsford, New York 10523, U.S.A.
CANADA	Pergamon of Canada, Suite 104, 150 Consumers Road, Willowdale, Ontario M2J 1P9, Canada
AUSTRALIA	Pergamon Press (Aust.) Pty. Ltd., P.O. Box 544, Potts Point, N.S.W. 2011, Australia
FRANCE	Pergamon Press SARL, 24 rue des Ecoles, 75240 Paris, Cedex 05, France
FEDERAL REPUBLIC OF GERMANY	Pergamon Press GmbH, 6242 Kronberg-Taunus, Pferdstrasse 1, Federal Republic of Germany

First edition 1979

British Library Cataloguing in Publication Data

International Cancer Congress, 12th, Buenos Aires, 1978
Advances in medical oncology, research and education.
Vol.4: Biological basis for cancer diagnosis
1. Cancer - Congresses
I. Title II. Fox, Margaret III. Canonico, A
616.9'94   RC261.A1   79-40469
ISBN 0-08-024387-8
ISBN 0-08-023777-0 Set of 12 vols.

In order to make this volume available as economically and as rapidly as possible the authors' typescripts have been reproduced in their original forms. This method unfortunately has its typographical limitations but it is hoped that they in no way distract the reader.

Printed and bound at William Clowes & Sons Limited Beccles and London

Contents

Biological Changes in Human Cancer

Foreword

This book contains papers from the main meetings of the Scientific Programme presented during the 12th International Cancer Congress, which took place in Buenos Aires, Argentina, from 5 to 11 October 1978, and was sponsored by the International Union against Cancer (UICC).

This organisation, with headquarters in Geneva, gathers together from more than a hundred countries 250 medical associations which fight against Cancer and organizes every four years an International Congress which gives maximum coverage to oncological activity throughout the world.

The 11th Congress was held in Florence in 1974, where the General Assembly unanimously decided that Argentina would be the site of the 12th Congress. Argentina was chosen not only because of the beauty of its landscapes and the cordiality of its inhabitants, but also because of the high scientific level of its researchers and practitioners in the field of oncology.

From this Assembly a distinguished International Committee was appointed which undertook the preparation and execution of the Scientific Programme of the Congress.

The Programme was designed to be profitable for those professionals who wished to have a general view of the problem of Cancer, as well as those who were specifically orientated to an oncological subspeciality. It was also conceived as trying to cover the different subjects related to this discipline, emphasizing those with an actual and future gravitation on cancerology.

The scientific activity began every morning with a Special Lecture (5 in all), summarizing some of the subjects of prevailing interest in Oncology, such as Environmental Cancer, Immunology, Sub-clinical Cancer, Modern Cancer Therapy Concepts and Viral Oncogenesis. Within the 26 Symposia, new acquisitions in the technological area were incorporated; such acquisitions had not been exposed in previous Congresses.

15 Multidisciplinary Panels were held studying the more frequent sites in Cancer, with an approach to the problem that included biological and clinical aspects, and concentrating on the following areas: aetiology, epidemiology, pathology, prevention, early detection, education, treatment and results. Preferred Papers were presented as Workshops instead of the classical reading, as in this way they could be discussed fully by the participants. 66 Workshops were held, this being the first time that free communications were presented in this way in a UICC Congress.

The Programme also included 22 "Meet the Experts", 7 Informal Meetings and more
than a hundred films.

METHODOLOGY

The methodology used for the development of the Meeting and to make the scientific
works profitable, had some original features that we would like to mention.

The methodology used in Lectures, Panels and Symposia was the usual one utilized
in previous Congresses and functions satisfactorily. Lectures lasted one hour each.
Panels were seven hours long divided into two sessions, one in the morning and one
in the afternoon. They had a Chairman and two Vice-chairmen (one for each session).
Symposia were three hours long. They had a Chairman, a Vice-chairman and a Secretary

Of the 8164 registered members, many sent proferred papers of which over 2000 were
presented. They were grouped in numbers of 20 or 25, according to the subject, and
discussed in Workshops. The International Scientific Committee studied the abstracts
of all the papers, and those which were finally approved were sent to the Chairman
of the corresponding Workshop who, during the Workshop gave an introduction and
commented on the more outstanding works. This was the first time such a method had
been used in an UICC Cancer Congress.

"Meet the Experts" were two hours long, and facilitated the approach of young professionals to the most outstanding specialists. The congress was also the ideal place
for an exchange of information between the specialists of different countries during
the Informal Meetings. Also more than a hundred scientific films were shown.

The size of the task carried out in organising this Congress is reflected in some
statistical data: More than 18,000 letters were sent to participants throughout the
world; more than 2000 abstracts were published in the Proceedings of the Congress;
more than 800 scientists were active participants of the various meetings.

There were 2246 papers presented at the Congress by 4620 authors from 80 countries.

The Programme lasted a total of 450 hours, and was divided into 170 scientific
meetings where nearly all the subjects related to Oncology were discussed.

All the material gathered for the publication of these Proceedings has been taken
from the original papers submitted by each author. The material has been arranged
in 12 volumes, in various homogenous sections, which facilitates the reading of the
most interesting individual chapters. Volume XII deals only with the abstracts of
proffered papers submitted for Workshops and Special Meetings. The titles of each
volume offer a clear view of the extended and multidisciplinary contents of this
collection which we are sure will be frequently consulted in the scientific libraries.

We are grateful to the individual authors for their valuable collaboration as they
have enabled the publication of these Proceedings, and we are sure Pergamon Press
was a perfect choice as the Publisher due to its responsibility and efficiency.

Argentina   Dr Abel Canónico
March 1979   Dr Roberto Estevez
                                        Dr Reinaldo Chacon
                                        Dr Solomon Barg

                                        General Editors

Introduction

The multidisciplinary attack on the problem of malignant disease is well illustrated in this volume. Many of the contributions are aimed at understanding the changes which occur in malignant cells at a molecular level and their biological significance. Such changes are thought to be the result of altered gene expression resulting in changes in the numbers and identity of proteins found in malignant cells both within the nucleus and cytoplasm and expressed on the cell surface.

At a clinical level alterations in gene expression in malignant cells result in paraneoplastic syndromes; this topic, the possible usefulness of "tumour markers" in monitoring the response of neoplastic disease to therapy, and the problems of screening for sub-clinical cancer, are also well covered.

March 1979   MARGARET FOX

Cell Biology and Cancer

Control of DNA Synthesis in Normal and Cancer Cells

José Mordoh

*Department of Cancerology, Fundación Centro de Investigaciones Médicas
Albert Einstein, Luis Viale 2831, (1416) Buenos Aires, Argentina*

ABSTRACT

DNA replication in eukaryotic cells is a complex process involving many different steps, the nature of which is still poorly understood. The present knowledge on eukaryotic DNA polymerases is briefly reviewed, and evidence is presented suggesting that in stimulated lymphocytes there are two distinct DNA polymerases-α. The utility of cancer cells as natural mutants to elucidate some aspects of DNA biosynthesis is illustrated, and the presence of an altered nuclear DNA polymerase in a case of acute lymphoblastic leukemia is reported. The presence of genetic diseases and in vitro conditional mutants with alterations in DNA replication is discussed. The role of the different factors involved in DNA synthesis may be investigated through the analysis of in vitro systems: permeabilized cells, isolated nuclei, subcellular extracts. Experiments on permeabilized lymphocytes are reported demonstrating that deoxyribonucleoside triphosphates may enter these cells and that dCTP is a precursor in vitro both to DNA and to phosphatidyl–dCMP.

INTRODUCTION

DNA replication in eukaryotic cells is a highly complex process involving many different metabolic reactions, highly coordinated between them. In spite of the effort dedicated to their study the nature of many of these reactions and how they are regulated is far from understood. The knowledge in this field, which has been recently reviewed by Sheinin, Humbert and Pearlman (1978), lays behind that of DNA replication in prokaryotes, where the last 10 years have witnessed a remarkable progress in our understanding of DNA replication. An essential factor which contributed to the achievements in the latter field was the extensive use of genetics which through the obtention of conditional mutants of DNA synthesis and its manipulation permitted the analysis of the intervening factors in DNA replication (Hirota and others, 1972).

Conditional mutants in eukaryotic cells are more difficult to obtain and characterize, and the role of the different factors involved in DNA synthesis has been studied mainly through the analysis of a great variety of cellular systems ranging from normal cells to tumor cells either growing in vivo or which have been transformed in vitro. The emerging picture from these studies suggest that the concept of units of

3

DNA replication or replicons initially proposed for prokaryotes (Jacob, Brenner and
Cuzin, 1963) may also apply to eukaryotes. There is already genetic, biochemical
and biophysical evidence that indicates that the simple genomes of the viruses of
the eukaryotic cells (e.g. papovaviruses, adenoviruses and herpes viruses) can be
classified as replicons. Although the replicons of the eukaryotic genome cannot
still be identified, we are able to define replication units. They consist of a
segment of DNA double helix varying from 10-100 μm lenght and operationally defined
from origin to terminus. The replication units appear to be tandemly arranged within the chromosomal DNA in clusters composed of 2 to 250 units. The DNA synthesis
is initiated at an origin within the replication unit and proceeds bidirectionally
by the movement of two replication forks toward the two distant termini.

With respect to the role of the different factors involved in eukaryotic DNA replication, the diversity of systems utilized for its study obviously makes it difficult
to interpret the information obtained since many observed characteristics may be peculiar to one type of cell or be determined by its growth conditions and may not be
applicable to other cells. This inconvenient appears specially when DNA replication
is analyzed in cells which have undergone a cancerous transformation and where, almost by definition, a mutation(s) has occurred somewhere in the chain of events controlling cell division. However, since cancer cells are "natural mutants" their
analysis could help to understand some features of DNA synthesis in their normal
counterparts, and it would be preferable that experimental systems be used where
this correlation is possible. Also, since many chemotherapic agents act through
the inhibition of DNA synthesis at some step, knowledge gained on any existing difference between normal and cancer cells could be useful to design more effective
and selective chemotherapic agents or to obtain better results with the existing
ones. The work which will be presented here will deal with two aspects of DNA synthesis. Our present knowledge on DNA polymerases will be briefly reviewed, and data from our laboratory will be presented demonstrating how the use of cancer cells
as "spontaneous mutants" may help to clarify some obscure points. The second aspect to be treated refers to the use of in vitro systems for the analysis of DNA
synthesis.

                    RESULTS

DNA Polymerases in Eukaryotic Cells
During the past few years considerable information has accumulated concerning the
type and number of DNA polymerases in eukaryotic cells, and the field has been recently reviewed (Weissbach, 1977). Due to the diversity of eukaryotic tissues
studied there was a great variety of nomenclatures for DNA polymerases, and in
1975 it was decided to establish a uniform system of nomenclature (Weissbach and
others, 1975). Only the enzyme classes representing distinct entities were included, and were named with Greek letters according to the order of discovery. In
this system were not included the reverse transcriptases or RNA tumor virus associated DNA polymerases, neither the virus induced DNA polymerases. Four polymerase
classes were identified:

1) DNA polymerase-α. It is the high molecular weight (> 100.000) DNA polymerase, first identified in calf thymus extracts almost 20 years ago (Bollum, 1960).
This enzyme is mainly detected in the cytoplasmic extracts of growing cells, but

when non aqueous solvents are used to break the cells, most of the activity is
found in the cell nucleus. The α -polymerase is particularly active in copying "activated" double stranded DNA, and it is inhibited when sulfhydryl groups are blocked. It has recently been purified to near homogeneity and was shown to be a dimer composed of two dissimilar subunits of 76.000 and 66.000 daltons present in
equimolar ratio (Fisher and Korn, 1977).

2) DNA polymerase-β: It is the low molecular weight enzyme (30.000–50.000) detected mainly in nuclear extracts (Weissbach and others, 1971). It is an ubiquitous
enzyme in the animal kingdom but it is absent in bacteria, plants and protozoa
(Chang, 1976). This enzyme is resistant to the blocking of sulfhydryl groups and
in the presence of an activated DNA template has a significant ability to incorporate a single deoxynucleoside triphosphate in the absence of the other three depending on the DNA: enzyme ratio (Franze de Fernández, Mordoh and Fridlender, 1975).

3) DNA polymerase-γ. This is the most recently described DNA polymerase that co-
pies preferently $An:dT_{\overline{15}}$ rather than natural or synthetic DNA templates (Fridlender
and others, 1972), and it is inhibited by sulfhydryl blocking compounds.

4) Mitochondrial (mt) DNA polymerase. This enzyme is separable from the others and
it is so named for its subcellular localization (Meyer and Simpson, 1968). However,
recent studies suggest that this enzyme may be a form of DNA polymerase-γ (Bolden,
Noy and Weissbach, 1977).

The physiological role of each of the DNA polymerases is still unclear. Most of the
studies performed to ascribe a role to the DNA polymerases have been correlative,
consisting in the measure of DNA polymerase activities under varying conditions of
growth or quiescence. In general, it has been found that in growing cells the predominant activity is the DNA polymerase-α while in resting cells the predominant
activity belongs to DNA polymerase-β (Weissbach, 1977).

Our studies on the control of DNA replication have been mainly done using the system
of human peripheral blood lymphocytes. While these cells are normally resting, they
can be induced to proliferate by a variety of substances such as phytohemagglutinin
(PHA) (Nowell, 1960). The DNA polymerase activities of non stimulated lymphocytes
were analyzed by DE52 column chromatography. In the cytoplasmic fraction (Fig. 1A)
the presence of two peaks of activity were observed, CI_n and CII_n, which eluted at
0.07 M NaCl and 0.13 M NaCl respectively. The soluble nuclear fraction showed a
single peak of activity, designed as NI_n, which did not adsorb to DE52 (Fig. 1B).

When the DNA polymerases from stimulated lymphocytes were analyzed by DE52 column
chromatography, the pattern shown in Fig. 2 was generally observed. In the cytoplasm
there was a single peak of activity (CII_s) eluting at 0.12 M NaCl (Fig. 2A) while in
the soluble nuclear fraction two peaks of activity appeared (Fig. 2B): NI_n which
did not adsorb to DE52, while the second peak, NII_s, eluted at 0.07 M NaCl.

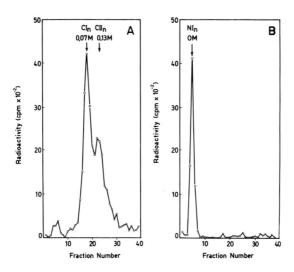

Fig. 1. DNA polymerase DNA dependent activities from non stimulated lymphocytes. The cytoplasmic (A) and nuclear soluble fractions (B) were chromatographed on DE52 cellulose (data from Fridlender and others, 1974).

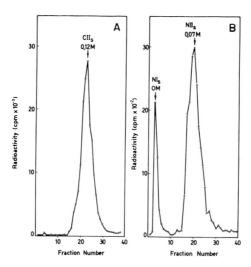

Fig. 2. DNA polymerase DNA dependent activities from stimulated lymphocytes. The cytoplasmic (A) and nuclear soluble fractions (B) were chromatographed on DE52 cellulose (data from Fridlender and others, 1974).

In some preparations of stimulated lymphocytes, however, two peaks of DNA polymerase activity were detected in the cytoplasm, CI_s and CII_s, eluting from the DE52 column at 0.07 M NaCl and 0.14 M NaCl respectively (Fig. 3A), while in the nuclear soluble fraction, besides the NI_s and NII_s enzymes, a small peak of activity eluting
at 0.12 M ($NIII_s$) was also observed (Fig. 3B).

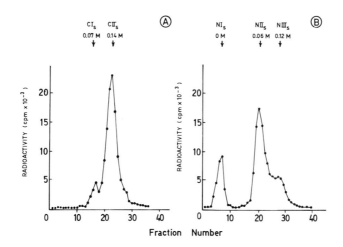

Fig. 3.   DNA polymerase DNA dependent activities from stimu-
           lated lymphocytes. The cytoplasmic (A) and nuclear
           soluble fractions (B) were chromatographed on DE52
           cellulose.   The measurement of the enzyme activity
           was performed as described by Fridlender and others
           (1974).

It is generally assumed that the DNA polymerase-α located in the cytoplasm and the
nucleus is the same enzyme (Weissbach, 1975) and recent reports suggest that the cytoplasmic enzyme is found there because it leaks from the nuclei when aqueous media
are used to homogeneize the cells (Foster and Gurney, 1976; Herrick, Spear and
Veomett, 1976). Our results, however, demonstrated a reproducible difference in the
chromatographic behaviour between the cytoplasmic CII_s and NII_s enzymes (Fig. 2A and
2B). In some preparations (Fig. 3) these two enzyme activities eluting at about
0.07 M NaCl and 0.14 M NaCl appeared both in the cytoplasm and in the nucleus although in inverse proportions. These activities could not be distinguished by their
salt requirements or template specificity (Fridlender and others, 1974) neither by
their sedimentation properties, where they behaved as DNA polymerase-α (Mordoh,
Fridlender and Virasoro, unpublished results). When these enzymes were further purified through a phosphocellulose column, they still showed a small difference in
their chromatographic behaviour (Medrano and Mordoh, unpublished results).

At this point the doubt existed if they were in fact two distinct DNA polymerases
or if they were the same enzyme, one of them complexed with substances which altered its chromatographic behaviour.

Strong evidence that these enzymes are in fact different proteins came from studies
performed on patients with acute lymphoblastic leukemia (Mordoh and Fridlender,
1975). The chromatographic analysis of the DNA polymerases isolated from leukemic
cells revealed in general a similar pattern to that of stimulated lymphocytes.   In
the cytoplasm there was a main peak of activity eluting from the column at 0.12 M
NaCl (CII_1) with a small shoulder of activity eluting at a concentration of 0.07 M
NaCl (Fig. 4A).   In the nuclear extract two peaks were observed, one not adsorbing
to the column and the other eluting at 0.07 M NaCl (Fig. 4B).

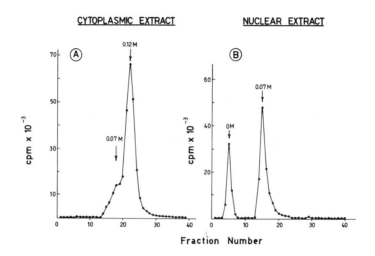

Fig. 4.   DNA polymerase DNA dependent activities from leuke-
          mic cells. The cytoplasmic (A) and nuclear soluble
          fractions (B) were chromatographed on DE52 cellulo-
          se (data from Mordoh and Fridlender, 1975).

When the requirements of the NII enzyme isolated from leukemic cells were compared
with those of the same enzyme isolated from normal stimulated lymphocytes, it was
found that they were generally similar.   In one patient, however, there was a striking difference in the KCl effect (Table 1).   While the normal enzyme was strongly
inhibited by 0.2 M KCl, the enzyme isolated from the nuclei of leukemic cells was
not affected by this salt concentration.   This effect suggested a difference between the normal and the leukemic enzymes.   When the KCl effect was studied in more
detail, a marked difference between the NII DNA polymerases from normal and leukemic cells was observed (Fig. 5A).   Since the NII enzyme had an altered sensitivity
to KCl, this peculiarity could be used to determine if the nuclear and cytoplasmic
DNA polymerases were in fact the same protein.   The CII_1 DNA polymerase is fully
inhibited by KCl in a manner similar to the cytoplasmic and nuclear enzymes isolated from normal cells.   However, when the small shoulder of activity eluting at
0.07 M (CI_1) was analyzed, the salt response mimics that of the NII_1 enzyme (Fig.
5B).

TABLE 1.   Requirements of the NII nuclear DNA polymerase.
The enzymes used were the peak activities obtained after
DEAE-cellulose column chromatography.

Reaction mixture	Normal enzyme	Leukemic enzyme
	% Activity	
Complete	100	100
Omit bovine serum albumin	0	1.9
Omit dithiothreitol	2.5	9.5
Omit dATP, dCTP, dGTP	27	39
Omit Mg^{++}, add 0.5 mM Mn^{++}	25	26
Plus 0.2 M KCl	31	112
Omit activated DNA, plus native DNA (62 µg)	5	6
Omit activated DNA, plus heated DNA (62 µg)	2	3

These results suggest that the cytoplasmic DNA polymerase CI_1 and the nuclear DNA polymerase NII_1 are the same enzyme, and that the cytoplasmic CII enzyme is a different protein.

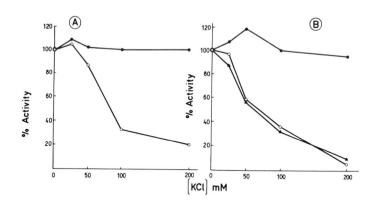

Fig. 5.   Effect of KCl on DNA polymerase activity from normal PHA stimulated lymphocytes and leukemic cells.
Reactions were carried out using lyophilized enzymes. KCl was added at the indicated concentrations.
A. Nuclear DNA polymerase: o NII_S; ● NII_1. B. Cytoplasmic enzymes: ● CI_1; o CII_1; ▲ CI_S (Mordoh and
Fridlender, 1975).

When the normal and leukemic enzymes were challenged by antiserum anti-DNA polymera-se-α (kindly provided by DR. A. Weissbach) the leukemic NII enzyme was resistant to it (Fig. 6).

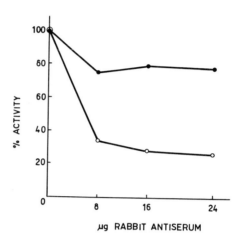

μg RABBIT ANTISERUM

Fig. 6.   Effect of antibody on NII DNA polymerases.   The lyophilized enzymes were mixed with 130 μg bovine serum
albumin and 80 nmoles Hepes buffer, pH 7.5, in a total volume of 15 μl and incubated 20 min. at room
temperature with varying amounts of antibody against
HeLa cytoplasmic DNA polymerase-α.   Afterwards, the
enzymes were assayed for activity.   o NII$_s$; • NII$_1$.
(Mordoh and Fridlender, 1975).

These findings provide support to the notion that at least in stimulated lymphocytes and leukemic lymphoblasts there are two different DNA polymerase-α: one activity elutes from DEAE at about 0.12 M NaCl and is recovered usually in the cytoplasm; the other DNA polymerase-α elutes from DEAE at 0.07 M NaCl and is detected in the nu-clear fraction.   In order to explain the discrepancy with the results indicating identity between the cytoplasmic and nuclear enzymes with respect to the reactivity towards antibody against DNA polymerase-α (Spadari, Muller and Weissbach, 1974) it might be assumed that the high MW DNA polymerases have very similar properties and that they share some common peptides.   In view of these results, and taking into ac-count the reports suggesting that the presence of the cytoplasmic DNA polymerase-α is an artifact due to the homogeneization procedures usually employed, the following scheme is proposed (Fig. 7).   In the nuclei of growing cells there would normally be three distinct DNA polymerases: The NI DNA polymerase-β; the NII DNA polymerase-α and the NIII DNA polymerase-α.   The first two would be firmly attached to the chro-matin and would not be dislodged by the usual homogeneization procedures.   The NIII enzyme would be loosely attached to nuclear structures, leaking from the nuclei when the cells are disrupted.

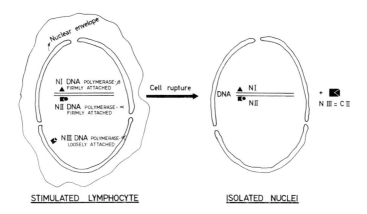

Fig. 7.   Scheme of the distribution of eukaryotic DNA polymerases.

The significance of the alteration of the NII enzyme in patients with acute lymphoblastic leukemia is difficult to assess. Springgate and Loeb (1973) showed that
cell free extracts from patients with acute lymphatic leukemia had a DNA polymerase
activity that copied a synthetic template with a higher level of infidelity than the
normal enzyme. It is tempting to correlate the alteration of the NII enzyme with
the disturbance of DNA replication in leukemic cells, but the generality of these
observations will have to be extended.

Genetic studies in DNA replication.

The importance of the availability of mutant cells with specific and well characterized defects in DNA replication has already been stressed, and example of the utility of the analysis of cancer cells as natural mutants has been shown above. There
are also a number of recessively inherited human disorders, where the affected individuals are cancer prone (German, 1972). Three of these disorders - xeroderma pig-
mentosum (XP), ataxia telangiectasia (AT) and Fanconi's anemia (FA) - are associated
with defects in the ability of cells to repair certain kinds of physical or chemical
damage to their DNA (Setlow, 1978). A number of human genetically determined diseases where the cells have a defect in DNA synthesis is shown in Table 2. The analysis and comprehension at the molecular level of the alterations in the repair of
DNA and in the normal process of chromosome replication which take place in these
diseases will undoubtedly contribute to understand the normal processes of DNA replication and the relationship between unrepaired DNA damage and carcinogenesis.

A number of eukaryotic conditional mutants affected in DNA replication have been
isolated (Sheinin, Humbert and Pearlman, 1978). These can be subdivided into mu-

tants that block the entry into the S phase or which block directly DNA synthesis. Again, much work is still needed before a coherent picture of the factors involved in DNA synthesis is obtained.

TABLE 2. Human diseases with mutations affecting DNA replication

Disease	Function affected	References
Xeroderma pigmentosum (XP)	Repair replication	Cleaver and Bootsma (1975)
Ataxia telangectasia (AT)	Repair replication	Hand (1977); Lehman and Stevens (1977)
Fanconi's anemia (FA)	Repair replication	Fujiwara, Tatsumi and Sasaki (1977); Sasaki and Tonomura (1973)
Bloom's syndrome (BS)	Repair replication and elongation of intermediates in DNA replication	Gianelli and others (1977)
Megaloblastic anemia (MA)	Elongation of intermediates in DNA replication	Hoffbrand and others (1976)

In vitro DNA replication. The advantages of studying a biochemical process in vitro is that the components of the reaction can be varied at will and the role of each one may be investigated. However, when purified cell components are used, many of the features imposed by the structural organization of the cell are lost. A degree of compromise between intact cells and extremely purified cell components must then be achieved. In the search of such a compromise, DNA synthesis has been studied in permeabilized whole cells, in lysates of whole cells, in isolated nuclei and in subnuclear preparations. Studies performed in our laboratory have demonstrated that nuclei isolated from non stimulated lymphocytes were able to synthesize DNA almost as efficiently as nuclei isolated from stimulated lymphocytes (Fridlender, Medrano and Mordoh, 1974). This observation suggested that the lack of available precursors could be a limiting step of DNA synthesis in non stimulated lymphocytes. However, since the rate of DNA synthesis in isolated nuclei was low as compared to in vivo rate, the possibility also existed that DNA synthesis of nuclei from stimulated cells could be greatly diminished. This slow rate could be atributed to two major factors: the loss or inactivation during isolation of some intranuclear substances essential for DNA replication (Herrick, Spear and Veomett, 1976; Foster and Gurney, 1974)or the lack of cytoplasmic factors which would be required for DNA replication (Jazwinski, Wang and Edelman, 1976; Jazwinski and Edelman, 1976). The use of cells permeabilized may help to answer some questions on the regulation of

DNA synthesis. When permeabilized lymphocytes are used, deoxyribonucleoside triphosphates may enter the cell and DNA is synthesized with an efficiency of about 50
percent respect to <u>in vivo</u>. Proteins of a molecular weight about 30.000 are also
able to enter permeabilized lymphocytes (Pszenny and Mordoh, unpublished results).
An aspect of the cellular changes induced by permeabilization is shown in Fig. 8.

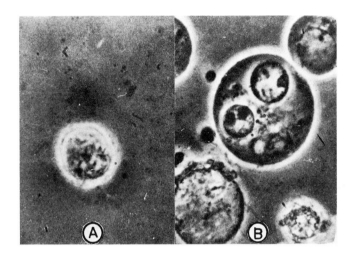

Fig. 8.   Effect of permeabilization on RAJI lymphoblastoid
          cells. Appearance to the phase contrast microscope
          of intact RAJI cells (A) or after standing for 30
          min. in 37° in the permeabilizing mixture (50 mM
          Hepes pH 7.9; 5 mM MgCl$_2$; 1 mM DTT; 0.5 mM ATP-Mg^{++};
          50 μM dNTPs) (B). Magnification: 1000 x

The metabolic alterations which take place in permeabilized cells may be helpful to
detect biochemical reactions which could otherwise escape notice. When DNA synthe-

TABLE 3.   dNTPs incorporation by permeabilized cells

Radioactive precursor	pmoles dNTP incorporated per 1 x 10^6 cells
(^{3}H)TTP	0.080
(^{3}H)dATP	0.154
(^{3}H)dCTP	2.76
(^{3}H)dGTP	0.45

sis was studied in permeabilized lymphocytes using deoxyribonucleotide triphospha-

tes as precursors, it was noticed that the incorporation of dCTP into an acid precipitable fraction was considerably higher than that of the other dNTPs (Table 3),
(Mordoh and Fridlender, 1977).

Product analysis demonstrated that (^3H)dCTP gave rise to DNA and to a compound solu-
ble in organic solvents. This compound has now been identified as phosphatidyl-dCMP
(Medrano and Mordoh, in press) and it has also been found to be synthesized in vivo
(Medrano and Mordoh, in preparation).

The system of permeabilized cells is now being actively studied (Berger and Johnson,
1976; Castellot, Miller and Pardee, 1978; Miller, Castellot and Pardee, 1978; Seki,
Lemamen and Mueller, 1975; Seki and Oda, 1977a, 1977b) and, together with the knowledge derived from the study of other subcellular systems, should provide valuable
information on the normal control of DNA synthesis and its alterations.

CONCLUSIONS

Our knowledge of DNA replication is still in the descriptive state. The proteins
involved are yet being characterized, and a better understanding of the role of histones, unwinding proteins and other chromatin proteins in the overall process must
still be acquired. The role of the different factors acting in DNA replication will
probably begin to be understood through the analysis of the different systems analyzed in this paper: cancer cells considered as natural mutants, genetic diseases
with known defects in DNA replication, in vitro produced conditional mutants, viral
infected cells, in vitro systems. Through this analysis it will be possible in a
not too distant future to identify the normal features of DNA replication and the
specific alterations taking place in cancer cells.

ACKNOWLEDGEMENTS

This work was supported by grant GM 19808 of the National Institutes of Health
(U. S. A.) and by grants from the Consejo Nacional de Investigaciones Científicas y
Técnicas (Argentina). José Mordoh is a Research Career Investigator of the latter
institution.

REFERENCES

Berger, N. A., and E. S. Johnson (1976). Biochim. Biophys. Acta, 425, 1-17.
Bolden, A., G. P. Noy, and A. Weissbach (1977). J. Biol. Chem., 252, 3351-3356.
Bollum, F. J. (1960). J. Biol. Chem., 235, 2399-2403.
Castellot, J. J., M. R. Miller, and A. B. Pardee (1978). Proc. Natl. Acad. Sci.
    USA, 75, 351-355.
Chang, L. M. S. (1976). Science, 191, 1183-1185.
Cleaver, J. E., and D. A. Bootsma (1975). Rev. Genet., 9, 19-38.
Fisher, P. A., and D. Korn (1977). J. Biol. Chem., 252, 6528-6535.
Foster, D. N., and T. Gurney (1976). J. Biol. Chem., 251, 7893-7898.
Franze de Fernández, M. T., J. Mordoh, and B. Fridlender (1975). Biochem. Biophys.
    Res. Commun., 65, 1409-1417.
Fridlender, B., M. Fry, A. Bolden, and A. Weissbach (1972). Proc. Natl. Acad. Sci.
    USA, 69, 452-455.
Fridlender, B., S. Virasoro, S. Blau, and J. Mordoh (1974). Biochem. Biphys. Res.

Commun., 60, 983-990.

Fridlender, B., E. Medrano, and J. Mordoh (1974). Proc. Natl. Acad. Sci. USA, 71, 1128-1132.

Fujiwara, Y., M. Tatsumi, and M. S. Sasaki (1977). J. Mol. Biol., 113, 635-649.

German, J. (1972). Progr. Med. Genet., 8, 61-101.

Giannelli, F., P. F. Benson, S. A. Pawsey, and P. E. Polani (1977). Nature, 265, 466-469.

Hand, R. (1977). Human Genet., 37, 55-64.

Herrick, G., B. B. Spear, G. Veomett (1976). Proc. Natl. Acad. Sci. USA, 73, 1136-1139.

Hirota, Y., J. Mordoh, I. Scheffler, and F. Jacob (1972). Fed. Proc., 31, 1422-1427.

Hoffbrand, A. V., K. Ganeshaguru, J. W. L. Hooton, and E. Tripp (1976). In A. V. Hoffbrand (ed.), Clinics in Hematology, Saunders, London, pp. 727-745.

Jacob, F., S. Brenner, and F. Cuzin (1963). Cold Spring Harbor Symp. Quant. Biol., 28, 329-348.

Jazwinski, S. M., and G. M. Edelman (1976). Proc. Natl. Acad. Sci. USA, 73, 3933-3936.

Jazwinski, S. M., J. L. Wang, and G. M. Edelman (1976). Proc. Natl. Acad. Sci. USA, 73, 2231-2235.

Lehman, A. R., and S. Stevens (1977). Biochim. Biophys. Acta, 474, 49-60.

Meyer, R., and M. Simpson (1968). Proc. Natl. Acad. Sci. USA, 61, 130-137.

Miller, M. R., J. J. Castellot, and A. B. Pardee (1978). Biochemistry, 17, 1073-1080.

Mordoh, J., and B. Fridlender (1975). Biochem. Biophys. Res. Commun., 67, 888-896.

Mordoh, J., and B. Fridlender (1977). Molec. Cell. Biochem., 16, 177-185.

Nowell, P. C. (1960). Cancer Res., 20, 462-466.

Sasaki, M. S., and A. Tonomura (1973). Cancer Res., 33, 1829-1836.

Seki, S., M. Lemahieu, and G. C. Mueller (1975). Biochim. Biophys. Acta, 378, 333-343.

Seki, S., and T. Oda (1977a). Biochim. Biophys. Acta, 476, 24-31.

Seki, S., and T. Oda (1977b). Cancer Res., 37, 137-144.

Setlow, R. B. (1978). Nature, 271, 713-717.

Sheinin, R., J. Humbert, and R. E. Pearlman (1978). Ann. Rev. Biochem., 47, 277-316.

Spadari, S., R. Muller, and A. Weissbach (1974). J. Biol. Chem., 249, 2991-2992.

Springgate, C. F., and L. L. Loeb (1973). Proc. Natl. Acad. Sci. USA, 70, 245-249.

Weissbach, A., A. Schlabach, B. Fridlender, and A. Bolden (1971). Nature New Biol., 231, 167-170.

Weissbach, A. (1975). Cell, 5, 101-108.

Weissbach, A., D. Baltimore, F. Bollum, R. Gallo and D. Korn (1975). Science, 190, 401-402.

Weissbach, A. (1977). Ann. Rev. Biochem., 46, 25-47.

Keywords: eukaryotes - DNA replication - DNA polymerases - lymphocytes - leukemic cells - permeabilized cells.

Control of Cell Proliferation and the Cell Cycle

R. Baserga

Department of Pathology and Fels Research Institute,
Temple University School of Medicine, Philadelphia, Pennsylvania, U.S.A.

ABSTRACT

The critical phase in the cell cycle for the control of cell proliferation is the G_0-G_1 period. It is at this stage that a cell decides whether to continue throughout the cell cycle or to go into a resting or a differentiating stage. A number of studies have been carried out on changes occurring in mammalian cells during the transition from the resting to the growing stage. These include changes in membrane transport, in the cytoplasm as well as in the nucleus. It should be said though that most of these changes, although they do accompany the transition from the resting to the growing stage, have not been rigorously shown to be necessary. Recent studies with virally coded proteins and with temperature sensitive mutants of the cell cycle have indicated, however, that at least three proteins can be isolated and purified that act on different steps of the G_0-G_1 phase of the cell cycle. These include the SV40 T antigen, RNA polymerase II and the T antigen coded by adenovirus 2. The identification of these three proteins as possible regulators of a cell cycle transition brings the study of the cell cycle to its truly molecular basis.

The details of these studies have been published recently:

Reference:

Rossini, M., J. Floros, R. Weinmann and R. Baserga. Adenovirus 2 induces the G_0 to S transition by a mechanism different from that of serum or polyoma. Cold Spring Harbor Symposium (in press).

Nuclei and Chromatin in Normal and Neoplastic Growth

R. Baserga

Department of Pathology and Fels Research Institute,
Temple University School of Medicine, Philadelphia, Pennsylvania, U.S.A.

ABSTRACT

When human diploid fibroblasts (WI-38 cells) in culture are maintained under conditions nonpermissive for growth (serum restriction), cell proliferation ceases but
the cells remain viable for extended periods of time. Under similar restrictive
conditions nonpermissive for growth, SV-40 transformed WI-38 fibroblasts (2RA cells)
die off at a rate of 10% per day. In resting WI-38 cells, the template activity of
isolated nuclei is related to both cell density and the length of time the cells
have been quiescent. In 2RA cells, nuclear template activity is related to time
after plating, regardless of cell density. The results are compatible with the
hypothesis that normal cells can enter a G_0 state more easily than transformed cells.
This, in turn, would allow normal cells to survive under conditions nonpermissive
for growth, whereas transformed cells gradually die off.

The details of these studies have been published recently:

Reference:

Schiaffonati, L., and R. Baserga. (1977). Different survival of normal and transformed cells exposed to nutritional conditions nonpermissive for growth. Cancer Res.
37:541-545.

Nonhistone Nuclear Proteins of Cancer Cells

**Harris Busch, Hiroshi Takami, Frances M. Davis, Rose K. Busch,
Benjamin C. Wu, William H. Spohn and Katari S. Raju**

*Department of Pharmacology, Baylor College of Medicine, Houston,
Texas 77030, U.S.A.*

CANCER CELLS AND GENETIC MECHANISMS IN CARCINOGENESIS

Cancer is a disease in which a dysplastic phenotype, represented by
uncontrolled cell growth and division, invasiveness and metastasis is
transmitted genetically or epigenetically to the daughter cells. The
earliest investigations on cancer which were purely morphological
suggested that this dysplasia primarily involved disordered biochemical genetics. Following the cell theory of Schleiden and Schwann
that "Omnis cellula e cellula", Virchow and his student Thiersch provided a genetic concept for cancer in their conclusion "Omnia cellula
e cellula ejusdem generis". Thus, the early conclusion that all
cells come from parental cells was extended to the idea that all cancer cells come from prior cancer cells except for the first cancer
cell. These statements of the 1860's were confirmed in elegant experiments of the 1930's by Furth and Kahn (1937) and later by Hosokawa (1950) and Ishibashi (1950) who showed that one cancer cell was
sufficient to produce cancer in a susceptible host.

GENETIC ANALYSIS OF CANCER CELLS

Although aberrations have been reported in chromosomes of individual
cancers, adequate evidence that there are differences in either the
specific chromosomes or the DNA of cancer cells has not yet been reported. Other than the translocated Philadelphia chromosomes which
may appear in myelogenous leukemia, no common clinical case of
chromosome aberration exists. If there were structural aberrations
in DNA, mutant proteins or specific gene deletions could have been
found unless such aberrations were in promoter or operator sequences.
At present, either because of limitations of methods or because such
events are very subtle, there is no convincing evidence for DNA
aberrations in cancer cells (despite the mutagenic effects of carcinogens). Efforts to prove viruses are causative in human neoplasia
have been fruitless in most studies although some reports of viral
genomes in human cancer cells (Ohno and Spiegelman, 1977) continue
to appear. So many neoplasms clearly have a chemical origin that it
is not necessary to postulate a viral etiology for human cancers; of
course, studies of the Burkitt and nasopharyngeal tumors may yet
lead to evidence for a viral etiology.

THE NUCLEAR PROTEINS

Evidence that cytoplasmic elements rather than DNA controlled the
cell phenotype emerged from studies of Gurdon (1974) who showed that
the nucleus was totipotent even up to stages of development of intestinal epithelial cells of frog tadpoles. Thus, the full information for development and differentiation of a whole frog is present
in the nucleus of each cell. The direct controls of gene function
are now generally considered to be the nonhistone nuclear proteins
(derived from cytoplasmic synthesis) which were shown years ago to be
heterogeneous (Busch et al, 1963) and later were directly implicated
by Gilmour and Paul (1969) as specifying RNA transcripts. The histones, which at one time were thought to control genes, are now being
largely relegated to structural roles in the "nu-bodies" or nucleosomes.

Some uncertainties exist in the "dogma" that the nonhistone proteins
control gene function. A definitive experiment has not yet been reported that shows the role of a specific nonhistone protein in the
production of a single special gene readout, although mixtures of
nonhistone proteins have been reported to serve that function. The
task of demonstrating such a specific function would seem experi-
mentally possible now but none of the methods reported to be adequate
for this task has worked thus far. This field is in great need of
diligent and elegant analytical studies.

Of the nuclear proteins, histones are present in greatest amounts,
i.e., each major histone species is present in amounts of approximately 2 pg (10^{-12} gram)/nucleus. Proteins C23-25, which are among
the most abundant of the more than 200 species of nucleolar nonhistone proteins, are present in amounts of approximately 10-100 fg
(10^{-15} gram) in nuclei and nucleoli. Such proteins are now readily
visualized by staining on 2D gels, particularly after fractionation
and purification. When ^{32}P and immunological methods are used, the
levels of detection are 10-100 fold greater, i.e. they approach 50
attagrams (10^{-18} gram)/nucleus. Such amounts begin to approximate
the levels probably important in gene control.

The combination of two-dimensional isoelectric focusing SDS gel
electrophoresis with successive extraction of nuclei of Novikoff
hepatoma and normal rat liver with (a) 0.075 M NaCl/0.025 M EDTA,
(b) 10 mM Tris, (c) 0.35 M NaCl, (d) 0.6 M NaCl, and (e) 3 M NaCl/
7 M urea provides an improved approach to analysis of the number and
types of nuclear proteins. Each fraction contained 108-200 spots,
of which (a) some were present in all of the fractions, (b) some were
present in more than one fraction, and (c) others were uniquely found
in one fraction. In the Novikoff hepatoma nuclei, 483 different
polypeptides were found; and 427 polypeptides were found in liver
nuclei.

In the Novikoff hepatoma, 18 protein spots (designated by molecular
weight/pI) were found in the various nuclear fractions that were not
found in the normal liver nuclei. In normal liver nuclei, 12 spots
were present in various nuclear fractions that were not found in the
Novikoff hepatoma.

These studies substantiate and extend earlier studies from this laboratory which showed differences in nuclear nonhistone proteins in

tumors and other tissues.

WHAT ARE THE NONHISTONE NUCLEAR PROTEINS?

The demonstration in this and other laboratories that there are hundreds of nuclear proteins composed of many species of enzymes, structural proteins and other polypeptides has led to concerted efforts to isolate, purify and determine the functions of these many protein species. First, methods were needed to separate and classify these proteins. Two systems are in use in our laboratory for two-dimensional analyses of these proteins, namely the "Orrick" system (Orrick et al, 1973) and the "O'Farrell" system (O'Farrell, 1975). In the former system, the acid-urea gel (first dimension) separates the proteins by charge, i.e. the proteins with the greatest positive charge migrate toward the cathode; in the latter system, the first dimension is isoelectricfocusing which separates the proteins on the basis of migration into regions in which their overall net charge is essentially zero. In both systems, the second dimension employs SDS gel electrophoresis.

TWO-DIMENSIONAL NUCLEAR PROTEIN "FINGERPRINTS"

Prior to the initial two-dimensional gel fingerprints of nucleolar proteins (Orrick et al, 1973), many experiments were carried out on one-dimensional SDS gels. The two-dimensional systems which employed both charge and molecular weight separations vastly improved the fractionation of these proteins (Busch et al, 1974). A series of proteins found in experimental hepatomas were absent from the non-tumor tissues used as controls (Busch et al, 1974). These chromatin proteins were designated CG', CH', Cg', CP and C15' (Busch et al, 1974; Ganpath et al, 1977; Yeoman et al, 1973). Subsequent studies on human and animal tumors as well as growing and nongrowing nontumor tissues led to the conclusion that tumors contain nonhistone protein Cg' and that protein CP' was markedly increased in tumors (Busch et al, 1974; Ganpath et al, 1977; Yeoman et al, 1973).

TUMOR PHOSPHOPROTEINS

Although the 2D gel systems represented a marked increase in the resolving properties of gel systems, they were still limited in their potential by the visibility of the protein spots which resolved protein amounts of 0.1-1 μg equivalent to 5-100 fg per nucleus. What became very important was to determine whether proteins of lower abundance, i.e. 0.1-1 fg/nucleus, could be visualized by labeling and autoradiographic methods (Ganpath et al, 1977; Olson et al, 1974). Comparisons were made of autoradiograms of ^{32}P-labeled nonhistone nuclear proteins of the normal, regenerating and thioacetamide-treated liver with the Novikoff hepatoma; this tumor was found to contain labeled proteins C5p, CMp, C13p, C21p and CU' (Ganpath et al, 1977) that were absent from other nuclei studied. This powerful probe is now being extended to much improved fractionation systems and to a broader group of tumor and nontumor tissues.

NUCLEAR ANTIGENS AND ONCOEMBRYONIC PROTEINS

Different antigens have been found in the nuclear and nucleolar proteins of tumors and nontumor tissues (Busch and Busch, 1977; Yeoman
et al, 1976). When corresponding studies were carried out on chromatin fractions, nuclear antigens (NAg) were found that were different from the nucleolar antigens (No-Ag). Because nuclear antigens
are present in large amounts, it became possible to isolate and characterize, at least in part, the nuclear antigen referred to as NAg-1
(Yeoman et al, 1976). Interestingly, this antigen is a nonhistone
glycoprotein which contains glucosamine. A surprising aspect of
chromatin antigen NAg-1 was the demonstration that it is a fetal protein (Yeoman et al, 1976); NAg-1 is present both in the cytoplasm and
the nucleus, but it is of particular interest because it was the
first fetal chromatin protein found in tumors.

Studies of the antigens in rat nucleoli with rabbit antibodies showed
that some tumor antigens were absent from the nontumor tissues and,
very importantly, the opposite was true (Busch and Busch, 1977).
More elegant analysis of the antigens showed that the Novikoff hepatoma nucleoli contained two antigens that were absent from the liver
and the liver contained four antigens that were absent from the tumor
(Busch and Busch, 1977). Because such results are of much potential
significance, these antigens are now being purified. At least one
of the tumor nucleolar antigens has been found to be present in fetal
liver, i.e. it is an "oncoembryonic antigen".

Such findings provided a basis for the concept (Busch, 1976) that
fetal chromatin proteins like NAg-1 or No-Ag 2, a nucleolar protein,
may be special stimuli that result in transcription and translation
of mRNA species for the cancer phenotype of (a) growth and cell
division, (b) invasiveness, and (c) metastasis.

HUMAN TUMOR NUCLEOLAR ANTIGENS

Following the demonstration that nucleolar antigens in Novikoff
hepatoma ascites cells and normal rat liver cells differed (Busch
and Busch, 1977; Davis et al, 1978) as shown by immunoprecipitation,
immunoelectrophoresis and absorption techniques, studies were then
made on the nucleolar antigens of human tumor cells. Rabbit antibodies (IgG) to HeLa cell nucleoli were preabsorbed with placental
nuclear extracts, and it was found that each of the human tumors
studied (Table 1) contained antigens which produced a bright nucleolar immunofluorescence with these antibodies as shown by the
double antibody technique (the second antibody was fluorescein
labeled goat antirabbit antibody). In further studies (Davis et al,
submitted), it has been found that the nontumor tissues studied did
not produce a positive immunofluorescence with this antibody (Table
1). This is the first demonstration of a common antigen in a variety
of human tumors that is not present in the nontumor tissues studied
thus far. The relationship of this antigen to the high concentration
of silver staining proteins in the nucleolus in telophase, the possible "short-circuiting" of G1 controls and possible diagnostic
approaches to human cancer remain to be elucidated.

TABLE 1   Immunofluorescence of Cells and Tissues with Antiserum to HeLa Cell Nucleoli[a,b]

	Positive	Negative
Biopsies from patients	Prostate carcinoma Thyroid carcinoma Adrenal cortical carcinoma Osteogenic Sarcoma Hairy cell leukemia (spleen) Colonic adenocarcinoma metastasis to liver Squamous cell carcinoma metastasis to spine	Prostate (hyperplastic) Thyroid (hyperplastic) Kidney Placenta Liver (cirrhotic) Liver-chronic hepatitis Bone marrow from 3 individuals
Human tumor transplant	Goldenberg tumor (GW39) Prostate carcinoma	
Human cell cultures	HeLa HEp-2 Mammary carcinoma	WI38 Fibroblasts, mammary
Subcellular fractions	Nucleoli (HeLa)	Nuclear matrix (HeLa)

[a]The antiserum had been absorbed with fetal bovine serum and with sonicated placental nuclei and was used at a 1:64 dilution in PBS.
[b]Davis et al, submitted.

ACKNOWLEDGMENTS

These studies were supported in part by the Cancer Center Grant CA-10893,P.1, awarded by the National Cancer Institute, DHEW, the Pauline Sterne Wolff Memorial Foundation, the Bristol-Myers Fund, and a generous gift from Mrs. Jack Hutchins.

REFERENCES

Busch, G. I., L. C. Yeoman, C. W. Taylor, and H. Busch (1974). Modified two-dimensional polyacrylamide gel electrophoresis systems for higher molecular weight nonhistone chromatin proteins from normal rat liver and Novikoff hepatoma ascites cells. Physiol. Chem. Phys., 6, 1-10.
Busch, H. (1976). A general concept for molecular biology of cancer. Cancer Res., 36, 4291-4294.
Busch, H., W. J. Steele, H. Mavioglu, C. W. Taylor, and L. Hnilica (1963). Biochemistry of the histones and the cell cycle. J. Cell. Comp. Physiol. (Suppl. 1) 62, 95-110.
Busch, R. K., and H. Busch (1977). Antigenic proteins of nucleolar chromatin of Novikoff hepatoma ascites cells. Tumori, 63, 347-357.
Davis, F. M., R. K. Busch, L. C. Yeoman, and H. Busch (1978). Differences in nucleolar antigens of rat liver and Novikoff

hepatoma ascites cells. Cancer Res., 38, 1906-1915.

Davis, F. M., F. Gyorkey, R. K. Busch, and H. Busch. A nucleolar antigen found in several human tumors but not in nontumor tissues. Submitted.

Furth, J., and M. C. Kahn (1937). The transmission of leukemia of mice with a single cell. Am. J. Cancer, 31, 276-282.

Ganpath, N., A. W. Prestayko, and H. Busch (1977). Comparison of nuclear nonhistone phosphoproteins of rat liver and Novikoff hepatoma. Cancer Res., 37, 1290-1300.

Gilmour, R. S., and J. Paul (1969). RNA transcribed from reconstituted nucleoprotein is similar to natural RNA. J. Mol. Biol., 40, 137-139.

Gurdon, J. B. (1974). The genome in specialized cells, as revealed by nuclear transplantation in amphibia. In H. Busch (Ed.), The Cell Nucleus, Vol. I, Academic Press, New York. pp. 471-489.

Hosokawa, K. (1950). Further research on transplantation of Yoshida sarcoma with a single cell and with cell-free tumor ascites. Gann, 41, 236-237.

Ishibashi, K. (1950). Studies on the number of cells necessary for the transplantation of the Yoshida sarcoma. Gann, 41, 1-14.

O'Farrell, P. H. (1975). High resolution two-dimensional electrophoresis of proteins. J. Biol. Chem., 250, 4007-4021.

Ohno, T., and S. Spiegelman (1977). Antigenic relatedness of the DNA polymerase of human breast cancer particles to the enzyme of the Mason-Pfizer monkey virus. Proc. Natl. Acad. Sci. USA, 74, 2144-2148.

Olson, M. O. J., W. C. Starbuck, and H. Busch (1974). The nuclear proteins. In H. Busch (Ed.), Molecular Biology of Cancer, Academic Press, New York. pp. 309-353.

Orrick, L. R., M. O. J. Olson, and H. Busch (1973). Comparison of nucleolar proteins of normal rat liver and Novikoff hepatoma ascites cells by 2-dimensional polyacrylamide gel electrophoresis. Proc. Natl. Acad. Sci. USA, 70, 1316-1320.

Yeoman, L. C., C. W. Taylor, and H. Busch (1973). Two-dimensional polyacrylamide gel electrophoresis of acid extractable nuclear proteins of normal rat liver and Novikoff hepatoma ascites cells. Biochem. Biophys. Res. Commun., 51, 956-966.

Yeoman, L. C., J. J. Jordan, R. K. Busch, C. W. Taylor, H. Savage, and H. Busch (1976). A fetal protein in the chromatin of Novikoff hepatoma and Walker 256 carcinosarcoma tumors that is absent from normal and regenerating rat liver. Proc. Natl. Acad. Sci. USA, 73, 3258-3262.

Chromatin Subunits in Nucleoli and Nucleolar Chromatin

Yoshihiro Tsutsui*, Cheng-Hsiung Huang and Renato Baserga

Fels Research Institute and the Department of Pathology,
Temple University School of Medicine, Philadelphia, Pa. 19140, U.S.A.

Chromatin subunits can be demonstrated in isolated nucleoli from sonicated hamster liver nuclei and have been characterized by immunological procedures and circular dichroism (CD). The length of the DNA repeating units of nucleolar chromatin is the same as that of nuclear chromatin, i.e. about 180 base pairs. Monomer, dimer+ trimer and multimer fractions were collected after micrococcal nuclease digestion of RNase digested nucleoli by an isokinetic sucrose gradient. These fractions were studied in complement fixation tests using antisera against hamster nonhistone protein (NHP)-DNA complex or hamster whole nucleoli. The higher the degree of polymerization of the subunits the more these subunits reacted with the anti NHP-DNA complex antibodies, while the antinucleolar antibodies reacted only with the multimer fraction.

Circular dichroism studies showed that the monomer, the dimer+trimer and the multimer had a molar ellipticity range of 1450-1600 deg.cm^2 dmole^{-1} at the positive peak (282 nm) indicating a marked reduction in molar ellipticity when compared to protein-free DNA. In going from monomer to the multimer, it was observed that a shoulder around 272 nm in the CD spectra became more pronounced, that the molar ellipticity at 225 nm, indicative of the protein α-helical structures, was reduced and that the crossover position was gradually shifted to a shorter wave length. In general these features of the CD spectra were similar to those observed in nuclear chromatin subunits.

Keywords. nucleoli/immunological procedures/circular dichroism/micrococcal nuclease digestion

INTRODUCTION

The nucleolus is an organelle that can be isolated in highly purified form from the nuclei of higher organisms. It constitutes 3.5 of the total genome (Steele, 1968; Busch and Smetana, 1970) and contains the genes for ribosomal RNA. However, less than 1% of the total nucleolar DNA is rDNA (McConkey and Hopkins, 1964), the rest being perinucleolar chromatin that is isolated as an integral part of DNA (Busch and Smetana, 1970).

Recently it has been established that the chromatin of eukaryotic organisms is composed of repeating subunits each containing about 200 base pairs of DNA (nucleosomes, ν-bodies) with a core of histones, apparently an octamer containing two each of histones H2A, H2B, H3, and H4 (Kornberg, 1974; Felsenfeld, 1975; Noll, 1974; van Holde, co-workers and colleagues, 1974; Oudet, Gross-Bellard and Chambon, 1975; Senior, Olins and Olins, 1975; Thomas and Kornberg, 1975). Todate there have been a few reports on subunits of chromatin containing ribosomal genes from Xenopus laevis (Reeves, 1975; Reeves and Jones, 1976), from Tetrahymena pyriformis (Mathis and Gorovsky, 1976; Piper and coworkers, 1976) and from Physarum polycephalum (Johnson and coworkers, 1976). However, there have been no reports on chromatin subunits of the mammalian nucleolus or nucleolar chromatin. In this paper we report the results of our studies on chromatin subunits of hamster liver nucleoli and nucleolar chromatin using immunological procedures and circular dichroism.

MATERIALS AND METHODS

Isolation of nucleoli from hamster liver. Perfused liver from Syrian hamster was minced and homogenized with a Potter Teflon homogenizer, 10 strokes in 0.25M sucrose 3.3mM $CaCl_2$, 0.2mM PMSF (Phenylmethyl Sulfonyl Fluoride). The homogenate was passed through four layers of cheese cloth. After washing, the nuclei were treated with 0.5% Triton X-100 in the same solution, and washed again. The nuclear suspension was layered over twice the volume of a 2.2M sucrose, 3.3mM $CaCl_2$ solution and centri fuged at 25,000 rpm for 60 min in a SW27 rotor of a Beckman L3-50 centrifuge to obtain a clean nuclear pellet. Nucleoli were prepared from nuclei essentially according to the procedure of Muramatsu and coworkers (1974) as modified by Huang and Baserga (1976). The nuclei were resuspended in 0.3M sucrose, and sonicated with a Branson Sonifier in a 25ml beaker, cooled in ice-water. The sonication was performed at a setting of 5 with an output of 70W at 15 sec intervals. Each soni cation was followed by a cooling time of about 30 sec. The completion of nuclear breakage was monitored by light microscopy. Usually the sonicated suspension was layered over twice the volume of 0.88M sucrose solution and centrifuged at 3300 rpm for 30 min in a PR-6 International Centrifuge for 30 min to collect nucleoli.

RNase digestion of nucleoli. Nucleoli were digested according to the procedure of Huang and Baserga (1976). The nucleolar pellet was resuspended in 50mM Tris HCl, pH 7.4, and incubated with 1 mg/ml ribonuclease A at 37°C for 2 hr with constant shaking. Before use the RNase A was incubated for 15 min at 85°C to inactivate contaminating DNase. After RNase digestion the nucleolar suspension was layered over twice the volume of 0.34M sucrose and pelleted at 3000 rpm for 20 min in a PR-6 International Centrifuge.

Preparation of nucleolar chromatin. Nucleolar chromatin was prepared basically according to the procedure of Bombik, Huang and Baserga (1977). The nucleolar pellet, after digestion with RNase, was suspended in 5% (wt/vol) sucrose in 10mM Tris HCl at pH 7.4, 0.5mM Mg acetate and 5M urea, and kept for 20 min with inter mittent pipetting at 2°C. This suspension was layered over 25% (wt/vol) sucrose in 10mM Tris HCl at pH 7.4, 0.5mM Mg acetate and 5M urea with a 1.0ml cushion of 2M sucrose, then centrifuged for 30 min at 15,000 rpm in a SW40 rotor of a Beckman L3-50 centrifuge. The band at the interlayer between the 25% sucrose solution and the cushion was collected and dialyzed overnight against the digestion buffer (see below) for micrococcal nuclease digestion or phosphate buffered saline (PBS) for immunological studies.

Micrococcal nuclease digestion. Digestions were carried out at DNA concentrations of about 15-20 A_{260} unit/ml in a solution containing 1mM Tris HCl, pH 8.0, 0.1mM CaCl and 250 units/ml of micrococcal nuclease at 37°C. Reactions were stopped by addition of 0.1M Na EDTA, pH 8.0 to 5mM (final concentration) at 2°C.

Gel electrophoresis of DNA. After digestion with micrococcal nuclease, DNA extra ction was carried out according to Axel and coworkers (1974). The reaction products were incubated with 200 µg/ml of Proteinase K (Merk) for 2 hr. Prior to use the proteinase was incubated at 37°C for 1 hr to inactivate contaminating DNase. The products were extracted two times with equal volumes of phenol equilibrated with

50mM Tris HCl (pH 8.0)-5mM EDTA and the DNA was precipitated with two volumes of 95% ethanol at -20°C overnight, then washed with 70% ethanol two times. Electrophoresis was carried out in 2.5% acrylamide (acrylamide/bisacrylamide, 19/1) and 0.5% agarose prepared according to Peacock and Dingman (1968), using an 11 cm-slab gel apparatus. The buffer system was also that described by Peacock and Dingman (1967). The gels were run at 75 V for 90 min then stained in 1.0 µg/ml ethidium bromide in electrophoresis buffer for 30 min. The gels were illuminated with ultraviolet light at 254 nm and photographed through a Kodak A red filter. DNA standards for electrophoresis were fragments from digests of SV40 DNA (Strain 776) with Haemophilus aegyptius restriction endonuclease (Hae III) (Lebowitz, Siegel and Sklar, 1974).

Isokinetic sucrose gradient. After digestion with micrococcal nuclease, sodium deoxycholate and Triton X-100 were added to the nucleolar samples to a final concentration of 0.5% each, according to Liew and Chan (1976). They were mixed by passage through a 25 7/8 gauge needle ten times at 2° (Simpson and Bustin, 1976) and layered over a 12ml isokinetic sucrose gradient containing 1mM Na EDTA, pH 7.0 with Ct=5%, Cr=28.8% and V_m=9.2ml, and centrifuged for 16 hr at 30,000 rpm in a SW40 rotor at 4°C, according to the procedure of Noll and Kornberg (1977). The gradient was collected from the bottom of the tubes and monitored for absorbance at 260nm with the use of a flow cell in a Gilford 2400-S spectrophotometer. The fractions were pooled and dialyzed extensively against 1mM Tris HCl, pH 8.0.

Gel electrophoresis of proteins. Proteins were analyzed in 15% acrylamide-sodium dodecyl sulfate (SDS) gel, according to Laemmli (1970) as modified by Weintraub, Palter and van Lente (1975). The fractions from an isokinetic sucrose gradient were extensively dialyzed against 1mM Tris HCl, pH 8.0, then lyophilized. The samples were suspended in 0.625M Tris HCl pH 6.8, 2% SDS, 10% glycerol, 5% 2-mercaptoethanol and 0.001% bromophenol blue. The samples were boiled for 1.5 min prior to being loaded on the gels. Electrophoresis was performed at 4mA/gel for 7 hr. The gels were stained in 0.1% Coomasie brilliant blue in methanol/acetate acid/water (5:1:5) overnight and destained in 5% methanol with 7.5% acetic acid (Thomas and Kornberg, 1975). The gels were scanned with a Gilford 2400-S spectrophotometer at 600 nm.

Preparation of nonhistone protein (NHP)-DNA complex from hamster liver nuclei.
NHP-DNA complex were prepared mostly by the procedure of Wakabayashi, Wang and Hnilica (1974). The nuclei prepared as described above were washed with 80mM NaCl-20mM EDTA, pH 7.5 extensively, and homogenized in cold water with a glass Dounce homogenizer, then spun through 1.7M sucrose in a SW40 rotor at 38,000 rpm for 90 min to obtain nuclear chromatin. The chromatin was extracted with 0.3M NaCl for 15 min and centrifuged at 38,000 rpm in a SW40 rotor for 30 min. The chromatin was dissociated in 2.5M NaCl-5M urea-50mM phosphate buffer, pH 6.0, and stirred on ice for several hours. The dissociated chromatin was spun down at 40,000 rpm in a 50 Ti rotor for 36 hr in a Beckman L3-50 centrifuge. The pellet (containing most of the DNA and the tightly bound NHP) was washed and dialyzed against 1.5mM NaCl-0.15mM sodium citrate, pH 7.0.

Immunological procedures. Preparation of antisera against hamster nucleoli and NHP-DNA complex was carried out by immunizing rabbits, as previously described (Tsutsui, Chang and Baserga, 1977). Immunofluorescent studies were also performed as previously described (Tsutsui, Chang and Baserga, 1977). Quantitative microcomplement fixation reaction was performed according to the method of Wasserman and Levine (1961) in a total volume of 1.4ml per reaction mixture. The amount of antigens was expressed in terms of DNA. DNA was determined by the procedure of Burton (1956), or absorbance at 260 nm after dissociation of samples in 2M NaCl-5M urea, assuming that 1 OD unit at 260 nm equals 50µg DNA.

Circular dichroic measurements. Circular dichroic (CD) studies were carried out as
previously described (Huang and Baserga, 1976). A modified JASCO Model J40 Recording Spectropolarimeter with a short sample to photomultiplier distance was used.
Samples in 10mM Tris, HCl, pH 8.0 with absorbance at 260nm of less than 1.1, were
measured in a fused 1-cm, 1-ml jacketed quartz cuvette from Hellma Co. Nucleolar
samples measured in this type of cuvette showed little optical activity (CD) above
300nm, indicating an absence of differential light scattering effect between the
left-and right-handed polarized lights (Urry and Krivacic, 1970; Glaser and Singer,
1971; Gordon, 1972; Dorman and Maestre, 1973; Schneider, 1973).   The nucleolar
subunit preparations were reasonably clear ($A_{320}/A_{260}<0.03$), since similar CD spectra
were obtained upon dilution of the sample to 1/2 for measurements in the 250-300nm
region and to 1/6 in the 210-250nm region, or using cuvettes with either 10mm or
1mm light path for the 210-250nm region. Therefore, the absorption flattening
effect (Duysens, 1956; Glaser and Singer, 1971; Gordon, 1972; Schneider, 1973),
may not be very significant. Scanning was repeated 3 to 5 times for the same
sample to minimize the random noise. Data on CD were expressed as molar ellipticity
$[\theta]$nm, in degree cm^2, $dmol^{-1}$ of DNA-P residues in the 250-300 nm region and amino
acid residue in the 210-250nm region, assuming a mean residue weight of 330 for
DNA-P and 110 for amino acid residue. Concentration of DNA was calculated from
absorbance at 260nm and that of proteins from absorbance at both 260nm and 230nm
(Tuan and Bonner, 1969).

Materials

Micrococcal nuclease (16,927 units/mg) and RNase A were purchased from Worthington,
Freehold, N.J. Proteinase K was purchased from E. Merk, Darmstadt. Hae III was
purchased from New England Bio-Lab, Beverly, Ma. SV40 DNA was purchased from
Bethesda Res.Lab. Inc., Rockville, Md. Ethidium bromide and calf thymus histones
were from Sigma Chem.Co., St. Louis, Mo. Sucrose and urea (ultra-pure) were from
Schwarz/Mann, Orangeburg, N.Y. Sheep red blood cells and antisheep hemolysin were
from Flow Lab., Rockville, Md. Guinea pig complement was from GIBCO, Grand Island,
N.Y. All other chemicals were of the highest grade available.

RESULTS

Purity of nucleolar preparations. We have already discussed, in a previous paper
from this laboratory (Huang and Baserga, 1976) the criteria used to determine the
purity of our nucleolar preparations. They are highly purified by electron microscopy and chemical composition. By hybridization techniques, they are enriched
(in respect to nuclei) in rDNA about twenty-fold, and their product of transcription hybridizes to nucleolar DNA and is effectively competed out by ribosomal RNA,
but not by other species of RNA (Whelly, Ide and Baserga, 1978). It should also
be emphasized that the question asked in this paper is whether nucleoli, as an
organelle like mitochrondria, and not rDNA, have a nucleosome structure?

DNA repeats of nucleoli and nucleolar chromatin. The polyacrylamide gel patterns
of fragments obtained by micrococcal nuclease digestion of untreated nucleoli or
RNase digested nucleoli, were similar to those of nuclei (Fig.1,A,B and C). Even
in the case of nucleolar chromatin prepared according to Bombik, Huang and Baserga
(1977), DNA repeat subunits were detected, although a small amount of DNA was
smeared throughout the gel (Fig.1D). On the other hand, extranucleolar chromatin
(after sonication of nuclei), gave only faint bands and mostly a continuous distribution of DNA fragments throughout the gel (Fig.1E). No difference could be detected in the size of the DNA digestion fragments between nucleoli and nuclei.
Although kinetic studies are desirable, we have omitted them from the present paper,
whose main purpose is not to quantitate but to establish the presence of subunits
in nucleoli and in nucleolar chromatin. The length of the DNA repeating unit in

both nuclei and nucleoli is about 180 base pairs according to the calculations of Noll and Kornberg (1977), which gave the size of a complete repeating unit irrespective of the extent of degradation of the bridge regions. This figure is not dissimilar to the figure of ~ 196 base pairs obtained by Compton, Bellard and Chambon (1976) from nuclear chromatin of Syrian hamster liver.

Fig 1.

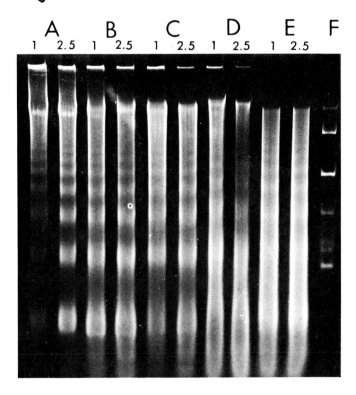

Fig. 1. 2.5% polyacrylamide - 0.5% agarose gel electrophoresis of micrococcal nuclease digests of hamster liver nuclei (A), nucleoli (B), nucleoli after RNase digestion (C), nucleolar chromatin prepared according to Bombik, Huang and Baserga (1977), (D), extranucleolar chromatin (E) and Hae III restriction fragments of SV40 DNA (F). Micrococcal nuclease digestion was performed in a concentration of 250 units/ml at 37°C for 1 min in each sample. SV40 DNA was digested with Haemophilus aegyptius restriction endonuclease (600 units/ml) at 37°C for 16 hr.

Fractionation of nucleolar chromatin subunits by isokinetic sucrose gradient. A typical fractionation pattern of nucleolar chromatin subunits after micrococcal nuclease digestion is shown in Fig.2A. The yield of the fractions was increased three times by treating the nucleolar subunits products with detergents, as described by Liew and Chan (1976). The subunit patterns in the fractionated gradients were basically the same whether micrococcal nuclease digested nucleoli were pretreated with RNase or not. We collected three different fractions from the gradient, as shown in Fig. 2A, for gel electrophoresis of the DNA fragment (Fig. 2B). The

first fraction contained monomers, the second fraction contained almost only dimer
and trimer and the third fraction contained multimers beyond the trimer. They were
designated as "monomer". "dimer+trimer" and multimer" respectively. The size of
the pooled monomers can easily be calculated from Figg. 2B and 1.

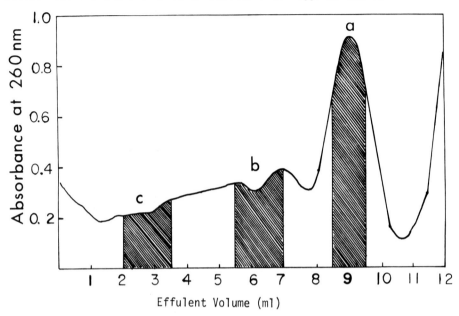

Fig.   2A.   Fractionation pattern of micrococcal nuclease
               digests of RNase digested nucleoli on 12 ml of
               an isokinetic sucrose gradient. RNase digested
               with micrococcal nuclease (250 units/ml) at 37°C
               for 2.5 min. Fractions were collected from the
               shaded areas as the monomer (a), the dimer+trimer
               (b) and the multimer fraction (c).

Since nucleoli contain a large amount of RNA and ribonucleoproteins besides nucleolar chromatin, we examined the protein pattern of the three fractions obtained from
the nucleoli either with or without RNase digestion, using 15% acrylamide-SDS gel
electrophoresis (Fig. 3). All fractions from intact or RNase digested nucleoli have
histones H2A, H2B, H3 and H4 (Fig.3A). More than thirty protein bands, in addition
to histones, could be detected in the monomer and the dimer+trimer fractions in intact nucleoli, while the multimer fraction had fewer bands than the other two fractions (Fig.3B). On the other hand in fractions from RNase digested nucleoli all
nonhistone bands became extremely weak and several of these bands disappeared. RNase
digestion per se caused a very small amount of protein to be lost, less than 10% of
the total (Huang and Baserga, 1976). Most of the nonhistone proteins were lost
during the preparation of subunits. Without RNase digestion, histone H1 was clearly
present in the dimer+trimer fraction and the multimer fraction. In fractions from
RNase digested nucleoli, H1 appeared only in trace amounts in the dimer+trimer
fraction and in the multimer fraction, while undetectable in the monomer fraction
(Fig.3B).

Complement fixation of nucleolar chromatin and its subunits to antisera against
hamster liver nucleoli and hamster NHP-DNA complex. Specificity of antinucleolar
antibody was determined by immunofluorescence. Nucleoli of hamster derived cultured

a   b   c

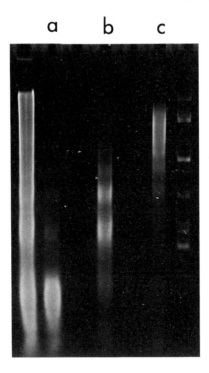

Fig. 2B. Polyacrylamide gel electrophoresis of the corres-
          ponding fractions from Fig. 2A (a,b,c.) The first
          sample shows DNA from unfractionated nuclease
          digest of RNase digested nucleoli. The last sample
          is Hae III restriction fragments.

cells (AF8 cells) were strongly stained and nuclear chromatin was weakly stained
with the antinucleolar antiserum, and no cytoplasmic staining was observed (Fig.4).
Antibodies against histones or nucleoplasmic nonhistone proteins did not preferentially react with nucleoli (Tsutsui, Chang and Baserga, 1977). As shown in
Fig.5A the reactivity of nucleoli in complement fixation tests to the antinucleolar
antiserum was not reduced after RNase digestion of nucleoli, and even after urea
treatment. This indicates that the antigenic determinants of the nucleoli versus
antinucleolar antibody are in the nucleolar chromatin rather than in RNA-protein
complexes that are removed by urea treatment (Bombik, Huang and Baserga, 1977).
Both antinucleolar and anti-NHP-DNA complex antisera reacted more strongly with
nucleolar chromatin than untreated nucleoli (left shift). Although anti-NHP-DNA
complex antibodies reacted the same with nucleolar chromatin as with nuclear chromatin (Fig.5B), antinucleolar reacted more strongly with nucleolar chromatin than
with nuclear chromatin (Fig.5A).

Three fractions of nucleolar chromatin subunits (monomer, dimer+trimer and multimer)
prepared by isokinetic sucrose gradients were tested with antinucleolar antibodies
and anti-NHP-DNA complex antibodies (Fig.6). In the case of anti-NHP-DNA complex
antibodies the order of reactivity of the fractions to the antibody was multimer,
dimer+trimer and monomer fraction, respectively. Even though very slightly, the
monomer fraction did react with the anti-NHP-DNA complex antibody. When the antinucleolar antibodies were reacted with the fractions, the monomer and dimer+trimer
fraction did not react at all, while the multimer fraction did react with the anti-

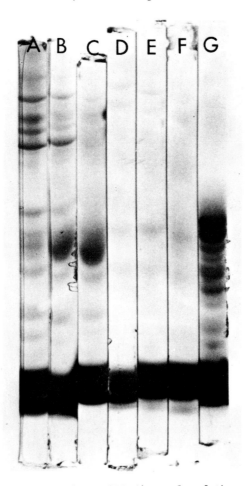

Fig. 3A.   15% acrylamide - SDS disc gels of the proteins from
the isokinetic sucrose gradient fractions collected
as shown in Fig. 2A. Nucleosome fractions were prepared from either untreated nucleoli (A: monomer;
B: dimer+trimer; C: Multimer) or RNase-digested
nucleoli (D: monomer; E: dimer+trimer; F: multimer).
These fractions and calf thymus histones (G) were
electrophoresed according to the procedure of
Weintraub, Palter and van Lente (1975).

body if the amount of the antigen was increased (Fig.6A). The intensity of the
reactions of the three fractions were the same whether obtained from intact or
RNase digested nucleoli (data not shown).

Circular dichroic studies. The conformation of nucleolar chromatin subunit preparations obtained from brief digestion by micrococcal nuclease of hamster liver
nucleoli was studied by CD. Figure 7 shows the positive CD bands in the 250-300nm
region of the monomer and the dimer+trimer obtained from nucleoli without RNase
digestion. The monomer had two positive peaks at 273nm and 268nm (4070 deg.cm^2
dmol^{-1} for both), a shoulder around 282nm and a cross-over at 265nm. A small negative band at 298nm was also seen. Compared to the monomer, the dimer+trimer

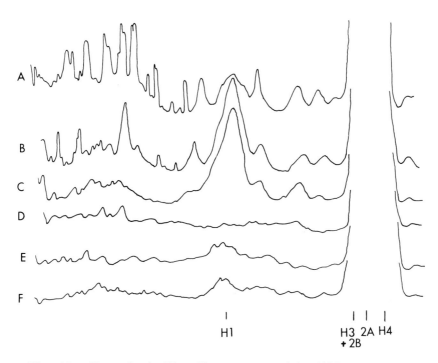

A

B

C

D

E

F

|
H1

| | |
H3 2A H4
+ 2B

Fig. 3B. The gels in Fig. 3A were scanned by Gilford spectro-
          photometer at 600nm after staining in 0.1% Coomasie
          brilliant blue, as described in Materials and Methods

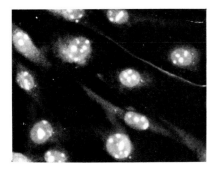
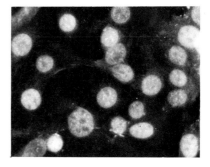

Fig. 4. Immunofluorescence of AF8 hamster nuclei reacted with
         antibodies against nonhistone protein-DNA complexes
         from hamster liver (right) and with antibodies against
         hamster liver nucleoli (left). The methodologies for
         the preparation of antibodies and the immunofluorescence
         technique are given in Materials and Methods.

preparation had a smaller positive band with two peaks, one at 272nm ($[\theta]$=2700) and
the other at 279nm ($[\theta]$=2500), a shoulder at 265nm, a small negative peak at 297nm
and a cross-over at 258nm. The difference in CD ellipticity between monomer and
the dimer+trimer is remarkable. However, if these preparations were digested with
RNase (data not shown) the magnitude of CD band was greatly reduced in both. The
CD band of the monomer peaked at 278 nm with a cross-over at 261nm and a small

negative peak at 298.   After RNase digestion, the CD of the dimer+trimer became
similar to that of the digested monomer.   It should be noted at this point that,
under the conditions of RNase digestion used in these experiments, more than 90%
of the nucleolar RNA is digested, as shown by radioactivity measurements as well as
by the CD ratio, ([θ]$_{265nm}$/[θ]$_{280nm}$.),   (Bombik, Huang and Baserga, 1977).
Thus it is obvious that RNA, which is almost as abundant in nucleoli as DNA, contri
butes significantly to the CD of the nucleolar subunit preparations.

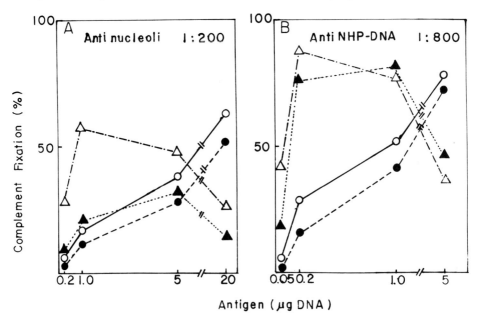

Fig. 5.   Complement fixation of nucleoli of hamster liver
          (○), nucleoli after RNase digestion (●) and
          nucleolar chromatin (△) prepared according to
          Bombik, Huang and Baserga (1977), and nuclear chrom-
          atin (▲) prepared as described in Materials and
          Methods.   A: with antinucleolar antiserum (1 : 200);
          B: with antihamster NHP-DNA complex antiserum (1 : 800).

Subunit preparations were then prepared from nucleoli devoid of RNA by RNase digestion, as previously described by Huang and Baserga (1976).   The positive CD bands
of the monomer, the dimer+trimer and the multimer preparations are shown in Fig.8.
Some differences in CD among them were observed.   The monomer showed a positive
peak at 283nm ([θ]=1590) and a cross-over at 267 nm.   No obvious shoulder was seen.
The CD of the dimer+trimer peaked at 283nm ([θ]=1550) with a shoulder around 272nm
and a cross-over at 266nm.   The CD of the multimer had a peak at 282nm ([θ]=1450)
with an enhanced shoulder at 272nm and a cross-over at 264nm.   All three preparations, especially the monomer, had a very small negative CD band around 300nm.   For
comparison, CD of the RNase digested nucleoli, either from HeLa cells (Huang and
Baserga, 1976) or hamster liver cells (not shown), usually had a peak at 282-283nm
([283]=700-1200) with a cross-over at 261-262 nm.

The negative CD bands in 210-250nm region of the three subunit preparations from
the RNase digested nucleoli, all expressed with respect to amino acid residue concentration, are shown in Fig.9.   The magnitude of the CD bands for all three preparations were different.   The molar ellipticity at 225nm, which is an indication
of the α-helix content of proteins (Chen, Yang and Martinez, 1972; Chou and Fasman

1974) was -9000, -5600 and -4300 for the monomer, the dimer+trimer and the multimer, respectively.

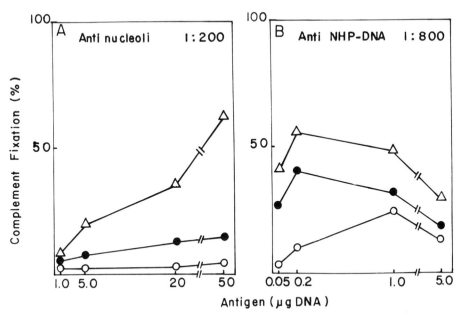

Fig. 6. Complement fixation of nucleolar chromatin subunits
(the monomer (O), the dimer+trimer (●) and the
multimer fractions (Δ), obtained from an isokinetic
sucrose gradient as shown in Fig. 2A. A: with antinucleolar antiserum (1 : 200); B: with antihamster
NHP-DNA complex antiserum (1 : 800).

DISCUSSION

The present study provides evidence that the nucleolus of mammalian cells has
chromatin subunit structure. In our procedure for the isolation of nucleoli,
vigorous sonication is necessary and sonication is known to cause shearing of
chromatin (Baserga and Nicolini, 1976). Noll, Thomas and Kornberg (1975) reported
that chromatin prepared by conventional methods involving shearing did not maintain
its chromatin subunit structure. Our results show that the extranucleolar chromatin
obtained after sonication and removal of the nucleoli lost most of its subunit
structure in terms of DNA repeats, although a few slight bands could still be detected. Under the same conditions, the presence of chromatin subunits could still
be detected in our nucleolar preparations. It is worth mentioning that chromatin
subunits were also detected in the nucleolar chromatin prepared according to Bombik,
Huang and Baserga (1977), which preserves some of the function of intact nucleoli,
although the nucleolar chromatin goes through a sucrose gradient with 5M urea to
remove most of the proteins and the RNA digests by RNase. Admittedly, our results
with polyacrylamide gels only indicate the existence of subunits in nucleolar
chromatin and do not give any quantitative information as to the yield of subunits
after sonication. However, in favor of a substantial preservation of the subunit
structure in nucleolar chromatin is the finding by CD of very low θ_{max} values in
intact and RNase digested nucleoli (Huang and Baserga, 1976). If extensive shearing had occurred, besides a smear in polyacrylamide gels, we would have observed a
much higher CD signal, since shearing causes a marked increase in the maximum positive ellipticity of chromatin (see below).

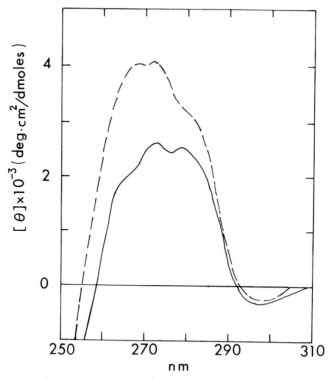

Fig. 7.   Positive CD spectra (250-310 nm of the monomer (----)
          and the dimer+trimer (———) isolated from nucleoli.
          All values are expressed in molar ellipticity in con-
          centrations of DNA-P estimated from absorbance at 260nm.

For analytical studies it is necessary to isolate chromatin subunits from nucleoli
by isokinetic sucrose gradient as done with nuclei or nuclear chromatin (Noll, 1974;
Finch, Noll and Kornberg, 1975; Noll and Kornberg, 1977). Compared to nuclei or
nuclear chromatin, nucleoli have two characteristics which must be taken into consideration. One is that nucleoli are small and yield few subunits for analysis.
The other is that nucleoli have almost the same amount of RNA as DNA and a protein/
DNA ratio of 7-8:1 (Busch and Smetana, 1970; Schmid and Sekeris, 1975), while in
chromatin isolated from whole nuclei, RNA is less than 5% of DNA and the protein/DNA
ratio is 2:1 (Baserga and Nicolini, 1976). We were able to increase the yield of
subunits by treating them with detergents, as described by Liew and Chan (1976).
For the second problem we found it important to digest nucleoli with RNase before
micrococcal nuclease digestion. By this procedure most of the RNA (checked by CD)
and most proteins (checked by acrylamide-SDS gels) were removed from the nucleoli
and the subunit fractions.

Busch and coworkers (1974) first reported that antinucleolar antisera can be produced
in rabbits immunized with isolated whole nucleoli. These antisera had some degree
of tissue specificity and tumor specificity by immunofluorescence and complement
fixation. However, the antigenic determinants of nucleoli to their antisera are
not yet known. Our results indicate that the antinucleolar antiserum reacted with
nucleolar chromatin from which most of the RNA and proteins had been removed.
Therefore, the antigenic determinants of nucleoli to the antiserum seem to be mostly
in nucleolar chromatin. The anti-NHP-DNA complex antisera are known to be tissue
specific (Wakabayashi, Wang and Hnilica, 1974; Chiu and coworkers, 1975) and species

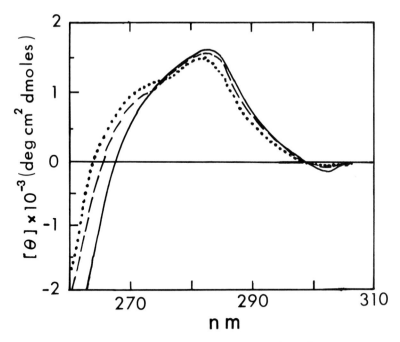

Fig. 8.   Positive CD bands of the monomer (———), the dimer+
trimer (----) and the multimer (····) obtained after
micrococcal nuclease digestion of RNase digested
nucleoli. Same conditions as in Fig.7.

specific (Zardi, and coworkers, 1974; Tsutsui, Suzuki and Iwai, 1976). According
to Chiu and coworkers (1975) the nonhistone proteins in the NHP-DNA complex consist
of 2-3 major low molecular weight proteins (not histones) and several minor high
molecular weight proteins, a finding we confirmed in our laboratory (data not shown).
The present results showing that anti-NHP-DNA complex antiserum reacted with both
nuclear and nucleolar chromatin in almost the same degree would suggest that the
antiserum does not recognize the difference between the two kinds of chromatin.

An immunological analysis of chromatin subunits has been reported by Simpson and
Bustin (1976), using antihistone antibodies. Since it would be of interest to relate chromatin subunits to the structure of chromatin (Mandel and Fasman, 1976;
Lawrence, Chan and Piette, 1976), we have investigated the relationship of nonhistone proteins to the subunit structure with the use of anti-NHP-DNA complex and
antinucleolar antisera. Although complement fixation depends on the class of antibodies in the serum, this is not too important in our experiments, because the same
antiserum was used for all the antigens. Even so, the extent of complement fixation is still highly dependent upon the arrangement as well as the number of antigenic sites, so that precise conclusions cannot be drawn from our data. However,
it can be stated that in our studies the higher the degree of polymerization of
the subunits, the more these subunits reacted with the anti-NHP-DNA complex antiserum. The antinucleolar antiserum reacted only with the multimer subunits. This
seems to be reasonable if nonhistone proteins are assumed to be located on the
bridge portion between the subunits. However, in acrylamide-SDS gels we could not
find obvious differences in the amount of nonhistone proteins between the subunit
fractions obtained from RNase digested nucleoli. It is possible that immunological
reactions can recognize a difference which is not detected in the ordinary staining
gels.

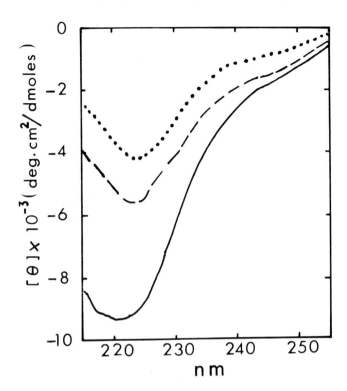

Fig. 9.   CD bands in 210-250nm region of the monomer (———),
the dimer+trimer (————) and the multimer (·····)
obtained after micrococcal nuclease digestion of
treated nucleoli.   All molar ellipticities are
expressed in concentrations of amino acid residue.

Circular dichroism has been used to probe the conformational states of DNA and proteins in complexes such as intact nuclei (Wagner and Spelsberg, 1971; Olins and
Olins, 1972; Chiu and Baserga, 1975), nuclear chromatin (Simpson and Sober, 1970;
Shih and Fasman, 1970; Johnson, Chan and Hanlon, 1972; Bartley and Chalkley, 1973;
Chang and Li, 1974; Hjelm and Huang, 1975; Baserga and Nicolini, 1976), isolated
nucleoli (Huang and Baserga, 1976; Bombik, Huang and Baserga, 1977), and nuclear
subunits (Rill and van Holde, 1973; Sahasrabuddhe and van Holde, 1974; Ramsay-Shaw
and coworkers, 1974; Mandel and Fasman, 1976; Lawrence, Chan and Piette, 1976;
Whitlock and Simpson, 1976; Olins and coworkers, 1977).   In these studies, when
compared to free DNA in aqueous solution with ($[\theta]_{275}$=8000), the positive CD bands
of all these complexes in the 250-300nm region were found greatly reduced, although
to different extents due to the protein-DNA interactions.   The subunit preparations
(from monomer up to pentamer) obtained from nuclear chromatin exhibited an ellipticity range at 282nm of 1300-2000 (Mandel and Fasman, 1976; Lawrence, Chan and Piette,
1976), which is lower than that of sonicated chromatin (4000-5000) and unsonicated
chromatin (2200-3300) (Huang and Baserga, 1976; Nicolini and Baserga, 1975; Lewis,
Dubuysere and Rees, 1976).   This in itself is an indication that little shearing
has occurred in the preparation of nucleoli and nucleolar subunits.   The CD bands
of the nuclear chromatin subunit preparations also showed a gradual blue-shift (to
short wave-lengths) in cross-over points, and an enhancement of the shoulder around
275nm from dimer up (Lawrence, Chan and Piette, 1976).   These subunits, up to trimer,
showed a similar positive peak around 282nm (Lawrence, Chan and Piette, 1976;

Mandel and Fasman, 1976) and a negative peak around 295 (Lawrence, Chan and Piette, 1976). To explain the differences in CD bands between the nuclear chromatin and its subunit preparations, it was suggested that upon organization of chromatin from subunits, some interactions between subunits occurred, resulting in a change of CD spectrum towards that of the native chromatin (Mandel and Fasman, 1976; Lawrence, Chan and Piette, 1976). Mandel and Fasman (1976) suggested more specifically that the higher molar ellipticity of chromatin than of subunits might reflect an increase in macromolecular asymmetry due to an asymmetric assembly of the subunits into chromatin at the tertiary structural level, e.g. superhelical array.

It is apparent from this study that changes in features of the positive CD band of the nucleolar subunit preparations, such as the magnitude, the shape and the peak and cross-over positions, were similar to those observed in nuclear chromatin subunit preparations. The gel electrophoretic patterns of the proteins and the DNA fragments of subunit preparations from both nuclear chromatin and RNase digested nucleoli were also similar.

It was concluded from a previous study (Huang and Baserga, 1976) that CD of the RNase digested nucleoli represented the true conformational state of DNA in the intact nucleoli. The present study indicates that all three subunit preparations had a positive ellipticity at 282nm falling within a range of 1450-1600, which was higher than that of 700-1200 exhibited by the RNase digested nucleoli. Furthermore, there was a gradual blue-shift in the position of the cross-over point, being at 267nm for the monomer, 266nm for the dimer+trimer, 264nm for the multimer and 262nm for the RNase digested nuclei. It should be noted at this point that the subunits were obtained from RNase digested nucleoli, i.e. RNA-free. Furthermore, the presence of residual RNA would not explain the spectral differences among subunit preparations (Fig.8). If the shoulder around 270nm and the blue-shift of the cross-over were due to higher RNA amounts in higher oligomers, then the molar ellipticity of these higher oligomers should be higher than that of monomers in the 275-280nm region, since the CD signal of RNA in this region is still higher than that of DNA. To explain these differences an interpretation similar to that for nuclear chromatin (Mandel and Fasman, 1976) may be used. The reduction in CD of the nucleoli may represent a loss of conformational asymmetry, as a result of the formation of tertiary structures of the subunit assembly through interactions of subunits. Alternatively, the reduction of CD ellipticity may come from a change in double-helical structure of part of the DNA molecules, such as a B to C type helical transition, as a result of interactions among subunits in nucleoli. Simultaneous contributions from both are also possible, since changes in CD band may come from changes in conformational asymmetry at both the secondary (double-helix) and the tertiary (folding or package) structural levels. Thus, in subunits, proteins markedly reduce the positive CD band of the subunits and in nucleoli proteins reduce the CD band of nucleoli further. As discussed previously (Huang and Baserga, 1976) the RNase digested nucleoli tend to aggregate, unlike subunit preparations. Thus the contribution to CD suppression from absorption flattening (Duysens, 1956; Glaser and Singer, 1971; Gordon, 1972; Schneider, 1973) cannot be ruled out.

The α-helix content of proteins, as measured by CD ellipticity at 225nm (Fig.9) was reduced as the number of the repeating subunits increased. Further studies are needed for a reasonable explanation. Assuming a similar extent of staining gel electrophoretic pattern of proteins in nucleolar subunits obtained from RNase digested nucleoli (Fig.3B) revealed that about 90% of proteins are histones, except histone H1. Most of H1 histone molecules in all three subunit preparations were lost, probably due to endogenous protease activity. Therefore, the difference among the subunit preparations in amount of histone H1, which exhibits much less helical structure than the other four histones (Bartley and Chalkley, 1973; Shih and Fasman, 1970) cannot account for the difference in total α-helix content. Somehow, upon increasing the number of subunit structures, the oligomers are organized in such a way that histones have a less α-helical structure. To our knowledge no comparative CD study on the proteins of nuclear chromatin subunit structure has bee reported.

Acknowledgments.

This work was supported by USPHS Research Grant CA-12923 and Wistar Contract AG-00378 from the National Institutes of Health. C.H. Huang is a Special Fellow of the Leukemia Society of America.

REFERENCES

Axel, R., W. Melchior, B. Sollner-Webb, and G. Felsenfeld (1974). Specific sites of interaction between histones and DNA in chromatin. Proc. Nat. Acad. Sci. USA 71, 4101-4105.

Bartley, J., and R. Chalkley (1973). An approach to the structure of native nucleo-histone. Biochemistry 12, 468-474.

Baserga, R., and C. Nicolini (1976). Chromatin structure and function in prolifer-ating cells. Biochim. Biophys. Acta 458, 109-134.

Bombik, B.M., C.H. Huang and R. Baserga (1977). Isolation of transcriptionally active chromatin from mammalian nucleoli. Proc. Nat. Acad. Sci. USA 74, 69-73.

Burton, K. (1956). A study of the conditions and mechanism of the diphenylamine reaction for the calorimetric estimation of deoxyribonucleic acid. Biochem. J. 62, 315-323.

Busch, H., and K. Smetana (1970). The Nucleolus. Academic Press, New York. pp.626

Busch, R.K., I. Daskal, W.H. Spohn, M. Kellermayer and H. Busch (1974). Rabbit antibodies to nucleoli of Novikoff hepatoma and normal liver of the rat. Cancer Res. 34, 2362-2367.

Chang, C., and H.J. Li (1974). Urea perturbation and the reversibility of nucleo-histone conformation. Nucleic Acids Res. 1, 945-958.

Chen, Y.H., J.T. Yang and H.M. Martinez (1972). Determination of the secondary structures of proteins by circular dichroism and opitcal rotatory dispersion. Biochemistry 11, 4120-4131.

Chiu, J.H., S. Wang, H. Fujitani and L.S. Hnilica (1975). DNA-binding chromosomal nonhistone proteins. Isolation, characterization, and tissue specificity. Biochemistry 14, 4552-4558.

Chiu, N., and R. Baserga (1975). Changes in template activity and structure of nuclei from WI-38 cells in the prereplicative phase. Biochemistry 14, 3126-3132.

Chou, P.Y., and G.D. Fasman (1974). Prediction of protein conformation. Biochemistry 13, 222-245.

Compton, J.L., M. Bellard and P. Chambon (1976). Biochemical evidence of vari-ability in the DNA repeat length in the chromatin of higher eukaryotes. Proc. Nat. Acad. Sci. 12, 4382-4286.

Dorman, B.P., and M.F. Maestre (1973). Experimental differential light-scattering correction to the circular dichroism of bacteriophage T2. Proc. Nat. Acad. Sci. USA 70, 255-259.

Duysens, L.N.M. (1956). The flattening of the absorption spectrum of suspensions, as compared to that of solutions. Biochim. Biophys. Acta 19, 1-12.

Felsenfeld, G. (1975). Strings of pearls. Nature 257, 177-178.

Finch, J.T., M. Noll and R.D. Kornberg (1975). Electron microscopy of defined lengths of chromatin. Proc. Nat. Acad. Sci. USA 72, 3320-3322.

Glaser, M., and S.J. Singer (1971). Circular dichroism and conformations of membrane proteins. Studies with red blood cell membranes. Biochemistry 10, 1780-1787.

Gordon, D.J. (1972). Mie scattering by optically active particles. Biochemistry 11, 413-420.

Hjelm, R.P. Jr., and R.C.C. Huang (1975). The contribution of RNA and nonhistone proteins to the circular dichroism spectrum of chromatin. Biochemistry 14, 1682-1688.

Huang, C.H., and R. Baserga (1976). Circular dichroic studies of the DNA and RNA of Nucleoli. Biochemistry 15, 2829-2836.

Johnson, E.M., V.C. Littau, V.G. Allfrey, E.M. Bradbury and H.R. Matthews (1976). The subunit structure of chromatin from physarum polycephalum. Nucleic Acids Res. 3, 3313-3329.

Johnson, R.S., A. Chan and S. Hanlon (1972). Mixed conformations of deoxyribonucleic acid in intact chromatin isolated by various preparative methods. Biochemistry 11, 4347-4358.

Kornberg, R.D. (1974). Chromatin structure: A repeating unit of histones and DNA. Science 184, 868-871.

Laemmli, U.K. (1970). Cleavage of structural proteins during the assembly of the head of bacteriophage T4. Nature (London) 227, 680-685.

Lawrence, J.J., D.C.F. Chan and L.H. Piette (1976). Conformational state of DNA in chromatin subunits. Circular dichroism, melting and ethidium bromide binding analysis. Nucleic Acids Res. 3, 2879-2893.

Lebowitz, P., W. Siegel and J. Sklar (1974). Hemophilus aegyptius restriction endonuclease cleavage map of the Simian virus 40 genome and its colinear relation with the Hemophilus influenzae cleavage map of SV40. J. Mol. Biol. 88, 105-123.

Lewis, E.A., M.S. Dubuysere and A.M. Rees (1976). Configuration of unsheared nucleohistone. Effects of ionic strength and of histone F1 removal. Biochemistry 15, 186-192.

Liew, C.C., and P.K. Chan (1976). Identification of nonhistone chromatin proteins in chromatin subunits. Proc. Nat. Acad. Sci. USA 73, 3458-3462.

Mandel, R., and G.D. Fasman (1976). Chromatin and nucleosome structure. Nucleic Acids Res. 3, 1839-1855.

Mathis, D.J., and A. Gorovsky (1976). Subunit structure of rDNA-containing chroma-
    Biochemistry 15, 750-755.

McConkey, E.H., and J.W. Hopkins (1964). The relationship of the nucleolus to the
    synthesis of ribosomal RNA in HeLa cells. Proc. Nat. Acad. Sci. 51, 1197-1204.

Muramatsu, M., Y. Hayashi, T. Onishi, M. Sakai, K. Takai and T. Kashiyama (1974).
    Rapid isolation of nucleoli from detergent purified nuclei of various tumor and
    and tissue culture cells. Exp. Cell Res. 88, 345-351.

Nicolini, C., and R. Baserga (1975). Circular dichroism and ethidium bromide bind-
    ing studies of chromatin from WI-38 fibroblasts stimulated to proliferate.
    Chem.-Biol. Interact. 11, 101-116.

Noll, M. (1974). Subunit structure of chromatin. Nature (London) 251, 249-251.

Noll, M., and R.D. Kornberg (1977). Action of micrococcal nuclease on chromatin
    and the location of histone H1. J. Mol. Biol. 109, 393-404.

Noll, M., J.O. Thomas and R.D. Kornberg (1975). Preparation of native chromatin
    and damage caused by shearing. Science 187, 1203-1206.

Olins, D.E., P.N. Bryan, R.E. Harrington, W.E. Hill and A.L. Olins (1977). Con-
    formational states of chromatin v bodies induced by urea. Nucleic Acids Res.
    4, 1911-1931.

Olins, D.E., and A.L. Olins (1972). Physical studies of isolated eucaryotic
    nuclei. J. Cell Biol. 53, 715-736.

Oudet, P., M. Gross-Bellard and P. Chambon (1975). Electron microscopic and bio-
    chemical evidence that chromatin structure is a repeating unit. Cell 4, 281-
    300.

Peacock, A.C. and C.W. Dingman (1967). Resolution of multiple ribonucleic acid
    species by polyacrylamide gel electrophoresis. Biochemistry 6, 1818-1827.

Peacock, A.C., and C.W. Dingman (1968). Molecular weight estimation and separation
    of ribonucleic acid by electrophoresis in Agarose-acrylamide composite gels.
    Biochemistry 7, 668-674.

Piper, P.W., J. Celis, K. Kaltoft, J.C. Leer, P.F. Nielson and O. Watergaard (1976).
    Tetrahymena ribosomal RNA gene chromatin is digested by micrococcal nuclease at
    sites which have the same regular spacing on the DNA as corresponding sites in
    the bulk nuclear chromatin. Nucleic Acids Res. 3, 493-505.

Ramsay-Shaw, B., J.L. Gorden, C.G. Sahasrabuddhe and K.E. van Holde (1974). Chroma-
    tographic separation of chromatin subunits. Biochem. Biophys. Res. Comm. 61,
    1193-1198.

Reeves, R. (1975). Ribosomal genes of Xenopus laevis: Evidence of nucleosomes
    in transcriptionally active chromatin. Science 194, 529-532.

Reeves, R., and A. Jones (1976). Genomic transcriptional activity and the structure
    of chromatin. Nature (London) 260, 495-500.

Rill, R., and K.E. van Holde (1973). Properties of nuclease-resistant-fragments of
    calf thymus chromatin. J. Biol. Chem. 248, 1080-1083.

Sahasrabuddhe, C.G., and K.E. van Holde (1974). The effect of trypsin on nuclease-resistant chromatin fragments. J. Biol. Chem. 249-152-156.

Schmid, W., and C.E. Sekeris (1975). Nucleolar RNA synthesis in the liver of partially hepatectomized and cortisol-treated rats. Biochim. Biophys. Acta 402, 244-252.

Schneider, A.S. (1973). Analysis of optical activity spectra of turbid biological suspensions. In C.H.W. Hirs and S.N. Timasheff (Eds.), Methods in Enzymol. 27D, 751-767.

Senior, M.B., A.L. Olins and D.E. Olins (1975). Chromatin fragments resembling ν bodies. Science 187, 173-175.

Shih, T.Y., and G.D. Fasman (1970). Conformation of deoxyribonucleic acid in chromatin: A circular dichroism study. J. Mol. Biol. 52, 125-129.

Simpson, R.T., and M. Bustin (1976). Histone composition of chromatin subunits studied by immunosedimentation. Biochemistry 15, 4305-4312.

Simpson, R.T., and H.A. Sober (1970). Circular dichroism of calf liver nucleohistone. Biochemistry 9, 3103-3109.

Steele, W.J. (1968). Localization of deoxyribonucleic acid complementary to ribosomal ribonucleic acid and preribosomal ribonucleic acid in the nucleolus of rat liver. J. Biol. Chem. 243, 3333-3341.

Thomas, J.O., and R.D. Kornberg (1975). An octamer of histones in chromatin and free in solution. Proc. Nat. Acad. Sci. USA 72, 2626-2630.

Tsutsui, Y., H.L. Chang and R. Baserga (1977). Cell-cycle dependent expression of proteins reacting with anti-human antiserum in a somatic cell hybrid between human and hamster cells. Cell. Biol. Int 1. Rep. 1, 301-308.

Tsutsui, Y., I. Suzuki and K. Iwai (1976). Immunofluorescent study of nonhistone protein-DNA complexes in cultured cells and lymphocytes. Exp. Cell Res. 101, 202-206.

Tuan, D.Y.H., and J. Bonner (1969). Optical absorbance and optical rotatory dispersion studies on calf thymus nucleohistone. J. Mol. Biol. 45, 59-76.

Urry, D.W., and J. Krivacic (1970). Differential scatter of left and right circularly polarized light by optically active particulate system. Proc. Nat. Acad. Sci. USA. 65, 845-852.

van Holde, K.E., C.G. Sahasrabuddhe, B.R. Shaw, E.F.J. Bruggen and A.C. Arnberg (1974) Electron microscopy of chromatin subunit particles. Biochem. Biophys. Res. Comm. 60, 1365-1370.

Wagner, T., and T.C. Spelsberg (1971). Aspects of chromosomal structure I. Circular dichroism studies. Biochemistry 10, 2599-2605.

Wakabayashi, K., S. Wang and L.S. Hnilica (1974). Immunospecificity of nonhistone proteins in chromatin. Biochemistry 13, 1027-1032.

Wasserman, E., and L. Levine (1961). Quantitative micro-complement fixation and its use in the study of antigenic structure by specific antigen-antibody inhibition. J. Immunol. 87, 290-295.

Weintraub, H., K. Palter and F. van Lente (1975). Histones H2a, H2b, H3, and H4 form a tetrameric complex in solutions of high salt. Cell 6, 85-110.

Whelly, S., T. Ide and R. Baserga (1978). Stimulation of RNA synthesis in isolated nucleoli by preparations of Simian virus 40 T antigen. Virology 88, 82-91.

Whitlock, J.P.Jr., and R.T. Simpson (1976). Preparation and physical characterization of homogeneous population of monomeric nucleosomes from HeLa cells. Nucleic Acids Res. 3, 2255-2266.

Zardi, L., J .C. Lin, R.O. Petersen and R. Baserga (1974). Specificity of antibodies to nonhistone chromosomal proteins of cultured fibroblasts. In B. Clarkson and R. Baserga (Eds.), Control of Proliferation in Animal Cells. Cold Spring Harbor Lab. pp.729-741.

Mitochondrial-Cytoplasmic Interactions in Protein Synthesis in the Walker Carcinosarcoma

N. F. González-Cadavid, L. Rodríguez E. and Z. Campos

Departamento de Biología Celular, Facultad de Ciencias,
Universidad Central de Venezuela, Caracas, Venezuela

ABSTRACT

Cancer cells contain mitochondria with deep structural and functional alterations accompanied by increase of circular DNA oligomers, decrease of electron carriers and respiratory enzymes, presence of replicating oncorna viruses, etc. The endoplasmic reticulum, where most mitochondrial proteins are made, is poorly developed and replaced by free ribosomes. Therefore, selection of mRNA coding for mitochondrial proteins in the cytoplasm, protein transport to the organelle, and the possible export of mitochondrial factors regulating the rate of translation on cytoribosomes, are processes likely to be disturbed in the cancer cell. We approached these questions by studying the influence of mitochondrial protein synthesis on cytoplasmic translation in Walker carcinosarcoma cells. We showed that they contain closed circular DNA, that it is transcribed in vivo to large and small rRNA, tRNA and poly A-containing RNA, and that their mini-ribosomes are similar to those of liver. However, mitochondrial protein synthesis was very low when cytoplasmic translation was blocked by cycloheximide, either in the solid tumour or in cell incubations, and in vitro in the isolated organelles. This reduced activity could be blocked in suspension cultures of ascites cells by chloramphenicol, and a significant decrease was observed in the rate of cytoplasmic protein synthesis. The inhibition was found at concentrations as low as 1 mM, was not counteracted by glucose, and was reflected in an impaired capacity of isolated ribosomes and soluble factors for mRNA translation. These results indicate that protein synthesis in tumour mitochondria is disarranged, but still may be required to regulate cytoplasmic protein synthesis through the possible release of translational inhibitors.

KEYWORDS

Mitochondria, protein synthesis, Walker carcinoma, chloramphenicol, coordination, regulation.

INTRODUCTION

The mitochondria of most cancer cells are characterized by a series of functional and structural alterations which, as most authors agree, are the result of the deep subcellular disarrangement occurring in the later stages of malignant transformation and proliferation, rather than being processes linked to earlier events

of carcinogenesis. Some of these changes are summarized in Table 1, with the per
tinent references given in the papers by Eboli and others (1976) and by González-
Cadavid and Pérez (1975, 1976). The general picture of a tumour cell corresponds
to a low respiration/high glycolysis type (Racker, 1974), and its mitochondria
are somehow similar to those of glucose -or anaerobiosis- repressed yeast cells.
This is reflected, as mitochondrial protein synthesis is concerned, in a very low
cytochrome aa₃/c ratio and decrease in succinate dehydrogenase, monoamino oxidase
and other enzymes (White and Tewari, 1973; White and Nandy, 1976; Sato and others,
1976).

TABLE 1 SUMMARY OF SOME ALTERATIONS OBSERVED

IN MITOCHONDRIA FROM CANCER CELLS

A) Morphological and ultrastructural alterations	B) Decrease in enzyme and electron carrier levels	C) Mecanochemical alterations
Decrease in number per cell Smaller size Irregular shape Fewer cristae Bizarre cristae configurations Vacuolization of the matrix Increased fragility during isolation Reduced buoyant density Population heterogeneity during centrifugation	a) Electron transport activity: NADH dehydrogenase and oxidase Succinate oxidase Cytochrome oxidase α-glycerophosphate oxidase and NADH-shuttle pathway b) Phosphorylating activity: ATPase c) Krebs cycle enzymes: Pyruvate carboxylase Succinate dehydrogenase d) Outer membrane enzymes: Adenylate kinase Rotenone-insens. NADH reductase	Impairment of respiratory rate and acceptor control ratio Low levels of ATP Loss of orthodox/condensed conformational transition and high amplitude swelling Failure to release accumulated Ca^{2+} and to accumulate K^+ Decrease of concanavalin binding

From the point of view of molecular biology, current interest is centered on some
early events taking place in mitochondria during cell transformation by oncogenic
viruses. Leukemic leucocytes have a high proportion of unicircular dimers and
higher oligomers of mitochondrial DNA (mtDNA), which correlates with the severity
and evolution of the disease (see e.g., Newman and Scaletti, 1975; Matsumoto, Pikó and Vinograd, 1976). Nass and coworkers (see e.g., D'Agostino and Nass, 1976)
have presented evidence that mtDNA synthesis in chick-embryo fibroblasts infected
with Rous sarcoma virus or with a thermosensitive mutant, is stimulated three to
five-fold over that in uninfected cells. These changes occur in the mutant infec
ted cells only at the permissive temperature. The stimulation of mtDNA synthesis
is also probably linked to the high content of mtDNA and RNA in neoplastic cells,
attributable to a higher rate of mitochondriogenesis due to rapid cell prolifera-

tion (see Marinozzi and others, 1977). Moreover, the formation of dimers and oli
gomers of mtDNA is temperature-dependent, correlating with the phenotypic manifes
tation of transformation, and apparently depends on the import into the organelle
of some cytoplasmically-made peptides. Suggestions that mitochondria play a signi
ficant role in the replication of oncogenic viruses and their cell-transforming ac
tion, are based on one side on the detection in the organelle of Gs antigens, viral
reverse transcriptase, and subviral particles (virosomes), and on the other side
on the blockade of virus replication and malignant transformation exerted by chloramphenicol and ethidium bromide (see for references González-Cadavid and Pérez,
1975, Neifakh, 1977), well known inhibitors of mitochondrial translation and trans
cription. Other reports dealing with the stimulation of mtDNA synthesis by cell
infection with oncogenic viruses (monkey cells with SV 40, 3T3 cells with polyoma,
Hela and mouse cells with herpes simplex) are listed by D'Agostino and Nass (1976).
These results agree with many reports on the electron microscopy observation of
intramitochondrial bodies assumed to be virus particles (Korb and Ríman, 1976; Marinozzi and others, 1977; Lunger and Clark, 1974; Szekely, Fisher and Schumacher,
1976), both in cell-lines and in human leukemic monoblasts and lymphoblasts, although in the latter case the inclusions have not yet been conclusively identified
histochemically.

The mitochondria of animal cells are semi-autonomous organelles containing the machinery for nucleic acid and protein synthesis, but with a small genome of about
10^6 dalton which codes for the organelle tRNAs, rRNAs, and poly A-containing RNAs
and for only a limited amount (about 10 %) of their proteins. The poly-peptides
made on mito-ribosomes can be separated in 10-12 bands by polyacrylamide gel elec
trophoresis with molecular weights ranging from 11 000 to 42 000. These bands are
assumed to correspond to the tree large peptides of cytochrome oxidase, four subunits of the oligomycin-sensitive ATPase, and at least one of the cytochrome b and
cytochrome c subunits (see Schatz, 1974, González-Cadavid 1974, Costantino and
Attardi, 1975). This means that most of the mitochondrial proteins are synthesized by cytoplasmic ribosomes and transferred to the organelle through soluble com
partments, such as the cytosol and the endoplasmic reticulum lumen (Sáez de Cordo
ba, Cohén and González-Cadavid, 1976). Therefore, the mitochondrial/cytoplasmic
coordination of protein synthesis must necessarily be based on regulatory mechanisms operating to and from the organelle. Most of the attention in this field
has been focused on the positive modulation of mitochondrial protein synthesis by
peptides manufactured by the cytoribosomes (Ibrahim and Beattie, 1976; Costantino
& Attardi, 1977).

We have approached the reverse situation, that is, the possibility that mitochondrial products play a significant role in the regulation of cytoplasmic translation, as a way to control the extra-mitochondrial formation of mitochondrial proteins, or even more general aspects of cell growth. The Walker carcinosarcoma
offers advantages for this type of study, because being originally a solid tumour,
it can be converted into ascites cells able to propagate in culture; and containing the deeply altered mitochondria already described as characteristic of highly
malignant tumours. If one considers that the cytoplasmic ribosomes are mainly
free in the cytoplasm, the carcinoma cells constitute the opposite situation to
that of a normal excretory cell such as the hepatocite. We have therefore chosen
both types of cells, in an effort to characterize the putative regulatory mechanisms through which mitochondria would affect cytoplasmic protein synthesis, and
to determine to what extent, if any, they are altered in the neoplastic cell.

The existence of translational regulation of cytoplasmic protein synthesis is a
well established fact (see review by Lodish, 1976), and it is thought that it may
be mediated in rapidly growing tumours through the defficiency of specific isoac-
cepting tRNAs (Lerman and others, 1976). Other plausible models of translational

control have been formulated (Pitot, 1974), where differentiation and oncogenic transformation are seen as extragenomic alterations possibly exerted at the level of translation. Some speculations have been advanced on the putative export of mitochondrial proteins, detected by chloramphenicol-sensitive labelling of protein in microsomes of Neurospora crassa, which might act as repressors of nuclear genes and be even one of the functional basis in animal cells for the linkage of the organelle to cellular transformation (Makclin and others, 1977), but a similar mechanism at the translational level is also possible (González-Cadavid, Dorta and Pérez, 1978). An ultimate goal of the present work, is therefore to investigate whether it is possible, by interfering with mtDNA transcription and translation, to slow down preferentially malignant cell proliferation as compared to the normal process.

RESULTS AND DISCUSSION

Our first aim was to determine to what extent endogenous protein synthesis was disarranged in the abnormal cell mitochondria, and we started to look for the identification of the components of the machinery required for autonomous replication, transcription and translation of the organelle genome. This is important, because it is known that 'petite' mutants of yeast may lack functionally or even structurally recognizable mitochondrial DNA and still have mitochondrial membranes not very different from the normal ones. The activity of mitoribosomes is neither essential for the formation of the organelle structure, although it is required for the integration of the cytochrome oxidase or ATPase complexes and of the hydrophobic type of other cytochromes such as $\underline{b}$ or $\underline{c_1}$ (Storrie and Attardi, 1973 a, b).

In the case of tumour mitochondria, one has to extreme precautions for purification because, due to their heterogeneity in size and density, it is usually difficult to remove ribosomes or endoplasmic reticulum fragments, lysosomes and peroxysomes, by simple differential centrifugation. Our laboratory developed a procedure which yielded a very small fraction of the total mitochondrial population with reasonable purity as assessed by electron microscopy and enzyme markers (González-Cadavid and Pérez, 1975, 1976). Cytochrome oxidase estimations gave a calculated recovery of only 7 % of the total mitochondrial protein, the latter amounting to about 10 % of the tumour cell protein.

When we tried to isolate closed circled DNA from these mitochondria by applying conventional phenol-based procedures we did not succeed. However we obtained an excellent separation of (^{3}H) thymidine labelled DNA I (corresponding to the native molecules) when disrupting the organelle with sodium dodecyl sulphate in the presence of a high concentration of ethidium bromide, followed by CsCl centrifugation with the same agent (Fig. 1). The closed twisted circles were readily apparent on electron microscopy with the Kleinshmidt technique.

The various forms of mitochondrial RNA, that is, tRNA, rRNA and poly A-containing RNA, were also detected in carcinoma mitochondria, and analysed by polyacrylamide gel electrophoresis and sucrose gradient centrifugation. The electrophoretic peaks 21 Se and 16 Se (16 and 14 S, respectively) were assumed to correspond to the large and small subunits of mitochondrial ribosomes, whereas the 4 Se (4S) peak contained the tRNAs. The ^{32}P -labelled fraction retained on poly U Sepharose from the crude phenolic RNA extract, was equated to mRNA since all other RNA species lack poly A (Fig. 2). The ribosomal RNAs are correctly assembled into large and small subunits of 'mini' ribosomes with sizes nearly identical to those of the liver sub-structures (30, 40 and 56 S, respectively). All these RNA species, with the possible exception of some tRNAs, are coded by mit DNA, since their synthesis is resistant to actinomycin D at doses that block nuclear DNA transcription into cytoplasmic rRNA. (González-Cadavid and Pérez, 1976).

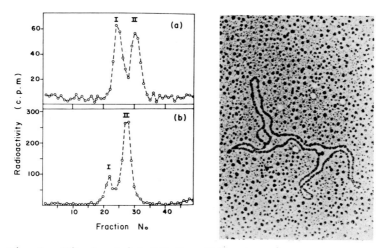

Fig. 1. Mitochondrial DNA from Walker carcinoma.

Left panel: separation by cesium chloride gra -
dient centrifugation of forms I (closed circles)
and II (open circles and linear molecules) labeled with (^{3}H) thymidine. Right panel: Electron
micrograph (kindly taken by Dr. Pedro Lava-Sán-
chez) of molecules in peak 1.

The real test for the functionality of this machinery in protein synthesis is the
assesment of the incorporation of radioactive amino acids into mitochondrial pro
teins under conditions of blockade of cytoplasmic protein synthesis, or in the iso
lated organelles. The first experiments were carried out in vivo by injecting in
creasing doses of cycloheximide until inhibition up to 98 % in the labelling of
microsomal protein by (^{14}C) leucine was obtained. The extent of cycloheximide re
sistant incorporation was then measured in both the Walker carcinoma and the liver
purified mitochondria. Whereas in the normal tissue about 10 % of the mitochon -
drial proteins were made on ribosomes insensitive to this antibiotic (that is,
endougenous to the organelle), in the tumour this fraction decreased to only 2.5%.

The isolated mitochondria from the tumour were even less active, since the incorpo
ration was about 10-fold lower than in the case of liver (Fig. 3). Besides, only
60 % was sensitive to chloramphenicol as compared to nearly 90% in liver; therefore, if only the cycloheximide-resistant, chloramphenicol-sensitive, protein syn
thesis was considered, the difference between the tumour and normal mitochondria
amounted to 15-fold. However, since the nearly total inactivity of the carcinoma
organelles could be due to increased fragility of their membranes, this question
was re-examined in incubations of ascites cells.

The ascites form of the tumour was obtained by inoculating the solid tumour fragments in the peritoneal cavity to allow a 2-3 days growth. Cells were then collected, freed from contaminating erythrocytes by hypotonic shock and suspended in
Spinner flasks in either Earle's-5% dialyzed calf serum for immediate short-time
incubations (0-4 h), or in Dulbecco 10% heat inactivated calf serum for more prolonged incubations, or for cell cultures. The latter were maintained for several
months with an average duplication time of 17 h.

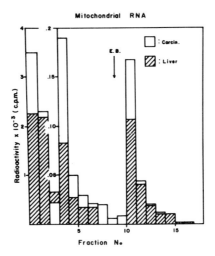

Fig. 2.   Mitochondrial poly A-containing RNA from Walker
carcinosarcoma and liver.

A phenol extract of mitochondrial ^{32}P-labeled RNA
was chromatographed on poly-U Sepharose. The frac‾
tion containing poly-A started to emerge at the
arrow.

In 1/2 and 2 h incubations with 100 ug/ml of cycloheximide, chloramphenicol inhited
by 80% the incorporation into proteins from the purified mitochondria, and the endogenous synthesis thus estimated amounted to 5 % of the total mitochondrial proteins. This is only half of the similar value in normal cells, but still showed
that the deeply disarranged carcinoma organelles can carry out protein synthesis,
albeit the acrylamide gel electrophoretic profile was very heterogenous, with no
distinct peaks visible in contrast to the situation in the absence of cycloheximide.

Having established that the tumour mitoribosomes are functional and normally inhibited by chloramphenicol, we set up to determine whether their blockade has any
affect on cytoplasmic protein synthesis, and on malignancy as measured by the in
vivo proliferation of the tumour cells. For this purpose we incubated in different
experiments cells recently isolated from the peritoneal cavity, and cultured cells,
with increasing concentrations of chloramphenicol for long periods (20 and 30 h),
and measured the incorporation of (^{3}H) leucine into total cell protein as an indi‾
cation of how cytoplasmic protein synthesis was affected (since mitochondrial syn‾
thesis accounts for less than 1% in this process). It was evident that even very
low concentrations of chloramphenicol ($\leq$10 ug/ml) inhibited cytoplasmic protein
synthesis by at least 10%, and that at 200 ug/ml the inhibition was 25-40% (Fig.
4). This is the concentration that assures a complete blockade of mitochondrial
protein synthesis, even of that fraction resistant to lower doses (Storrie and
Attardi, 1973 a). The inhibition is not due to a direct interference of the drug
with NADH dehydrogenase, since addition of glucose at various concentrations does
not counteract inhibition (see Freeman, Patel and Haldar, 1977, for references).
HeLa cells can grow for up to 5 days in 200 ug/ml chloramphenicol without gross
effects on mitochondrial number or general size or on the amount of inner membrane
per mitochondrion, but the morphology is considerably altered leading to fewer and
concentric cristae rolled in whorled or myelin-like configuration. Mitochondrial
protein synthesis and cell growth recovers quite rapidly after chloramphenicol

removal (Storrie and Attardi, 1973 a, b). Also, in mouse liver the administration of chloramphenicol induces the appearance of matrix-enriched megamitochondria with greatly reduced inner membrane enzyme activities (Wagner and Rafael, 1977).

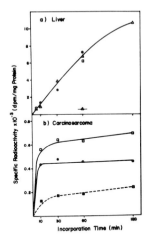

Fig. 3.   Time course of endogenous protein synthesis by isolated mitochondria from liver and Walker carcinoma.

Liver: o; □ ; △: cycloheximide-resistant incorpor. -▲-: cycloheximide and chloramphenicol-resistant incorp.; Carcinoma:□ : cycloheximide-resistant in corpor.; o: cycloheximide and chloramphenicol-re-sistant incorp.; ▨--- ▨ : chloramphenicol sensi-tive incorpor.

From the start of the incubation with chloramphenicol, treated cells incorporate less (^{3}H) leucine than the controls, and since leucine pools are not significantly modified, this indicates a lower rate of protein synthesis (Fig. 4). This was con firmed by direct protein estimation of cells incubated in tubes. The decrease in protein synthesis is more considerable than the slight inhibition of DNA synthesis shown by an 8-12% reduction in (^{3}H) thymidine incorporation (decreasing slopes are caused by radioactive precursor depletion and not by arrest of DNA synthesis). Besides the duplication time is increased leading to a corresponding decrease in cell number in the second generation time. Therefore, cells contain less protein, and in fact they are smaller than the controls.

We assume that the decrease in cytoplasmic protein synthesis observed in the car-cinoma cells treated with 200 ug/ml of chloramphenicol is a consequence of the blockade of mitochondrial protein synthesis rather than due to unspecific effects derived from chloramphenicol interference with cell respiration. This would point to a tight coupling of cytoplasmic and mitochondrial translation which could lead to a preferential inhibition of the cytoplasmic synthesis of mitochondrial pro-teins. After a long-term labelling with (^{3}H) leucine (20 h), mitochondrial pro-teins were immunoprecipitated from the three soluble cell compartments using spe cific antisera. Cells treated with chloramphenicol showed the usual 25 % decrease in cumulative total protein radioactivity, whereas the mitochondrial proteins in the matrix compartment were reduced by 45 %, with no corresponding accumulation in the cytosol or the endoplasmic reticulum lumen.

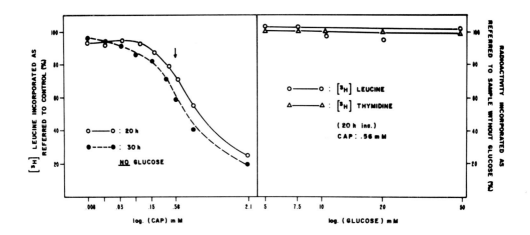

Fig. 4.   Inhibition of cytoplasmic protein synthesis in
Walker carcinoma cells with mitochondrial translation blocked by chloramphenicol.

Left panel: Log dose-response to the drug in 20
and 30 h incubations. Arrow shows 0.56 mM (0.2
ug/ml). Right panel: Lack of effect of added
glucose on the inhibition exerted by 0.2 ug/ml
chloramphenicol.

Do these results mean that in the cell there are mitochondrial signals which can
traverse the inner and outer membranes and switch off cytoplasmic protein synthesis at the transcription or the translation level? We believe so, and from the
two possibilities, we have chosen to examine the latter. Previous work from our
laboratory demonstrated that purified mitochondria from both Walker carcinoma and
rat liver contain easily extractable, small size, factors that can inhibit protein
synthesis in vitro by cytoplasmic ribosomes from both tissues. These inhibitors
penetrate into intact cells, blocking both cytoplasmic and mitochondrial protein
synthesis (González-Cadavid, Dorta, and Pérez, 1978), and are in part free in the
matrix or bound to macromolecules. The latter can be released by heating or high
ionic strenght. We have estimated them in liver mitochondria and calculated that
the passage of only 5% to the cytoplasm would suffice for inhibiting cytoplasmic
protein synthesis by 50%. Preliminary estimations in carcinoma mitochondria show
a considerably reduced content. For the moment, we have not yet detected and estimated the inhibitory factors in the cytoplasm from either normal or carcinoma
cells, and therefore we ignore whether their lower mitochondrial content is conco
mitantly accompanied by a similar decrease in the cytoplasmic concentration in
tumour.

Chloramphenicol inhibition of cytoplasmic protein synthesis in intact normal and
carcinoma cells causes a 20-30% decrease in the ability of isolated cytoplasmic
ribosomes to translate polyuridilic acid in vitro into polyphenylalanine. The
pH5 fraction from the chloramphenicol-treated cells, when tested at different pro
tein concentrations in a translation system with liver ribosomes, exhibits a different curve to that from the normal cells, suggesting the presence of an inhibitor. Preliminary experiments with the concentrated supernatant from heat-treated
dialyzed cell sap support this assumption. We have no idea yet on whether the

putative inhibitors in the cytosol and/or the ribosomes, would be the same as the inhibitory factors described so far in normal and in carcinoma mitochondria. The fact that inhibitory factors apparently increase in the cytoplasm of tumour cells with mitochondrial translation blocked by chloramphenicol would be due to a facilitated passage of these factors to the cytoplasm, derived from a more considerable alteration in the chloramphenicol inhibited organelle.

A certain degree of translational inhibition in tumour cells as compared to normal ones is not necessarily incompatible with a higher overall rate of protein synthesis, depending primarily on the release of transcriptional regulatory mechanisms. On the contrary, it would provide firstly, a way for manufacturing less mitochondrial proteins for conditions where they are required in lower amounts and in more general and speculative terms, for modulating cell growth according to the functional and structural integrity of the mitochondria. This is not illogical, considering that the final stages of tumour growth lead gradually to deeper alteration of the organelle and a slower rate of cell replication and protein synthesis. Additional work is necessary to clarify the mechanisms by which mitochondrial nucleic acid and protein synthesis are related to cytoplasmic protein synthesis. Whether this interaction is altered and to what extent it may affect the uncontrolled malignant growth, remains to be elucidated.

REFERENCES

Avadhani, N.G., Hansel, G., Ritter, C., and Rutman, R.J. (1976). Cancer Biochem. Biophys., 1, 167-174.

Costantino, P., and Attardi, G. (1975). Identification of discrete electrophoretic components among the products of mitochondrial protein synthesis in HeLa cells. J. Mol.Biol., 96, 291-306.

Costantino, P., and Attardi, G. (1977). Metabolic properties of the products of mitochondrial protein synthesis in HeLa cells. J.Biol. Chem., 252, 1702-1711.

D'Agostino, M.A., and Nass, M.M.K. (1976). Specific changes in the synthesis of mitochondrial DNA in chick embryo fibroblasts transformed by Rous sarcoma viruses. J. Cell. Biol., 71, 781-794.

Eboli, M.L., Galeotti, T., Dionisi, O., Longhi, G., and Terranova, T. (1976). Shuttles for the transfer of reducing equivalents in Ehrlich ascites tumour cells. Arch. Biochem. Biophys., 173, 747-749.

Egilson, V., Evans, I.H., and Wilkie, D. (1976). Primary antimitochondrial activity of carcinogens in Sacharomyces cerevisiae. in Th. Bücher and others (ed). 'Genetics and biogenesis of chloroplasts and mitochondria', Elsevier/North Holland Biomedical Press, Amsterdam. The Netherlands.

Freeman, K.B., Patel, H., and Haldar, D. (1977). Inhibition of deoxyribonucleic acid synthesis in Ehrlich ascites cells by chloramphenicol. Mol. Pharmacol., 13, 504-511.

González-Cadavid, N.F. (1974). The biosynthesis of mitochondrial cytochromes. Sub Cell. Biochem., 3, 275-309.

González-Cadavid, N.F., and Pérez, J.L. (1975). Electrophoretic and centrifugation behaviour of mitochondrial ribonucleic acid from Walker 256 carcinosarcoma. Biochem. J., 146, 361-363.

González-Cadavid, N.F., and Pérez, J.L. (1976). Identification of the products of mitochondrial transcription in the Walker carcinosarcoma by the use of actinomycin D and ethidium bromide. Cancer Res., 36, 1754-1760.

González-Cadavid, N.F., Dorta, B., and Pérez, J.L. (1978). Isolation and partial characterization of protein synthesis inhibitors present in mitochondria from rat liver and Walker carcinosarcoma. Biochem. Biophys. Acta, submitted for publication.

Ibrahim, N.G., and Beattie, D.S. (1976). Regulation of mitochondrial protein synthesis at the polyribosomal level. J. Biol. Chem., 251, 108-115.

Korb, J., and Ríman, J. (1976). Presence of intramitochondrial bodies in avian leukemic myeloblasts. Europ. J. Cancer, 12, 959-961.

Lerman, M.I., Pilipenko, N.N., Ugarova, T.Y., Sokolova, E.S., Vinnizky, L.I., and

Phishkova, Z.P. (1976). The limiting effect of transfer RNA's on the rate of pro
tein synthesis in cell extracts of rapidly growing tumours. Cancer Res., 36, 2995
3000.

Lodish, H.F., (1976). Translational control of protein synthesis. Ann. Rev.Biochem
45, 39-72.

Lunger, P.D., and Clarck, H.F. (1974). Ultrastructural studies of cell-virus inte
action in reptilian cell lines. II. Distribution, incidence, and factors enhancing
the production of intramitochondrial virions. Natl. Cancer Inst.Monograph, 53, 533
540.

Macklin, W.B., Meyer, D.J., Woodward, D.O., and Erickson, S.K. (1977). Chloramphenicol-sensitive labelling of protein in microsomes of Neurospora crassa. Nature,
269, 447-450.

Marinozzi, V., Derenzini, M., Nardi, F., and Gallo, P. (1977). Mitochondrial inclusions in human cancer of the gastrointestinal tract. Cancer Res., 37, 1556-1563.

Matsumoto, L., Pikó, L., and Vinograd, J. (1976). Complex mitochondrial DNA in ani
mal thyroids. A comparative study. Biochem. Biophys Acta, 432, 251-266.

Miyaki, M., Yatagai, K., and Ono, T. (1977). Strands breaks of mammalian mitochondrial DNA induced by carcinogens. Chem. Biol. Interactions, 17, 321-329.

Neifakh, S.A. (1977). Mitochondrial genes and cell heredity. Molec & Cell Biochem.,
14, 5-10.

Newman, D.C. and Scaletti, J.V. (1975). Topological forms of mitochondrial DNA in
AKR mice. J. Natl. Cancer Inst., 55, 1219-1221.

Pitot, H. (1974). Neoplasia: a somatic mutation or a heritable change in cytoplasmic membranes? J. Natl Cancer Inst., 53, 905-911.

Racker, E. (1974). History of the Pasteur effect and its pathobiology. Molec. and
Cell Biochem., 5, 17-23.

Reitz, R.C., Thompson, J.A., and Morris, H.P. (1977). Mitochondrial and microsomal
phospholipids of Morris hepatoma 7777. Cancer Res., 37, 561-567.

Sáez de Córdova, C., Cohén, R. and González-Cadavid, N.F. (1977). Synthesis of
haem and cytochrome c prosthetic group from α-aminolaevulinate by the cell sap
from rat liver. Biochem. J., 106, 305-313.

Sato, N., Hagihara, B., Kamada, T., Abe, H., Senoh, H., and Kitagawa, M. (1976).
An abnormal ratio of cytochromes in the respiratory chain of mouse and human myelo
mas. Biochem. Biophys. Acta, 423, 557-572.

Schatz, G., and Mason, T.L. (1974). The biosynthesis of mitochondrial proteins.
Ann. Rev. Biochem., 43, 51-87.

Storrie, B., and Attardi, G. (1973 a). Mode of mitochondrial formation in HeLa
cells. J. Cell Biol., 56, 833-838.

Storrie, B., and Attardi, G. (1973 b). Expression of the mitochondrial genome in
HeLa cells. XV. Effect of inhibition of mitochondrial protein synthesis on mitochondrial formation. J. Cell Biol., 56, 819-831.

Szekely, I.E., Fischer, D.R., and Schumacher, H.R. (1976). Leukemic mitochondria
II. Acute monobastic leukemia. Cancer, 37, 805-811.

Wagner, T., and Rafael, J. (1977). Biochemical properties of liver megamitochondria induced by chloramphenicol or cuprizone. Exp. Cell Res., 107, 1-13.

White, M.T., and Tewari, K.K. (1973). Structural and functional changes in Novikoff hepatoma mitochondria. Cancer Res., 33, 1645-1653.

White, M.T., and Nandi, S. (1976). Biochemical studies on mitochondria isolated
from normal and neoplastic tissues of the mouse mammary gland. J. Natl. Cancer
Inst., 56, 65-73.

Role of Cyclic Nucleotides in the Expression of Malignancy and Differentiated Functions in Nerve Cells

K. N. Prasad

Department of Radiology, University of Colorado Medical Center,
4200 East 9th Avenue, Denver, Colorado 80262, U.S.A.

ABSTRACT

The purposes of this study were to identify the loci of control of malignancy of nerve cells, and to discover agents which would selectively kill tumor cells. Using clonal lines of neuroblastoma (NB) cells in culture, we have identified at least one possible locus of control of malignancy, namely a defect in adenosine 3',5'-cyclic monophosphate (cyclic AMP) system. An increase in the cellular cyclic AMP in certain NB cells increases the expression of differentiated functions and decreases the malignancy, whereas cyclic GMP was ineffective. There are NB cells which either do not respond or partially respond to cyclic AMP indicating the existence of additional sites of control of malignancy in different cells and even within the same cell. The expression of individual differentiated function is not linked with the expression of tumorigenicity. However, when several of these are increased in a coordinate fashion, the malignancy is decreased or abolished. In vitro data suggest that three naturally occurring substances, butyric acid, ascorbic acid and vitamin E, may have a role in the managements of human neuroblastomas. Sodium butyrate causes cell death and enhances the expression of some differentiation in NB cells. Sodium butyrate increases the level of cAMP and decreases the activity of lactate dehydrogenate. Sodium ascorbate at nonlethal concentrations increases the growth inhibitory effect of ionizing radiation and certain chemotherapeutic agents, but it markedly reduces the cytotoxic effect of methotrexate and DTIC. The mechanism of sodium ascorbate-effect on NB cells is not mediated by cyclic AMP. Vitamin E causes an inhibition of cell division and an extensive morphological differentiation of NB cells in culture. The mechanism of this effect is unknown.

KEYWORDS

Neuroblastoma, cyclic AMP, malignancy, differentiation, butyric acid, ascorbic acid, vitamin E.

INTRODUCTION

The relationship between the regulation of malignancy (capacity of cells to form tumor in syngenic host) and differentiation is not well understood. The expression of abnormal differentiation may be the result of malignant transformation of normal cells. The spontaneous transformation from normal to cancer cells probably occurs in the body as a result of exposure to ionizing radiation, viruses, chemical carcin-

ogens, or any combination of these agents; but these transformed cells do not alwa
establish themselves in the host. This may be due to the fact that the cellular r
pair mechanism of the host corrects the defect and/or the host's immune system kil
the transformed cells. Thus, the environment of the host's body exerts considerab
selection pressure on the first transformed cells. The transformed cells respond
to this pressure by undergoing additional mutations, thus creating additional independent loci of control of malignancy. Such tumor cells then can escape the
host's cellular repair system, as well as the host's immune surveillance mechanism.
These transformed cells would continue to grow in the host and eventually become
clinically detectable. During the tumor growth, cancer cells probably continue to
acquire more independent sites of control of malignancy at a rather low rate. Thus
the tumor tissues which are commonly used for investigation consist of cells which
may contain independent multiple sites of regulation of oncogenicity. Even a
single cell may have more than one locus of control of tumorigenicity. Many tumor
therapeutic agents which are known to be carcinogenic must induce many more independent sites of control of malignancy at a high rate among surviving tumor cells.
These survivors may contain more complex mechanisms of regulation of malignancy
than those found before the treatment. Invariably, such tumors are known to respond very poorly to all the therapeutic agents. Therefore, it would be important
to identify all sites of control of malignancy in order to stop the progression of
the neoplasm in a highly selective manner.

Because of the existence of multiple sites of control of malignancy within a single
cell or within a group of cells in the tumor mass, the relationship between the
expression of malignancy and differentiated functions becomes very complex. The
identification of one site of control may allow only partial expression of differentiated functions in the tumor cells. Based on several studies, the following
assumptions can be made with regard to possible relationship between differentiatio
and malignancy. (1) The malignant properties acquired by the cells are probably
due to mutational events, and these properties are dominant and heritable from one
cell generation to another. (2) Some properties of cancer cells are unique to
malignancy; some are similar to those of embryonic cells, and some are characteristi
of differentiated cells. Some genomes of embryonic features re-express in the cance
cells derived from "differentiated" cells, and many features of "differentiated"
cells continue to express at varying degrees in spite of malignant transformation.
Some genomes of embryonic features continue to express in cancer cells derived from
embryonic cells, but some genomes of differentiated functions express at varying
degrees in spite of malignant transformation of embryonic cells. (3) A malignant
cell may be transformed to a "differentiated" and nonmalignant state but may retain some characteristics of tumor cells (e.g., tumor specific antigen and abnormal number of chromosomes). Conversely, a cell may express many differentiated
functions at varying degrees, mostly at low levels, but may still be malignant.

Using clonal lines of mouse and human neuroblastoma (NB) cells in culture we have
identified at least one possible locus of control of malignancy; namely, a defect
in adenosine 3',5'-cyclic monophosphate (cyclic AMP) system. An increase in the
cellular cyclic AMP in certain NB cells increases the expression of differentiation
and decreases the malignancy, whereas cyclic GMP is ineffective (Prasad and Hsie,
1971; Prasad, 1975; Prasad and Sinha, 1978). The percentage of cAMP-sensitive cells
may vary from one individual to another and from one stage of tumor to another in
the same individual. There are NB cells which do not respond to cyclic AMP, indicating that other independent loci of control of tumorigenicity must exist in
these cells. In addition, some NB cells become only partially differentiated after
the elevation of intracellular levels of cyclic AMP, suggesting that multiple sites
of control of malignancy must exist in the same cell. Hence, additional sites of
control of tumorigenicity or agents which kill tumor cells without significantly
affecting the normal cells must be discovered before any further improvement in
the treatment of this neoplasm can be expected. We have identified three naturally

occurring substances, namely, butyric acid, ascorbic acid and vitamin E$_1$ which causes growth inhibition and/or elevated levels of differentiation in NB cells in culture when used individually. However, these agents, when used in combination with X-irradiation and certain chemotherapeutic agents, enhance the growth inhibitory effect of the individual agent.

The regulation of individual differentiated function and its relationship with the expression of malignancy are discussed below.

Regulation of Neurites

A mature and nonmalignant neuron contains well-defined axons and dendritic processes. The neurites that are extended in NB cells appear similar in appearance to the axons and dendrites of normal neurons (Ross and co-workers, 1975). Although these processes are electrically excitable and are capable of generating action potentials (Nelson and co-workers, 1969; Ross and co-workers, 1975), cells having such processes may not express many of the biochemically differentiated functions (Prasad, 1973; Prasad and Kumar, 1974). The neurites in mouse and human NB cells are formed after treatment of cells with various agents, some of which do not increase the level of cellular cyclic AMP. One can make the following conclusions with respect to the regulation of neurite formation in NB cells: (1) Various agents induce neurites by promoting the organization of microtubules and microfilaments (Prasad, 1975). (2) The expression of neurites does not require the synthesis of new RNA (Prasad, 1975; Miller and Ruddle, 1974). (3) Neurite formation can be initiated in the absence of new protein but soon reaches a point beyond which de novo synthesis of protein is required (Schubert and co-workers, 1971). The expression of neurites in NB cells involves more than one mode, one of which is cyclic AMP mediated (Prasad, 1975; Prasad and Sinha, 1978). (4) The inhibition of cell division is not a prerequisite for the expression of neurites; on the contrary, the neurites are formed in the dividing NB cells (Prasad, 1975). However, a more elaborate network of neurites is established following inhibition of cell division. (5) The expression of neurites appears to be independent of malignancy, since the neurites of varying sizes may be formed in the dividing neuroblast cells (Prasad and Sinha, 1978). A NB cell may permanently stop cell division without the expression of long neurites. (6) The neurites are also expressed in the absence of any increase in the expression of many biochemically differentiated functions.

Regulation of Neurotransmitter Metabolizing Enzymes

A mature and nonmalignant neuron expresses the activities of neural-specific enzymes at high levels; but in the NB cells they are expressed at low levels (Prasad and Kumar, 1974). An elevation of the intracellular level of cyclic AMP always increased tyrosine hydroxylase (TH) (Prasad and Kumar, 1974; Richelson, 1972), choline acetyltransferase (CAT) (Prasad, 1975), and acetylcholinesterase (AChE) (Prasad, 1975; Kates, Winterton, Schlesinger, 1971). The TH activity increased after treatment of human NB cells with 5-bromodeoxyuridine (Prasad, 1975) and after treatment of mouse NB cells with 5-(3,3-dimethyl-1-triazeno)-imidazole-4-carboxamide (DTIC) (Culver and co-workers, 1977). These agents do not increase cyclic AMP levels. Similarly, the activities of CAT and AChE are increased in cells treated with X-irradiation, 6-thioguanine, and 5'-AMP which inhibit cell division but do not increase cyclic AMP (Prasad, 1975). Thus, the activities of TH, CAT and AChE are regulated by at least two modes, one of which is mediated by cellular cyclic AMP. Unlike TH activity, the activities of CAT and AChE are inversely related to growth rate. The morphological differentiation and activities of TH, CAT, and AChE are independently regulated in the sense that the expression of one can be increased in the absence of the other two. Since the differentiated cells in which most of the differentiated functions are increased in a coordinate manner lose the tumorigenicity, it is possible that a defect in

the cyclic AMP system may be responsible for malignant transformation as well as
for expression of low activities of neural-specific enzymes, but the expression of
malignancy and low enzyme activity may be only casually related. For example, a
mutant clone of NB cells isolated from tyrosine-free medium contains tyrosine
hydroxylase activity that is similar to that observed in the brain (Breakefield
and Nirenberg, 1974). The activities of acetylcholinesterase and choline
acetyltransferase can be increased in cells that maintain tumorigenicity (Prasad,
1973).

Catechol-o-methyltransferase (COMT) degrades catecholamines in mammalian cells and
the enzyme activity is not regulated by cyclic AMP (Prasad, 1975).

Pyruvate Kinase and Lactic Acid Dehydrogenase

We have shown (Sakamoto and Prasad, 1972) that NB cells are relatively more sensitive to inhibitors of anaerobic glycolysis. It is well known that a shift from
anaerobic glycolysis to aerobic glycolysis occurs during differentiation of nerve
cells. Therefore, the question arose whether cyclic AMP- or X-ray-induced differentiated NB cells would show a decrease in anaerobic glycolysis. This was studied
by measuring lactate dehydrogenase (LDH) activity in control and differentiated
cells (Prasad and co-workers, 1978). The activity of LDH (converts pyruvate to
lactic acid) increased by about two-fold in cells treated with prostaglandin E_1
(PGE_1), inhibitor of cyclic nucleotide phosphodiesterase (R020-1724), and X-
irradiation (600 rads) in comparison to that observed in untreated or ethyl
alcohol-treated control.(Table 1).

TABLE 1   Effect of Various Agents on Lactate Dehydrogenase
           (LDH) and Pyruvate Kinase (PK) Activities in Mouse
           Neuroblastoma Cells in Culture

| | Specific activity unit/mg protein | |
Treatment	LDH	PK
Control (untreated)	$0.39 \pm 0.10^*$	1.61 ± 0.16
Control (alcohol)	0.31 ± 0.08	0.56 ± 0.05
Prostaglandin E_1	1.04 ± 0.16	1.49 ± 0.21
R020-1724	0.82 ± 0.04	1.44 ± 0.18
X-irradiation	0.92 ± 0.06	2.34 ± 0.22

*Standard deviation

PGE_1 (10 µg/ml), R020-1724 (200 µg/ml), X-irradiation (600 rads), and
ethyl alcohol (final concentration 1%) were added 24 hours after plating.
The enzyme activity was determined three days after treatment. Each
value represents an average of three samples $\pm$ SD. (Prasad and co-workers,
1978)

The pyruvate kinase (converts phosphophenolpyruvate to pyruvate) activity markedly
decreased in ethyl alcohol-treated cells in comparison to untreated cells (Table
1); however, this decreases in enzyme activity was prevented in the presence of
elevated cellular cyclic AMP. X-irradiation of NB cells which does not increase
cellular cyclic AMP enhanced the pyruvate kinase (PK) activity. Therefore, the
activity of LDH and PK may be regulated by more than one mode, one of which is
cyclic AMP mediated. This suggests that at least for the criterion of type of
respiration, the differentiated neuroblastoma cells continue to maintain a high
rate of anaerobic glycolysis in culture.

Synthesis and Phosphorylation of Chromosomal Proteins

The synthesis and phosphorylation of chromosomal proteins have been implicated to be important events in the control of cell proliferation and differentiation. Therefore, the synthesis of histone and phosphorylation of histone and nonhistone proteins were studied in cyclic AMP-induced "differentiated" NB cells. We found that the synthesis of histone (Fig. 1a) and phosphorylation of H_1-histone were decreased in differentiated cells (Lazo, Ruddon and Prasad, 1976).

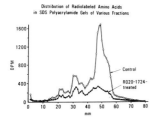

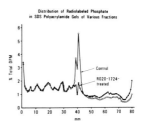

Fig. 1a. Distribution of radiolabeled amino acids in SDS polyacrylamide gels of various histone fractions (0.25 N HCl fraction) from control and cyclic AMP-induced "differentiated" mouse neuroblastoma cells. Control and treated cells were labeled with ^{14}C- or ^3H-amino acids for 2 hours. Total DPM ^{14}C=25,133; ^3H= 8,975. Gels were run for 17.5 hours at 6 ma/gel.

Fig. 1b. Distribution of radiolabeled phosphate in SDS polyacrylamide gels of various histone fractions (0.25 N HCl fraction) from control and cyclic AMP-induced "differentiated" mouse neuroblastoma cells. Control and treated cells were labeled with ^{32}P or ^{33}P for 2 hours. Total DPM ^{32}P=108,670. Gels were run for 21 hours at 6 ma/gel. (Lazo, Prasad and Ruddon, 1976).

Since the above changes occur at the time of inhibition of cell division and DNA synthesis (Prasad and Kumar, 1974), they may be important biological signals for the dividing neuroblasts to turn off cell division. The occurrence of histone synthesis and phosphorylation of H_1-histone may be necessary biological events for the proliferating system (differentiated or embryonic); but for the embryonic nerve cells, which must eventually stop cell division, a continuation of these events after a specified time during development may be indicative of malignant change.

We have reported that there was no prominent change in the synthesis or phosphorylation of nonhistone chromosomal proteins in cyclic AMP-induced "differentiated" cells (Lazo and co-workers, 1976). Other investigator has been unable to demonstrate any significant changes in nonhistone chromosomal proteins during development of rat brains. However, we have found a small decrease in the synthesis and a small increase in phosphorylation of 40,000 dalton peptides in cyclic AMP-induced "differentiated" cells. The significance of this change in nonhistone protein is unknown. It has been suggested (Elgin and co-workers, 1973) that a nonhistone protein of the 40,000-50,000 dalton range may be involved in DNA replication in mammalian cells. If this is true, the changes in the synthesis and phosphorylation of 40,000 dalton peptides in the "differentiated" cells may be a reflection of the inhibition of DNA synthesis that occurs in these cells (Prasad and Kumar, 1974).

Reduction in the Tumorigenicity of Differentiated Cells

The tumorigenicity of differentiated cells is markedly reduced or completely abolished, depending on the experimental conditions (Prasad, 1973). For example, in an uncloned cell line or a clonal line (NBP$_2$) analogs of cyclic AMP, RO20-1724 (phosphodiesterase inhibitor), and PGE$_1$ only partially reduced the tumorigenicity of "differentiated" cells, whereas the combination of PGE$_1$ with either analogs of cyclic AMP or a phosphodiesterase inhibitor completely abolished malignancy of NB cells. Of the mice that failed to develop tumors after subcutaneous injection of "differentiated" cells, 30% rejected the malignant cells (0.25 x 10^6) administered subcutaneously (Prasad and co-workers, 1976a). This suggested, for the first time that the differentiated NB cells may act as a strong antigen against malignant NB cells.

Regulation of the Intracellular Level of Cyclic AMP

Since cyclic AMP is one of the important factors in regulating the expression of malignancy and differentiation in NB cells, it would be important to identify the defect in a particular step involved in the metabolism of this cyclic nucleotide. Many exogenous and endogenous factors affect the intracellular level of cyclic AMP. These include relative activity of adenylate cyclase and cyclic AMP phosphodiesterase, response of adenylate cyclase to neurotransmitters, and levels of cyclic AMP binding proteins. Therefore, the study of each step involved in the metabolism of cyclic AMP is important.

Adenylate cyclase activity. The basal level of adenylate cyclase activity and the sensitivity of adenylate cyclase to neurotransmitters in homogenates vary from one clone of mouse NB cells to another (Prasad and Gilmer, 1974; Prasad and Kumar, 1974; Prasad and co-workers, 1975c). In homogenates of cyclic AMP-induced "differentiated" NB cells, we have made the following observations: (1) The sensitivity of adenylate cyclase to dopamine, norepinephrine (Fig. 2a), and acetylcholine increases; (2) the sensitivity of adenylate cyclase to PGE$_1$ and guanosine triphosphate (GTP) does not change; (3) GTP potentiates the PGE$_1$-stimulated adenylate cyclase activity (Fig. 2b); and (4) high concentrations of calcium, magnesium, and manganese inhibit adenylate cyclase activity.

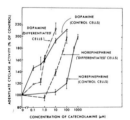   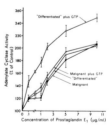

Fig. 2a   Fig. 2b

Fig. 2a and Fig. 2b.   Changes in adenylate cyclase activity in homogenates of control and cyclic AMP-induced "differeniated" mouse neuroblastoma cells. Dopamine and norepinephrine (2a), PGE$_1$ and GTP (2b) were added to homogenates immediately before assaying the enzyme activity. The basal activities of adenylate cyclase were considered 100% control values; the adenylate cyclase values of treated homogenates were expressed as percentage of control. Each value represents an average of 8 to 12 samples. The bar at each point is standard deviation.(Prasad & co-workers, 1974; 1975c)

Thus, the decrease in the sensitivity of adenylate cyclase to neurotransmitters, ions, and GTP appears to be associated with malignancy; however, these may be secondary lesions, since the stimulatory effect of dopamine and norepinephrine on the cyclic AMP level in the malignant cells cannot be measured (Table 2) until the activity of cyclic AMP phosphodiesterase is inhibited (Prasad and co-workers, 1974; Sahu and Prasad, 1975).

TABLE 2   Effect of Neurotransmitters and PGE_1 on Cyclic AMP Level in Neuroblastoma Clones

Treatment	Cyclic AMP Levels in Various Clones (pmoles/mg protein)			
	NBA_2 (1)	NBE^- (A)	$NBDB^-$	NBP_2
Control, dopamine, or norepinephrine	14 ± 2	19 ± 2	19 ± 4	11 ± 2
RO20-1724	48 ± 7	107 ± 5	25 ± 4	65 ± 8
PGE_1	20 ± 2	22 ± 2	56 ± 9	19 ± 2
RO20-1724 + dopamine	233 ± 14	139 ± 4	162 ± 49	66 ± 5
RO20-1724 + norepinephrine	191 ± 19	120 ± 11	122 ± 36	67 ± 4
RO20-1724 + PGE_1	2,803 ± 173	1,953 ± 118	2,426 ± 124	2,404 ± 212

*Standard deviation.

NBA_2 (1) contains tyrosine hydroxylase (TH) but no choline acetyltransferase (ChA); NBE^- (A) contains ChA but no TH; $NBDB^-$ contains neither TH nor ChA; NBP_2 contains both ChA and TH (Sahu and Prasad, 1975).

PGE_1 stimulates the intracellular level of cyclic AMP in varying degrees in most of the mouse clones (Gilman and Nirenberg, 1971; Prasad, 1973; Hamprecht and Schultz, 1973; Blume and co-workers, 1973; Sahu and Prasad, 1975), but in one clone (NBE^-) it does not increase the cyclic AMP level significantly until the phosphodiesterase activity is inhibited (Table 2). PGE_1 in combination with a phosphodiesterase inhibitor increases the cyclic AMP level more than that produced by the individual agent alone. A similar observation was made for adenosine (Prasad, 1975). Thus, the rate-limiting factor in the accumulation of cyclic AMP following the treatment of neuroblastoma cells with neurotransmitters, adenosine, and PGE_1 appears to be the level of cyclic AMP phosphodiesterase activity. Therefore, we have suggested that an increase in cyclic AMP phosphodiesterase activity in the dividing neuroblasts may be one of the early lesions of malignancy of nerve cells (Prasad and co-workers, 1974).

Cyclic AMP phosphodiesterase activity. The cyclic AMP phosphodiesterase activity is markedly increased (Prasad, 1973; Kumar and co-workers, 1975) in cyclic AMP-induced "differentiated" mouse NB cells in culture. This increase in enzyme activity was blocked by cycloheximide but not by actinomycin D. The activity of cyclic AMP phosphodiesterase also increases during exponential growth and reaches a maximal value at confluence (Sinha and Prasad, 1977). The increase in enzyme activity during growth period occurs without any change in the intracellular level of cyclic AMP and is blocked by both cycloheximide and actinomycin D. Thus, the activity of cyclic AMP phosphodiesterase in NB cells is regulated by at least two modes; namely, cyclic AMP and growth.

Binding of cyclic AMP with proteins. Since the intracellular levels of cyclic AMP and cyclic AMP phosphodiesterase activity increase in "differentiated" NB cells, the cells must develop the mechanism of protecting the formed cyclic AMP from the enzymatic hydrolysis. Indeed, the level of cyclic AMP binding proteins increases

by about 2-fold (Fig. 3) in cyclic AMP-induced "differentiated"neuroblastoma cells
(Prasad, 1976b). The protein-bound cyclic AMP is less susceptible to enzymatic
hydrolysis.

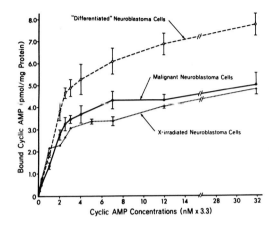
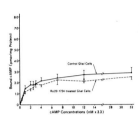

Fig. 3a   Fig. 3b

Fig. 3.   Binding of cyclic AMP with soluble proteins of neuroblastoma cells as a function of cyclic AMP concentrations (NB
cells 3a; glioma cells 3b). The incubation mixture contained
100 μg proteins. Each value represents an average of 6 samples.
Bars are S. D.

X-irradiation and 6-thioguanine increase total protein, inhibit cell division and
induce some differentiated functions (Prasad, 1973) in NB cells without changing
the cellular cyclic AMP; however, they do not elevate the level of cyclic AMP
binding proteins (Prasad and co-workers, 1976b). This indicates that neither the
inhibition of cell division nor the increase in total protein is sufficient to increase the levels of binding proteins. Thus, one of the mechanisms by which NB
cells could maintain a high intracellular level of cyclic AMP is to increase the
amount of binding proteins during differentiation. Glioma (C-6)and L-cells, after
treatment with PGE_1 or RO20-1724 fail to develop such a mechanism (Fig. 3b). This,
in part, may account for the reversibility of cyclic AMP effects on non-neural
tumor cells soon after the removal of a drug. Thus, there is a defect in the
regulation of cyclic AMP-binding protein in rat glioma cells in culture, or the
level of binding proteins in rat glioma cells is not regulated by cyclic AMP. The
increase in the levels of binding proteins in "differentiated" NB cells is associated with the irreversible effect of cyclic AMP, but this is not the cause of
irreversibility, since the increase in binding proteins occurs in dividing nerve
cells (24 hours after treatment with PGE_1). However, this may be one of the important events that is essential for maintaining the irreversible neural
differentiation.

Cyclic AMP-dependent phosphorylation. The binding of cyclic AMP with the regulatory
subunits results in dissociation of the regulatory proteins from the catalytic
units, with subsequent activation of the latter (Tao, Salas and Lipmann, 1970)
which then phosphorylate various proteins. If this is true during differentiation
of NB cells, the cyclic AMP-dependent phosphorylation activity should increase in
"differentiated" cells. Indeed, we have observed (Ehrlich and co-workers, 1977)
that the cyclic AMP-dependent phosphorylation of cytosol proteins markedly in-

creases, but cyclic AMP-independent phosphorylation of another protein decreases by about twofold in "differentiated" cells (Fig. 4).

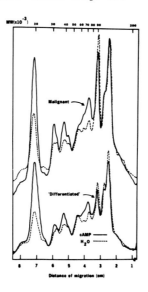

Fig. 4

Fig. 4. Autoradiogram tracing of phosphorylated proteins in the cytosol of malignant and cyclic AMP-induced "differentiated" neuroblastoma cells in culture. It should be noted that the incorporation of ^{32}P into proteins from gamma ^{32}P-ATP is a net result of the action of protein kinase(s) and phosphoprotein phosphatase(s) activities. (Ehrlich and co-workers, 1977)

There is also an increase in cyclic AMP-independent phosphorylation activity of two specific proteins in the crude nuclear fractions of "differentiated" cells. Thus, changes in phosphorylation activity are important biochemical events associated with the increase in differentiated functions.

Regulation of the intracellular level of cyclic GMP and its relationship to Malignancy. Mouse NB cells also have cyclic GMP (Prasad and co-workers, 1976b), the concentration of which is 100-fold less than cyclic AMP (Table 3).

TABLE 3   Effect of Various Agents on the Intracellular Level of Cyclic Nucleotides in Neuroblastoma Cells

Treatment	Dose (µg/ml)	Cyclic AMP Level (pmoles/g protein)	Cyclic GMP Level (pmoles/g protein)
Control		5,000 ± 400*	50 ± 7
Acetylcholine	100	5,300 ± 450	109 ± 12
R020-1724	200	29,000 ± 400	39 ± 6
Papaverine	25	32,000 ± 600	84 ± 9
PGE$_1$	10	8,500 ± 500	41 ± 8

*Standard deviation

(Prasad and co-workers, 1976b)

In addition to the presence of cyclic GMP phosphodiesterase, which is distinct
from cyclic AMP phosphodiesterase (Prasad and co-workers, 1975a), the extremely
low binding affinity of cyclic GMP with proteins (10 times less than cyclic AMP)
may in part account for the low intracellular level of cyclic GMP. Acetylcholine
increases the intracellular level of cyclic GMP by about twofold; however, it does
not significantly change the level of cyclic AMP. Acetylcholine does not anatago-
nize the effect of PGE₁ or RO20-1724 on differentiation and does not affect growth
rate or differentiation in mouse NB cells in culture (Prasad and co-workers, 1975c)
The addition of either exogenous cyclic GMP or N^2-2'0-dibutyryl cyclic GMP into
cultures of mouse or human NB cells inhibits cell division without causing differentiation and when added with PGE₁ or RO20-1724 fails to antagonize the expression
of differentiation (Prasad, 1975). These data suggest that cyclic GMP neither
has any role in regulating the expression of differentiated functions in NB cells
nor antagonizes the effect of cyclic AMP. The changes in cyclic GMP level are not
related to the expression of malignancy of nerve cells.

Hypothesis for the Malignancy of Nerve Cells

Figure 5 shows a diagrammatic model to explain the malignancy of nerve cells (1976a)
This model suggests that a mutation in the regulatory gene for cyclic AMP phosphodiesterase within a single and/or a group of dividing nerve cells may result from
exposure to viruses, chemical carcinogens, ionizing radiation, or any combination
of these agents; and this mutational change may increase phosphodiesterase activity
in mutated cells.

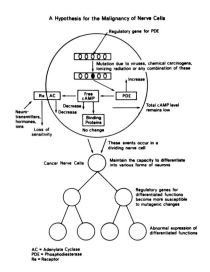

Fig. 5

Fig. 5. A diagrammatic model to explain the postulated
mechanism for the development of cancer of nerve cells.
Adenosine 3',5'-cyclic monophosphate = cAMP; cAMP phospho-
iesterase = PDE; adenylate cyclase = AC; receptor = Re;
dopamine = DA; norepinephrine = NE.

The high cyclic AMP phosphodiesterase activity could lead to low levels of cyclic AMP,
which in turn could cause low levels of adenylate cyclase activity and insensitivity c
adenylate cyclase to neurotransmitters. These changes might then prevent the expressic
of neuronal differentiated functions in the mutated nerve cell, causing it to become a
cancer cell. The regulatory genes for other differentiated functions in the daughter

cancer cells may consequently become more susceptible to mutagenic changes, which then may produce further molecular lesions. This may account for the fact that the NB cells obtained from a tumor differ quantitatively and qualitatively from one another with respect to expression of cellular properties and to sensitivity to different drugs. The mutated nerve cell appears to maintain the capacity to differentiate into various forms of nerve cells. This is supported by the fact that the NB contains four major types of nerve cells (Amano and co-workers, 1972; Prasad, 1973; Knapp and Mandell, 1974)--(1) adrenergic cells, (2) cholinergic cells, (3) sensory-like cells, and (4) serotonergic cells. However, the differentiated functions of these nerve cells are not adequately expressed, and therefore they continue to divide. Whether or not the first cancer nerve cell will lead to the formation of a detectable neoplasm depends on the host's repair system and immunological environment. If the host's repair mechanism and immunological response are normal, the mutated nerve cell may be repaired or rejected, and no malignant lesion will ever appear. On the other hand, if the host has unresponsive immune system or poor repair mechanisms, the malignant neoplasm may become detectable in a few months or years after the appearance of the first cancer cells. The following experimental data support the proposed hypothesis: (1) a raised intracellular level of cyclic AMP in some neuroblastoma cells irreversibly induces several differentiated functions that are characteristic of mature neurons (Prasad, 1975); (2) the inhibition of cyclic AMP phosphodiesterase activity reduce the oncogenicity of NB cells (Prasad, 1975); (3) although dopamine and norepinephrine-sensitive adenylate cyclases are demonstrable in vitro (Prasad and Gilmer, 1974), these agents do not increase the cyclic AMP level until the phosphodiesterase activity is inhibited (Prasad and co-workers, 1974; Sahu and Prasad, 1975); (4) a relatively high phosphodiesterase activity in NB cells is associated with low activity of adenylate cyclase and a low level of cyclic AMP (Prasad and co-workers, 1975c). Although the basal level of cyclic AMP phosphodiesterase activity in "differentiated" mouse NB cells increases (Prasad, 1973; Kumar and co-workers, 1975), the intracellular level of cyclic AMP also increases (Prasad and Kumar, 1974). This is due to an increased level of cyclic AMP-binding proteins (Prasad and co-workers, 1976b).

Serum as a Biological Tool for Identifying the Sites of Control of Malignancy

We have recently observed (Prasad, 1977; Prasad and co-workers, unpublished observations) that the extent of morphological differentiation, clumping, doubling time, and tyrosine hydroxylase activity varied depending upon the type of serum (Table 4).

TABLE 4   Growth Rate of Neuroblastoma Cells (NBP$_2$ Clone) in Various Sera

Type of Serum	% of Differentiated Cells	Doubling Time (hrs)	TH Activity	cAMP levels (pmole/mg protein)
Fetal Calf Serum (FCS)	11 ± 2*	19 ± 1*	74 ± 5*	7.6 ± 0.8*
Heat inactivated FCS	2 ± 0	20 ± 1	13 ± 3	6.8 ± 0.9
Dialyzed FCS	6 ± 1	>50	14 ± 1	6.3 ± 0.7
Agammaglobulin FCS	Toxic, poor growth			
Newborn Calf Serum (NBCS)	2 ± 0	23 ± 1	333 ± 63	17.2 ± 1.8
Heat inactivated NBCS	5 ± 0	20 ± 1	125 ± 28	12.9 ± 1.9
Agammaglobulin NBCS	2 ± 0	18 ± 1	42 ± 8	9.9 ± 0.4
Calf Serum (CS)	Toxic (complete lethality)			
Heat inactivated CS	66 ± 5	23 ± 1	101 ± 19	25 ± 3.2
Dialyzed CS	28 ± 3	24 ± 1	257 ± 61	14 ± 0.6
Agammaglobulin CS	77 ± 3	34 ± 7	580 ± 82	26 ± 3.0

*Standard error of mean

The % of morphological differentiation was determined 5 days
after plating. The doubling time was determined on the exponential portion of the curve. The level of cyclic AMP was
determined 4 days after plating. The tyrosine hydroxylase
(TH) activity was determined 4 days after plating, and the
enzyme activity was expressed as pmoles $^{14}CO_2/106$ cells/hr.
(From Prasad and co-authors, submitted for publication.)

In addition, the effect of PGE_1 and RO20-1724 on morphological differentiation
varied depending upon the serum type. The increase in neurite formation or TH
activity or decrease in the growth rate in various sera is not always associated
with a rise in cellular cyclic AMP. However, these data show that the extent of
spontaneous and drug-induced differentiation is highly dependent upon the type of
serum. Therefore, it is possible that change in the serum contents may in part
account for the spontaneous regression of NB tumor which is known to occur
occasionally.

Role of Cyclic AMP in Differentiation of Neuroblastoma Cells in Vivo

A recent study has shown (Imashuku and co-workers, 1977) that the spontaneously
occurring ganglioneuroma and sympathetic ganglia have eight times more cyclic AMP
than immature round cell neuroblastoma. One patient with immature neuroblastoma
who had been treated with papaverine showed a threefold higher cyclic AMP level.
Thus, cyclic AMP is one of the important factors which regulate the expression of
differentiation in vitro as well as in vivo. Obviously, additional sites of control must exist in the same or different neuroblastoma cells in vivo. Therefore,
a continued effort must be made to identify other loci of control of malignancy of
nerve cells.

Butyric Acid, Ascorbic Acid and Vitamin E

We have identified three naturally occurring substances, namely, butyric acid,
ascorbic acid and vitamin E, which cause varying degrees of growth inhibition and/
or elevated levels of differentiation in NB cell culture. In addition, these agents
potentiate the effect of certain tumor therapeutic agents on NB cells.

Sodium butyrate. Butyric acid, a 4-carbon fatty acid, occurs naturally in body.
Sodium butyrate (0.5 to 1.0 mM) appears to be either innocuous or produces reversible growth inhibition, and morphological and biochemical alterations in several mammalian cells in culture (Prasad and Sinha, 1976). However, it causes an extensive cell death in human neuroblastoma cells in culture and elevated levels of
differentiation. Sodium butyrate also enhances the growth inhibitory effect (due
to cell death and inhibition of cell division) of ionizing radiation and chemotherapeutic agents (Table 5).

TABLE 5   Effect of the Combined Effect of Sodium Butyrate and
           Therapeutic Agents on Neuroblastoma Cells in Culture

Treatment	No. of Cells x 10^4
Control	228 ± 18*
Sodium butyrate (0.5 mM)	53 ± 8
5-Fluorouracil (0.05 µg/ml)	163 ± 12
Sodium butyrate + 5-Fluorouracil	4.3 ± 1.5
X-irradiation (400 rads)	49 ± 7
X-irradiation + Sodium butyrate	7.0 ± 2
DTIC (20 µg/ml)	77 ± 13
Sodium butyrate + DTIC	25 ± 4
CCNU (20 µg/ml)	121 ± 11

Sodium butyrate + CCNU	11 ± 4
Vincristine (0.002 µg/ml)	89 ± 8
Sodium butyrate + Vincristine	15 ± 5
Adriamycin (0.008 µg/ml)	78 ± 10
Sodium butyrate + Adriamycin	14 ± 3
Methotraxete (0.1 µg/ml)	31 ± 4
Sodium butyrate + Methotrexate	12 ± 2

*Standard deviation

Neuroblastoma cells (50,000) were plated in plastic culture dishes. Drugs and X-irradiation were given 24 hours after plating. The drugs and medium were changed 2 days after treatments. Each value represents an average of at least 6 samples.

The mechanism of the effect of sodium butyrate involves more than one mode. We have identified two of these. Sodium butyrate inhibits anaerobic glycosis by reducing lactic acid dehydrogenase activity (Prasad, R. and co-workers, unpublished observation). NB cells are more sensitive to the inhibition of anaerobic glycolysis than other cell types (Sakamoto and Prasad, 1972). Therefore, sodium butyrate-induced cell death in NB cells may in part be due to inhibition of anaerobic glycolysis in these cells. Sodium butyrate also increases the cellular cyclic AMP, but this effect is not apparent until 3 days after treatment. Sodium butyrate neither inhibits cyclic AMP phosphodiesterase activity in vitro nor increases the intracellular level of cyclic AMP within an hour of treatment, indicating that the effect of sodium butyrate is possibly due to membrane changes which result in increased basal activity of adenylate cyclase (Prasad and Sinha, 1976). Indeed, the basal activity of adenylate cyclase in homogenates of sodium butyrate-treated NB cells increases (Prasad and Gilmer, 1974). These data led us to suggest sodium butyrate alone and in combination with other therapeutic agents may be useful in the management of human neuroblastomas. Sodium butyrate also increases growth inhibitory effect of cyclic AMP stimulating agents on human amelanotic melanoma cells in culture (Prasad and Sakamoto, 1978). Thus, the possibility exists that sodium butyrate may be useful in other neoplasms.

Sodium butyrate has been used clinically first by Dr. Tom Voute of Spinozastraat 51, Postgiro 2388, Amsterday, and then by Dr. L. Furman Odum of Children's Hospital in Denver (personal communication). Although the clinical value of sodium butyrate cannot be evaluated at this time, high doses (7-10 g per day) of sodium butyrate produce no clinically detectable toxic effect in patients with neuroblastomas.

Sodium ascorbate. The beneficial effects of high doses of ascorbic acid in advanced neoplasms has been reported (Cameron and Pauling, 1976). Sodium-L-ascorbate at non-lethal concentrations potentiates the growth inhibitory effect of 5-fluorouracil, X-irradiation (Table 6), bleomycin (3-fold), R020-1724 (75-fold), PGE_1 (3-fold), and sodium butyrate (3-fold) on NB cells, but did not produce such an effect on glioma cells.

TABLE 6   Effect of Sodium-L-Ascorbate in Combination with 5-FU or X-Irradiation on Neuroblastoma Cells in Culture

	Cell Number (% of control cultures)	
Treatment	Neuroblastoma	Glioma
Sodium-L-ascorbate	105 ± 9	98 ± 5
5-fluorouracil (5-FU)	62 ± 5	58 ± 6
Sodium-L-ascorbate + 5-FU	5.6 ± 2.0	45 ± 5
X-irradiation	28 ± 3	29 ± 3
Sodium-L-ascorbate + X-irradiation	1.8 ± 0.4	27 ± 3

Sodium-D-ascorbate (10 μg/ml)	96	± 6
5-FU + Sodium-D-ascorbate	4.6	± 1.4
Glutathione (25 μg/ml)	103	± 9
5-FU + glutathione	49	± 4

*Standard deviation

Sodium-L-ascorbate (5 μg/ml for NB, 100 μg/ml for glioma); 5-FU (0.08 μg/ml for NB; 0.3 μg/ml for glioma); X-irradiation (400 rads for NB and glioma).

sodium-L-ascorbate did not enhance the effect of vincristine, 6-thioguanine, adriamycin or CCNU except at higher drug doses (Prasad and co-workers, 1978). The potentiating effect of sodium-L-ascorbate in combination with 5-FU was seen even at a concentration of 1 μg/ml of culture medium. Sodium-D-isoascorbate was equally effective, indicating that the effect of sodium-L-ascorbate was not due to its vitamin property. Although glutathione, a reducing agent, was more toxic to NB cells than Sodium-L-ascorbate or Sodium-D-ascorbate, it failed to potentiate the effect of 5-FU at an equimolar concentration (Table 6). Thus, the effect of Sodium-L-ascorbate is not due entirely to its reducing property. Since sodium ascorbate inhibits catalase activity in vitro (Orr, 1967), it is possible that one of the mechanisms of sodium ascorbate-effect involves inhibition of catalase activity. The effect of sodium ascorbate on NB cells is not mediated via cyclic AMP. Sodium ascorbate completely prevented the cytotoxic effects of DTIC and partially (about 50%) prevented the effect of methotrexate on NB cells. The reasons for this effect is not known. However, it is possible that sodium ascorbate inactivates these drugs in vitro, and thereby reduces their effectiveness on cells. If such a phenomenon is also observed in vivo, a reduction in the sodium-L-ascorbate level in blood prior to the administration of methotrexate or DTIC may increase their effectiveness or may reduce the drug requirements for the same effect on tumor cells. Thus, it is very important that sodium ascorbate is combined with only those drugs with which the potentiating effects are observed.

Vitamine E. Unlike vitamin C, vitamin E increases the expression of morphological differentiation in mouse neuroblastoma cells (clone NBP$_2$) in culture. The extent of differentiation was as high as 98% (Table 7).

TABLE 7   Effect of Vitamin E on Morphological Differentiation and Growth Rate of Mouse Neuroblastoma Cells in Culture

Concentrations (U/ml)	% Morphological Differentiation	Cell Number X 104
Control	2 ± 0*	58 ± 7
0.02	2 ± 0	41 ± 3
0.04	5 ± 1	24 ± 5
0.05	15 ± 2	13 ± 2
0.06	93 ± 3	5.7 ± 1.6
0.07	98 ± 2	3.0 ± 1.2
0.1	all dead	

*Standard deviation

Cells (10^4) were plated in Falcon dishes (60mm), and Vitamin E was added 24 hrs after plating. The % morphological differentiation was determined 3 days after treatment. Each value represents an average of 6 samples.

The increase in morphological differentiation was associated with the inhibition of cell division. The effective concentration range of vitamin E in causing morphological changes was very narrow. at concentrations of 0.06 - 0.07 Units/ml, the effect on morphological differentiation was maximal, the concentrations higher

than these were toxic and lower than these were ineffective. The mechanism of
vitamin E-effect on NB cells is unknown.

Clinical Trial of Differentiating Agents

We have suggested (Prasad and co-workers, 1974) that the addition of differentiating
agents in the currently used therapeutic model may be useful in the management of
human neuroblastomas. Dr. L. Helson of Memorial Hospital, New York, has added pap-
verine and tri-fluoro-methyl-2-deoxyuridine in his treatment protocol, which involves vincristine and cytoxan but no ionizing radiation. Although a marked regression of tumor was observed in all patients over two years and stage IV
neuroblastoma and the conversion from neuroblastoma to ganglioneuroma was observed
in cases where biopsies were taken and examined (Helson, 1975), the response of
the previously untreated patients appears to be the best. Dr. Helson has indicated
(personal communication) that the median survival time of 25 treated patients was
about 18 months. Two out of 6 patients developed intracranial neuroblastoma at 30-
36 months after treatment.

CONCLUSIONS

Adenosine 3',5'-cyclic monophosphate (cyclic AMP) appears to be one of the important factors in induction as well as in regulation of several differentiated functions
in neuroblastoma cells in vivo and in vitro. A low level of cyclic AMP in dividing
nerve cells, which results from an increase in cyclic AMP phosphodiesterase
activity due to a mutation on the regulatory gene of this enzyme, may be responsible
for the expression of malignancy and "abnormal differentiation". Data show that
no one individual differentiated function is linked with malignancy. This is not
surprising because the expression of many of these functions is independently
regulated. However, when several of the differentiated functions express at maximal
levels and in a coordinate manner the tumorigenicity of such cells is abolished.
The increased level of cyclic AMP-binding proteins provides one of the important
intracellular mechanisms for protecting the formed cyclic AMP from enzymatic
hydrolysis during differentiation of neuroblastoma cells. Reduction in histone
synthesis and in H_1-histone phosphorylation may be an important biological signal
for the dividing neuroblasts to "turn off" cell division. If these events do not
occur, it might be indicative of malignant change. Three naturally occurring substances, butyric acid, ascorbic acid and vitamin E may be useful in the management
of neuroblastomas because they cause growth inhibition and/or differentiation and
increase the effect of ionizing radiation and certain pharmacological agents in a
highly selective manner.

ACKNOWLEDGMENTS

This work was supported in part by NIH grant ES NS01576, and in part by USPHS
NS-09230. We thank Marianne Gaschler for her technical help and Valerie Carlock
for her help in typing the manuscript.

REFERENCES

Amano, T., E. Richelson, and M. Nirenberg (1972). Neurotransmitter synthesis by
    neuroblastoma clones. Proc. Natl. Acad. Sci. USA, 69, 258-263.
Blume, A., C. Dalton, and H. Sheppard (1973). Adenosine mediated elevation of
    cyclic 3',5'-adenosine monophosphate concentrations in cultured mouse
    neuroblastoma cells. Proc. Natl. Acad. Sci. USA, 70, 3099-3102.
Breakefield, X.O., and M. W. Nirenberg (1974). Selection for neuroblastoma cells
    that synthesize certain transmitters. Proc. Natl. Acad. Sci. USA, 71,
    2530-2533.
Burdman, J.A. (1972). The relationship between DNA synthesis and the synthesis of
    nuclear proteins in rat brain during development. J. Neurochem., 19, 1459-1469
Culver, B., S.K. Sahu, A. Vernadakis, and K.N. Prasad (1977). Effects of 5-
    (3,3,-dimethyl-1-triazeno) imidazole-4-carboxamide (NSC 45388, DTIC) on
    neuroblastoma cells in culture. Biochem. Biophys. Res. Commun., 76, 778-783.
Ehrlich, Y.H., E. G. Brunngraber, P. K. Sinha, and K. N. Prasad (1977). Specific
    alterations in phosphyrylation of cytosol proteins from differentiating
    neuroblastoma cells grown in culture. Nature, 265, 238-241.
Elgin, S.C.R., J.B. Boyd, L.E. Hood, W. Wray, and F.C. Wu (1973). A prologue to
    the study of the nonhistone chromosomal proteins. Cold Spring Harbor Symp.
    Quant. Biol., 38, 821-833.
Hamprecht, B., and J. Schultz (1973). Stimulation by prostaglandin E_1 of adenosine
    3',5'-cyclic monophosphate formation in neuroblastoma cells in the presence
    of phosphodiesterase inhibitors. FEBS Lett., 34, 85-89.
Helson, L. (1975). Management of disseminated neuroblastoma CA, 25, 264-268.
Imashuku, S., S. Todo, T. Amano, F. Nakajima, and T. Kusunoki (1977). Preliminary
    studies on maturational therapy of neuroblastoma: Correlation between
    neurotransmitter synthesis and cyclic nucleotide levels in neuroblastoma
    tissues. J. Jap. Soc. Pediat. Surg., 13, 887-895.
Kates, J.R., R. Winterton, and K. Schlesinger (1971). Induction of acetylcholines-
    terase activity in mouse neuroblastoma tissue culture cells. Nature, 229,
    345-346.
Knapp, S., and A. J. Mandell (1974). Serotonin biosynthetic capacity of mouse
    C-1300 neuroblastoma cells in culture. Brain Res., 66, 547-551.
Kumar, S., G. Becker, and K.N. Prasad (1975). Cyclic AMP phosphodiesterase activity
    in malignant and cyclic AMP-induced "differentiated" neuroblastoma cells.
    Cancer Res., 35, 82-87.
Lazo, J.S., K.N. Prasad, and R.W. Ruddon (1976). Synthesis and phosphorylation of
    chromatin associated proteins in cAMP-induced "differentiated" neuroblastoma
    cells in culture. Exp. Cell Res., 100, 41-46.
Miller, R.A., and F.H. Ruddle (1974). Enucleated neuroblastoma cells form neurites
    when treated with dibutyryl cyclic AMP. J. Cell Biol., 63, 294-299.
Nelson, P., W. Ruffner, and M. Nirenberg (1969). Neuronal tumor cell with excitable
    membrane grown in vitro. Proc. Natl. Acad. Sci. USA, 64, 1004-1010.
Orr, C.W.M. (1967). Studies on ascorbic acid. Factors influencing the ascorbate-
    mediated inhibition of catalase. Biochemistry, 6, 2995-
Prasad, K.N. (1973). Role of cyclic AMP in the differentiation of neuroblastoma
    cell culture. In J. Schultz and H.G. Gratzner (Eds.), The Role of Cyclic
    Nucleotides in Carcinogenesis, Academic Press, Inc., New York. 207-237.
Prasad, K.N. (1975). Differentiation of neuroblastoma cells in culture. Biol. Rev.,
    50, 129-165.
Prasad, K.N. (1977). Differentiation and growth of neuroblastoma cells and serum
    types. Trans Am. Soc. Neurochem., 8, 87a.
Prasad, K.N., G. Becker, and K. Tirpathy. (1975a). Differences and similarities
    between guanosine 3',5'-cyclic monophosphate phosphodiesterase and adenosine
    3',5'-cyclic monophosphate phosphodiesterase activities in neuroblastoma
    cells in culture. Proc. Soc. Exp. Biol. Med., 149, 757-762.

Prasad, K.N., and K.N. Gilmer (1974). Demonstration of dopamine-sensitive adenylate cyclase in malignant neuroblastoma cells and change in sensitivity of adenylate cyclase to catecholamines in "differentiated" cells. Proc. Natl. Acad. Sci. USA, 71, 2525-2529.

Prasad, K.N., K.N. Gilmer, S.K. Sahu, and G. Becker (1975b). Effect of neurotransmitters, guanosine triphosphate, and divalent ions on the regulation of adenylate cyclase activity in malignant and adenosine cyclic 3',5'-monophosphate-induced "differentiated" neuroblastoma cells. Cancer Res. 35, 77-88.

Prasad, K.N., and A.W. Hsie (1971). Morphological differentiation of mouse neuroblastoma cells induced in vitro by dibutyryl adenosine 3',5'-cyclic monophosphate. Nature New Biol., 233, 141-142.

Prasad, K.N., and S. Kumar (1974). Cyclic AMP and the differentiation of neuroblastoma cells. In B. Clarkson and R. Baserga (Eds.), Control of Proliferation in Animal Cells, Cold Spring Harbor Laboratory, Cold Spring Harbor, New York. pp. 581-594.

Prasad, K.N., S. Kumar, G. Becker, and S.K. Sahu (1975c). Role of cyclic nucleotides in differentiation of neuroblastoma cells in culture. In B. Weiss (Ed.) Cyclic Nucleotides in Diseases, University Park Press, Baltimore, pp. 45-66.

Prasad, K.N., S.K. Sahu, and S. Kumar (1974). Relationship between cyclic CMP and differentiation of neuroblastoma cells in culture. In W. Nakahara, T. Ono, T. Sugimura, and H. Sugano (Eds.) Differentiation and Control of Malignancy of Tumor Cells, University of Tokyo Press, Tokyo. pp. 287-309.

Prasad, K.N., S.K. Sahu, and P.K. Sinha (1976a). Cyclic nucleotides in the regulation of expression of differentiated functions in neuroblastoma cells. J. Natl. Cancer Inst., 57, 619-631.

Prasad, K.N., P.K. Sinha, S.K. Sahu, and J.L. Brown (1976b). Binding of cyclic nucleotides with proteins in malignant and cyclic AMP-induced "differentiated" neuroblastoma cells in culture. Cancer Res., 36, 2290-2296.

Prasad, K.N., and A. Sakamoto (1978). Effect of sodium butyrate in combination with prostaglandin E_1 and inhibitors of cyclic nucleotide phosphodiesterase on human amelanotic melanoma ce-ls in culture. Experientia (in press).

Prasad, K.N., and P.K. Sinha (1976). Effect of sodium butyrate on mammalian cells in culture: A review, In vitro, 12, 125-132.

Prasad, K.N., and P.K. Sinha (1978). Regulation of differentiated functions and malignancy in neuroblastoma cells in culture. In G. F. Saunders (Ed.), Cell Differentiation and Neoplasia, Raven Press, New York pp. 111-141.

Prasad, K.N., J.C. Waymire, and N. Weiner (1972). A further study on the morphology and biochemistry of X-ray and dibutyryl cyclic AMP-induced differentiated neuroblastoma cells in culture. Exp. Cell Res., 74, 110-114.

Richelson, E. (1973). Stimulation of tyrosine hydroxylase activity in an adrenergic clone of mouse neuroblastoma by dibutyryl cyclic AMP. Nature New Biol., 242, 175-177.

Ross, J.R., J.B. Olmsted, and J.L. Rosenbaum (1975). The ultrastructure of mouse neuroblastoma cells in tissue culture. Tissue Cell, 1, 106-136.

Sahu, S.K., and K.N. Prasad (1975). Effect of neurotransmitters and prostaglandin E_1 on cyclic AMP levels in various clones of neuroblastoma cells in culture. J. Neurochem., 24, 1267-1269.

Sakamoto, A., and K.N. Prasad (1972). Effect of DL-glyceraldehyde on mouse neuroblastoma cell culture. Cancer Res., 32, 532-534.

Schubert, D., S. Humphreys, F. Vitry, and F. Jacob (1971). Induced differentiation of a neuroblastoma. Dev. Biol., 52, 514-546.

Sinha, P.K., and K.N. Prasad (1977). A further study on the regulation of cyclic nucleotide phosphodiesterase activity in neuroblastoma cells. Effect of growth. In Vitro, 13, 497-501.

Tao, M., M.L. Salas, and F. Lipmann (1970). Mechanism of activation by adenosine 3',5'-cyclic monophosphate of a protein phosphokinase from rabbit reticulocytes. Proc. Natl. Acad. Sci. USA, 67, 408-414.

Mechanisms of Reversion of Mammalian Sarcoma Virus Transformed Cells

S. Aaronson*, K. Porzig** and J. Greenberger***

*National Institutes of Health, National Cancer Institute,
Bethesda, Maryland 20014, U.S.A.
**Division of Oncology, Stanford University, School of Medicine,
Stanford, California 94305, U.S.A.
***Joint Center for Radiation Therapy, Boston, Massachusetts 02115, U.S.A.

ABSTRACT

Mammalian type-C RNA sarcoma viruses have arisen in nature by a mechanism involving recombination of a type-C helper leukemia virus with host cellular genetic information. The latter is believed to be responsible for the virus's transforming activity. Thus, sarcoma viruses provide a unique opportunity to study mechanisms by which normal or altered cellular genes may be involved in spontaneous neoplasia. Investigations aimed at defining viral and cellular functions required for expression of sarcoma virus functions have utilized a strategy involving the isolation and characterization of morphologic revertants of virus-transformed cells. Several distinct mechanisms of reversion have been demonstrated. These include both loss and reversible genetic alteration of the integrated virus genome. These findings imply the need for continued translation of viral transforming gene products for maintenance of the malignant state. Moreover, the lack of complementation between independent isolates of transformation-defective sarcoma virus mutants obtained from revertants of the latter type argues that a single viral gene function is responsible for initiation of the events leading to all of the profound alterations associated with the transformed cell.

Morphologic reversion has also been shown to result from a reversible cellular restriction to the expression of biologically functional sarcoma virus integrated within the host cell genome. The evidence indicates that this block is exerted at the level of viral RNA transcription of post-transcriptional processing but is specific to site at which the sarcoma virus is integrated. As such, this reversion mechanism provides a model for oncogenesis resulting from derepression of cellular genes that possess malignant potential.

INTRODUCTION

RNA-containing sarcoma viruses have been isolated from a number of mammalian species. In many cases, these viruses have been obtained from naturally occurring tumors (for review, see Aaronson and Stephenson, 1976). Sarcoma viruses cause cells to undergo striking alteration in their morphology and growth properties. These viruses are defective for their own replication and, thus, induce transformation of cells in the absence of detectable virus production (Aaronson and Rowe, 1970; Aaronson, 1973; Bassin, Tuttle and Fischinger, 1970; Henderson, Lieber and Todaro,

1974; Levy, 1971).

When sarcoma virus nonproducer cells are superinfected with helper leukemia virus, the productively infected cells release both helper virus and defective sarcoma virus in the helper virus envelope. Producer cells are far less neoplastic than nonproducer cells, due to the fact that the helper leukemia virus confers virion antigens to the virus-producing cell, which help the host to recognize and immuno- logically reject it (Stephenson and Aaronson, 1972; Strouk and co-workers, 1972). The lack of transplantation antigens associated with the nonproducer cell make these cells very useful as models for study of spontaneous neoplasia.

Molecular and immunologic studies have shown that mammalian sarcoma viruses contain genetic information of a portion of a helper virus (Aaronson, Bassin and Weaver, 1972; Barbacid, Stephenson and Aaronson, 1976; Benvensite, Scolnick, 1973; Dina, Beemon and Duesberg, 1976; Frankel, Neubauer and Fischinger, 1976; Hu, Davidson and Verma, 1977; Maisel and co-workers, 1973; Parks and co-workers, 1976; Scolnick, Goldberg and Parks, 1974) linked to some other nucleotide sequences (Anderson and Robbins, 1976; Frankel, Neubauer and Fischinger, 1976; Hu, Davidson and Verma, 1977; Maisel and co-workers, 1973; Scolnick, Goldberg and Parks, 1974). Accumulating ev- idence suggests that the latter are derived from the cellular genome of the species from which the sarcoma virus was initially isolated (Anderson and Robbins, 1976; Frankel, Neubauer and Fischinger, 1976; Scolnick, Goldberg and Parks, 1974). Since helper viruses do not, themselves, cause transformation of cells in culture, it is likely that the non-helper virus-related sequences of the sarcome virus code for its transforming functions. Thus, it is thought that mammalian sarcoma viruses have arisen by a mechanism involving recombination of a replicating helper virus with normal or altered cellular genes, the expression of which can cause transform- ation. The present review summarizes efforts aimed at elucidating sarcoma viral gene functions responsible for transformation as well as host cell functions necessary for expression of the malignant phenotype. Our strategy has involved the isolation of morphologic revertants of sarcoma virus nonproducer cells and the analysis of mechanisms responsible for reversion.

Selection of Revertants of Sarcoma Virus Transformed Cells

Methods for the isolation of revertants of sarcoma virus transformed cells have been devised to take advantage of the differences in growth properties of trans- formed and normal cells. Transformed cells are capable of multiplying on contact- inhibited cell monolayers (Aaronson and Todaro, 1968) or in suspension in semi- solid medium (Shin and co-workers, 1975; Stoker and co-workers, 1968) while the growth of normal cells is restricted under each of these conditions. Our technique for isolation of morphological revertants is based on a method used to increase the frequency of isolation of conditional lethal mutants of avian sarcoma virus (Wyke, 1973). The approach is to suspend single cells in semisolid medium containing agar or methyl cellulose. This allows only the transformed cells to replicate. Then an antimetabolite that kills actively dividing cells is added to the culture. After an appropriate time interval, the surviving cells are removed from the suspension, washed free of the antimetabolite and plated into petri dishes for subsequent selection of morphologically normal-appearing cells (Greenberger and Aaronson, 1974). This method can enrich for revertant cells in the populations by a factor of more than 100-fold.

The frequency at which revertants are isolated can be enhanced by prior exposure of the transformed cell population to a mutagen. In order to rigorously show that individual revertant clones result from separate mutagenizing events, it is neces- sary to obtain only a single revertant from a given stock of transformed cells. Since a particular mutagen may have a predilection for certain sites in the DNA, we have also used different mutagens to try to increase the range of mutations, and, thus, increase the number of viral and/or cellular gene functions that may be affected. A schematic diagram of the selection system is presented in Fig. 1.

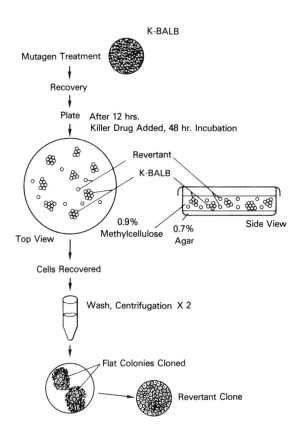

Fig. 1. Selection system for isolation of morphologic revertants of mammalian sarcoma virus-transformed cells.

In Vitro and In Vivo Properties of Morphologic Revertants

The methylcellulose selection technique has resulted in the isolation of a large number of morphologic revertants (Bensinger and co-workers, 1977; Greenberger and Aaronson, 1974). Table 1 compares in vitro growth characteristics of a series of revertants of a Kirsten murine sarcoma virus transformant of BALB/3T3, with the parental transformed and nontransformed cell lines, respectively. The revertants each demonstrated growth properties similar to those of BALB/3T3.

Their saturation densities ranged from 3 to 7×10^4 cells/cm^2, compared to 3×10^5 cells/cm^2 for the parental transformant, K-BALB. Most of the revertants and BALB/3T3 demonstrated no detectable colony formation in methylcellulose suspension medium (<0.001%). In contrast, K-BALB formed colonies with an efficiency around 10% under the same conditions. As shown in Table 1, none of the revertants formed tumors when inoculated into weaning BALB/c mice, while K-BALB was highly oncogenic.

S. Aaronson, K. Porzig and J. Greenberger

TABLE 5 Growth Characteristics of K-BALB Revertant Clones

Cell Line	Colony-formation[a] (% cells/colonies plated)		Retransformation[c] Frequency
	0.9% Methylcellulose	Tumor Formation[b] (10^6 cells inoculated)	
BALB/3T3	<0.001	0/10	$<10^{-8}$
K-BALB	10.0	9/10	-
R20	<0.001	0/10	10^{-7}-10^{-8}
R30	<0.001	0/10	10^{-6}-10^{-7}
R40	<0.001	0/10	$<10^{-8}$
R54	<0.001	0/10	10^{-6}-10^{-7}
R61	<0.001	0/10	$<10^{-8}$
R70	0.01	0/10	10^{-6}-10^{-7}
R80	<0.001	0/10	$<10^{-8}$
R90	<0.001	0/10	$<10^{-8}$
R100	<0.001	0/10	$<10^{-8}$

[a] Ten-fold dilutions of each cell line were plated into empty 50-mm petri dishes or were suspended in 0.9% methylcellulose and layered over a prehardened base of 0.7% agar in complete medium. Growing colonies were scored at 14 days.

[b] BALB/C mice (6 to 8 weeks old) were inoculated subcutaneously in the intrascapular area and observed weekly for 12 weeks. Tumors achieving a diameter of 0.5cm were scored as positive.

[c] Subclones of each revertant were grown to saturation in as many as 200-mm petri dishes as needed to detect the appearance of retransformed colonies. The retransformation frequency was calculated as the number of transformed colonies that appeared per number of calculated divisions required for the cells to reach that confluence. A frequency of $<10^{-8}$ reflects the absence of any retransformed colonies in 20 petri dishes containing cells grown to confluence. In reconstruction experiments, one K-BALB cell in a mixture containing 10^7 BALB/3T3 cells was readily detectable.

The stability of the revertant phenotype varied among individual revertant isolates. Spontaneous retransformation occurred at a frequency of 1 per 10^6 to 10^8 cell doublings for some, including R30, R54, and R70. Such retransformed foci closely resembled those induced by KiMSV. With other revertants, retransformation was not observed (TABLE 1).

Reversion Due to Loss of Sarcoma Viral Nucleotide Sequences

A DNA transcript of the sarcoma virus genome can be generated by reverse transcription and used as a molecular probe to determine the presence of complementary viral sequences within cellular DNA or RNA. This approach was used to analyze revertants that demonstrated no evidence of spontaneous retransformation. Such revertants also failed to yield sarcoma virus following helper virus superinfection. As shown in Fig. 2, cellular DNA of a representative revertant, R61, lacked sarcoma virus-specific DNA sequences that were readily detectable in the parental transformant (Bensinger and co-workers, 1977). Moreover, the extents of hybridization of the probe by revertant cellular DNA and RNA (Fig. 2) were no greater than that achieved with BALB/3T3 DNA and RNA, respectively. Similar findings have been reported for revertants of Moloney murine sarcoma virus transformed cells (Frankel and co-workers, 1976). It is not yet known whether the deletion of sarcoma virus information in this class of revertants results from chromosome loss or specific loss of all or a large portion of the viral genome.

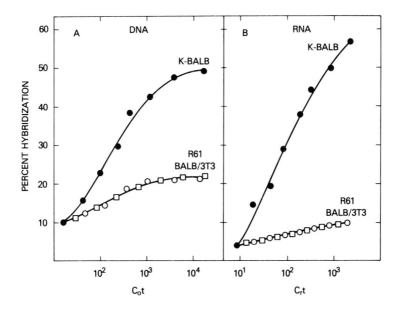

Fig. 2.   Molecular hybridization of Kirsten murine sarcoma virus (KiMSV) cDNA to A) cellular DNA and B) cellular RNA of virus transformed and revertant lines. Uninfected BALB/3T3 (□); K-BALB (●), a KiMSV nonproducer transformant of BALB/3T3; and R61 (○), a morphologic revertant subclone of K-BALB. The methods used have been previously reported (Bensinger and co-workers, 1977).

Reversion Due to Reversible Lesion in the Integrated Sarcoma Virus Genome

Among revertants demonstrating a low frequency of spontaneous retransformation, certain ones possessed properties representing a common phenotype. These revertants released very low titers of biologically active sarcoma virus following helper virus superinfection. Moreover, by infectious center analysis, wild-type sarcoma virus was rescuable from only a low fraction of the cell population, very similar to that which appeared morphologically transformed. However, when retransformants were cloned from the revertant population, sarcoma virus was rescuable from every cell (Bensinger and co-workers, 1977; Greenberger, Anderson and Aaronson, 1974).

As shown in Fig. 3, cellular DNA of a revertant, R30, possessing this phenotype, contained nucleotide sequences of the sarcoma virus. Moreover, the level of sarcoma virus-specific RNA in these cells was indistinguishable from that present in the parental transformant (Fig. 3). These findings suggested that the mechanism of reversion might involve a reversible lesion, such as a point mutation or small deletion, in the region of the integrated sarcoma virus coding for its transforming functions.

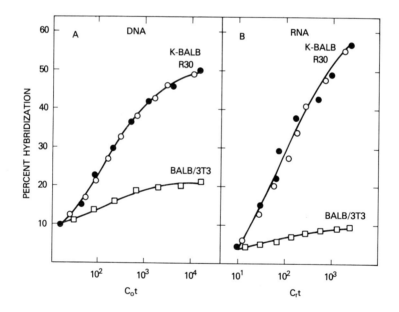

Fig. 3.   Molecular hybridization of Kirsten murine sarcoma
           virus (KiMSV) cDNA to A) cellular DNA and B) cel-
           lular RNA of virus transformed and revertant lines.
           Uninfected BALB/3T3 (□); K-BALB (●), a KiMSV
           nonproducer transformant of BALB/3T3; and R30
           (○), a morphologic revertant subclone of K-BALB.
           The methods used have been previously reported
           (Bensinger and co-workers, 1977).

Proof of this hypothesis was obtained in experiments demonstrating that virus rescued from such revertants contained disproportionally high levels of sarcoma virus
RNA compared to biologically active virus. It was possible to transmit transformation-defective virus to new cells. In cultures to which the defective virus was
transmitted, there was a low frequency of spontaneous restoration of the virus's
transforming ability. All of these findings established that a lesion in the integrated sarcoma virus, as opposed to a cellular block to virus expression, was the
mechanism responsible for reversion of this phenotype (Bensinger and co-workers,
1977; Greenberger, Anderson and Aaronson, 1974).

The above nonconditional sarcoma virus mutants have helped to demonstrate that the
continued presence of viral translational products is essential for maintenance of
the sarcoma virus-transformed state. Efforts have also been made to detect complementation between nonconditional sarcoma virus mutants obtained from independent
isolates of revertants containing genetically altered viruses. These studies have
been performed to determine whether one or more than one viral gene is required for
transformation (Bensinger and co-workers, 1977; Greenberger, Anderson and Aaronson,
1974). The lack of detectable complementation for expression of transformation by
these virus mutants implies that a single sarcome viral gene function is responsible for inducing the malignant phenotype in normal cells. As such, revertants
containing reversibly altered sarcoma viruses provide a model in which a small
alteration affecting a single gene can profoundly alter the phenotype of the cell,
causing it to be either malignant or normal.

Reversion Due to Cellular Regulation of Sarcoma Virus Gene Expression

Relatively little information is available concerning cellular functions required
for expression of the virus-transformed phenotype. There has been evidence obtained that morphologic reversion of sarcoma virus transformants can be associated
with cellular alterations (Boettiger, 1974; Den and co-workers, 1974; Krzyzek and
co-workers, 1977; Peebles, Scolnick and Howk, 1976; Stephenson, Reynolds and Aaronson, 1973). By selection techniques analogous to those utilized for isolation of
revertants due to viral genome alterations or loss, it has recently been possible
to isolate still another revertant phenotype, due to cellular control of viral
gene expression. From a clone of the mink-derived MvlLu cells, nonproductively
transformed by feline sarcoma virus (FeSV), revertant subclones were obtained and
shown to undergo spontaneous retransformation at low frequencies of 10^{-6}-10^{-8}.
Helper virus superinfection of these revertant cells resulted in rescue of biologically active sarcoma virus at very high efficiency. The rescued sarcoma virus
was capable of transforming new cells with one-hit kinetics, implying that reversion in this system was due to a cellular block to sarcoma virus expression rather
than to a genetic lesion in the transforming virus (Porzig, Barbacid and Aaronson,
in press).

Cellular levels of FeSV-specific RNA were compared in cells possessing revertant
and transformed phenotypes. As shown in Fig. 4, RNA of an FeSV transformed subclone, T61-1, hybridized 32% of FeLV cDNA with a $C_r t$ 1/2 of 6×10^0, while RNA of the
revertant subclone, R82-3, hybridized the same probe to an extent of only 7%, a
level indistinguishable from that of uninfected MvlLu cells. The restriction to
viral RNA expression in the revertant cells was dramatically reversed in a retrans-
formant subclone, RT90-4. As a control, the levels of endogenous mink viral RNA in
each cell line were found to be very similar (Fig 4). These results indicate that
reversion of the FeSV transformed phenotype in R82-3 cells was associated with a
specific, reversible restriction to FeSV RNA expression.

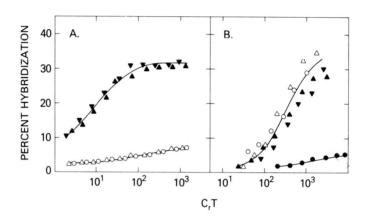

Fig. 4.   Virus-specific RNA in FeSV transformed nonproducer
          and morphological revertant MvlLu cells. Cellular
          RNAs were purified and used to hybridize A) FeLV
          viral cDNA, and B) mink endogenous viral cDNA.
          FeLV viral cDNA was hybridized to a final extent of
          90% by cellular RNA purified from FeLV-infected
          A673. Mink endogenous viral cDNA was hybridized
          to a final extent of 94% by cellular RNA purified
          from mink endogenous virus-infected canine fetal
          thymus cells. Cellular RNAs tested were from:
          FeSV transformed subclone T61-1 (▲); FeSV rever-
          tant subclone R82-3 (△); FeSV retransformant
          subclone RT90-4 (▼); uninfected MvlLu (○);
          and FeLV-infected kitten lung (●).

A marked reduction in viral RNA expression might result from inhibition at a transcriptional level. However, an increase in viral RNA processing could also account
for these findings. It was reasoned that enhanced viral RNA processing would be
likely to affect an additional copy of the same sarcoma virus. Thus, by this latter mechanism, the revertant cells should be resistant to superinfection with FeSV.
When a comparison was made of the susceptibilities of the revertant subclone and
normal MvlLu cells to transformation by exogenous FeSV, each was found to be com-
parably susceptible (Porzig and co-workers, in press). These findings argue that
the block to FeSV gene expression in the revertant cells was a specific one affecting transcription, although a mechanism involving cis-acting post-transcriptional
processing of viral RNA can not be excluded.

A reversible transcriptional restriction might be specific to the site at which the sarcoma viral genome is integrated or involve a larger region and, thus, affect transcription of other cellular genes as well. Recent studies have demonstrated that cell differentiation can be associated with internal rearrangement of cellular genetic sequences (Hozumi and Tonegawa, 1976). Such findings raise the possibility that the reversible alteration in sarcoma viral gene expression could result from a change in site of the integrated sarcoma viral genome. This last possibility should be amenable to investigation through the application of molecular hybridization and DNA blotting techniques.

In this reversion system, a reversible cellular alteration affecting expression of the integrated sarcoma virus markedly alters the growth properties and malignant phenotype of the cell. There is accumulating evidence that sarcoma viruses have originated by recombination between a type C helper virus and some cellular nucleotide sequences (Anderson and Robbins, 1976; Frankel, Neubauer and Fischinger, 1976; Scolnick and co-workers, 1973; Scolnick, Goldberg and Parks, 1974; Stehelin and co-workers, 1976). The latter are thought to be responsible for the virus's transforming activity. Whether these nucleotide sequences represent an altered cellular gene or a gene that may be normally expressed at a particular stage in differentiation is not resolved. According to the latter hypothesis, a cellular alteration that would lead to derepression of such a gene could lead to transformation. This class of revertants provides a model for this spontaneous transformation mechanism.

CONCLUSIONS

The present review has summarized evidence concerning virus and cellular interactions involved in the expression of sarcoma virus-induced transformation. These findings have been derived from investigations of mechanisms responsible for morphologic reversion of mammalian sarcoma virus transformed cells. Demonstration of reversion due to loss (Bensinger and co-workers, 1977; Frankel and co-workers, 1976) or genetic alteration (Bensinger and co-workers, 1977; Greenberger, Anderson and Aaronson, 1974) of the integrated sarcoma virus has helped to establish that continued expression of virus-coded translational products is required for maintenance of the transformed state. Moreover, the lack of complementation between nonconditional sarcoma virus mutants isolated from revertants of the latter type has implied that only a single sarcoma virus gene function is necessary for transformation (Bensinger and co-workers, 1977; Greenberger, Anderson and Aaronson, 1974). Finally, an important role of the cell in the expression of the malignant state has been elucidated through the discovery of a reversible cellular control that specifically affects the expression of sarcoma virus genes (Porzig, Barbacid and Aaronson, in press). The continuence investigation of processes by which the cell can restrict expression of viral genes with malignant potential should aid further in the development of approaches toward prevention of spontaneous neoplasia.

REFERENCES

Aaronson, S. A. and G. J. Todaro (1968). Basis for the acquisition of malignant potential by mouse cells cultivated in vitro. Science, 162, 1024-1026.

Aaronson, S. A. and W. P. Rowe (1970). Nonproducer clones of murine sarcoma virus transformed BALB/3T3 cells. Virology, 42, 9-19.

Aaronson, S. A., R. H. Bassin and C. Weaver (1972). Comparison of murine sarcoma viruses in nonproducer and S+L- transformed cells. J. Virol., 9, 701-704.

Aaronson, S. A. (1973). Biologic characterization of mammalian cells transformed by a primate sarcoma virus. Virology, 52, 562-567.

Aaronson, S. A. and J. R. Stephenson (1976). Endogenous Type-CRNA viruses of mammalian cells. Biochemica et Biophysica Acta, 458, 323-354.

Anderson, G. R. and K. C. Robbins (1976). Rat sequences of the Kirsten and Harvey murine sarcoma virus genomes: Nature, origin, and expression in rat tumor RNA. J. Virol., 17, 335-351.

Barbacid, M., J. R. Stephenson and S. A. Aaronson (1976). Gag gene of mammalian type-C RNA tumor viruses. Nature, 262, 554-559.

Bassin, R. H., N. Tuttle and P. J. Fischinger (1970). Isolation of murine sarcoma virus transformed mouse cells which are negative for leukemia virus from agar suspension cultures. Int. J. Cancer, 6, 95-107.

Bensinger, W. I., K. C. Robbins, J. S. Greenberger and S. A. Aaronson (1977). Different mechanisms for morphologicreversion of a clonal population of murine sarcoma virus-transformed nonproducer cells. Virology, 77, 750-761.

Benvensite, R. E. and E. M. Scolnick (1973). RNA in mammalian sarcoma virus transformed nonproducer cells homologous to murine leukemia virus RNA. Virology, 77, 750-761.

Boettiger, D. (1974). Reversion and induction of Rous sarcoma virus expression in virus transformed baby hamster kidney cells. Virology, 62, 522-529.

Deng, C. T., D. Boettiger, I. Macpherson and H. E. Varmus (1974). The persistence of expression of virus-specific DNA in revertants of Rous sarcoma virus-transformed BHK-21 cells. Virology, 62, 512-529.

Dina, D. K., K. Beemon and P. Duesberg (1976). The 30S Moloney sarcoma virus RNA contains leukemia virus nucleotide sequences. Cell, 9, 299-309.

Frankel, A. E., D. K. Haapala, R. L. Neubauer and P. J. Fischinger (1976). Elimination of the sarcoma genome from murine sarcoma virus transformed cat cells. Science, 191, 1264-1266.

Frankel, A. E., R. L. Neubauer and P. J. Fischinger (1976). Fractionation of DNA nucleotide transcripts from Moloney sarcoma virus and isolation of sarcoma virus-specific complementary DNA. J. Virol., 18, 481-490.

Greenberger, J. S., G. R. Anderson and S. A. Aaronson (1974). Transformation-defective virus mutants in a class of morphologic revertants of sarcoma virus-transformed nonproducer cells. Cell, 2, 279-286.

Greenberger, J. S. and S. A. Aaronson (1974). Morphologic revertants of murine sarcoma virus transformed nonproducer BALB/3T3: selective techniques for isolation and biologic properties In Vitro and In Vivo. Virology, 57, 339-346.

Henderson, I. C., M. M. Lieberand, G. J. Todaro (1974). Focus formation and the generation of "nonproducer" transformed cell lines with murine and feline sarcoma viruses. Virology, 60, 282-297.

Hozumi, N. and S. Tonegawa (1976). Evidence for somatic rearrangement of immuno-globulin genes coding for variable and constant regions. Proc. Natl. Acad. Sci. U.S.A., 73, 3628-3632.

Hu, S., N. Davidson and I. M. Verma (1977). A heteroduplex study of the sequence relationships between the RNAs and M-MLV. Cell, 10, 496-477.

Krzyzek, R. A., A. F. Lau, D. H. Spector and A. J. Faras (1977). Post-transcriptional control of avian oncornavirus transforming gene sequences in mammalian cells. Nature, 269, 175-179.

Levy, J. A. (1971). Demonstration of differences in murine sarcoma virus foci formed in mouse and rat cells under a soft agar overlay. J. Natl. Cancer Inst., 46, 1001-1007.

Maisel, J., V. Klement, M. M-C Lai, W. Ostertag and P. Duesberg (1973). Ribonucleic acid components of murine sarcoma and leukemia viruses. Proc. Natl. Acad. Sci. U.S.A., 70, 3536-3540.

Parks, W. P., R. S. Howk, A. Anisowicz and E. M. Scolnick (1976). Deletion mapping of Moloney type-C virus: polypeptides and nucleic acid expression in different transforming virus isolates. J. Virol., 18, 491-503.

Peebles, P. T., E. M. Scolnick and R. S. Howk (1976). Increased sarcoma virus RNA in cells transformed by leukemia viruses: model for leukemogensis. Science, 192, 1143-1145.

Scolnick, E. M., E. Rands, D. Williams and W. P. Parks (1973). Studies on the nucleic acid sequences of Kirsten sarcoma virus: a model for formation of a mammalian RNA-containing sarcoma virus. J. Virol., 12, 458-463.

Scolnick, E. M., R. J. Goldberg and W. P. Parks (1974). A biochemical and genetic analysis of mammalian RNA-containing sarcoma viruses. Cold Spring Harbor Symp. Quant. Biol., 39, 885-895.

Shin, S., V. H. Freedman, R. Risser and R. Pollack (1975). Tumorigenicity of virus-transformed cells in nude mice is correlated specifically with anchorage independent growth in vitro. Proc. Natl. Acad. Sci. U.S.A., 72, 4435-4439.

Stehelin, D., R. V. Guntaka, H. E. Varmus and J. M. Bishop (1976). Purification of DNA complementary to nucleotide sequences required for neoplastic transformation of fibroblasts by avian sarcoma viruses. J. Mol. Biol., 101, 349-365.

Stephenson, J. R. and S. A. Aaronson (1971). Murine sarcoma and leukemia viruses: genetic difference determined by RNA-DNA hybridization. Virology, 46, 480-484.

Stephenson, J. R. and S. A. Aaronson (1972). Genetic factors influencing type-C RNA virus induction. J. Exptl. Med., 136, 175-184.

Stephenson, J. R., R. K. Reynolds and S. A. Aaronson (1973). Characterization of morphologic revertants of murine and avian sarcoma virus-transformed cells. J. Virol., 11, 218-222.

Stoker, M., C. O'Neill, S. Berryman and J. Wazman (1968). Anchorage and growth regulation in normal and virus-transformed cells. Int. J. Cancer, 3, 683-693.

Strouk, V., G. Frunder, C. M. Fenyo, E. Lamon, H. Shuryak and G. Klein (1972). Lack of distinctive surface antigen on cells transformed by murine sarcoma virus. J. Exptl. Med., 136, 344-352.

Wyke, J. A. (1973). Complementation of transforming functions by temperature-sensitive mutants of avian sarcoma virus. Virology, 54, 28-36.

Oncornavirus-Related Non Virion Glycoproteins Associated with Cell Proliferation and Malignant Expression

M. Rieber, M. S. Rieber and M. Alonso

Center of Microbiology and Cell Biology,
Instituto Venezolano de Investigaciones Científicas, Apartado 1827, Caracas,
Venezuela

ABSTRACT

Antiserum to murine leukemia virus is able to recognize the presence of two components in the 100,000 dalton region and a 60,000 dalton component on the external surface of rat cells that express a transformed phenotype. "Normal" resting cells of the same origin reveal by the same reaction the presence of a 200,000 dalton external macromolecule not detected in the transformed or proliferating cells.

KEYWORDS

Growth control/antigenic surface glycoproteins/gel electrophoresis/oncornaviruses.

INTRODUCTION

A significant advance in the definition of molecular differences in cell surface components of normal and malignant fibroblasts took place with the discovery of a 200,000 dalton large external transformation-sensitive (LETS) glycoprotein or fibronectin, known to be absent or decreased in most transformed fibroblasts but present in the corresponding normal cells (see #5 for Review).

As there were early indications of important exceptions to the correlation between LETS absence and transformation (6), a number of recent studies have suggested a probable role of fibronectin in cell adhesion (15,1). As the presence or absence of iodination label in the 200,000 dalton region was not a sufficient indication of the growth properties of cultured cells, we have searched for additional criteria to differentiate normal from transformed cells. Recent reports from our laboratory have indicated that antiserum to murine leukemia virus can be used to detect transformation-associated glycoproteins different from those found in virus infected-untransformed cells and normal cells (11, 12). In order to continue our studies on growth-related macromolecules, we have further used a normal rat kidney system infected by a temperature-sensitive mutant of Rous Sarcoma virus, consisting of cells that display a malignant morphology and behaviour at 33° and revert to the normal phenotype at 37° (8, 10).

In such a system, we have further investigated possible antigenic relationships between transformed and normal cell surfaces. Our results show that the conversion of resting normal cells into proliferating and transformed cells is accompanied by the processing of preexisting normal surface proteins into antigenically related forms of lower molecular weight which remain on the surface of the proliferating populations.

MATERIALS AND METHODS

Cell Cultures. The temperature-sensitive cell line used in this study was a clone (NT$_3$-KR) from an isolate of NRK cells infected with the ts 339 temperature-sensitive mutant of B77 virus. These cells exhibited the characteristics of transformed cell at 33° and of the normal phenotype at 37° when propagated in Dulbecco's medium (Grand Island Biological Co., Grand Island, N.Y.; Catalog No. H-16) supplemented with 10% fetal calf serum, 10% tryptose phosphate broth (Difco Laboratories, Detroi Mich.), and 1% Dimethyl sulfoxide (Sigma Chemical Co., St. Louis, Mo.). No signifi cant change in the temperature-mediated phenotype was observed when the growth rate of cells was limited by seeding them in the above-described medium, supplemented wi just 0.5% serum.

Iodination. This was carried out (11) with cultures, seeded at 2.5 x 10^4 cells/sq cm, that were inoculated in 9-cm Petri dishes (NUNC, Denmark). For most experi- ments, cells were iodinated after a 3-day exposure to a medium supplemented with 0.5% serum, except where indicated. However, in all cases the cultures were washed 3 times with medium without serum and were washed subsequently 3 times with PBS-G that contained 5 mM glucose. Iodination was carried out in PBS-G, to which we added simultaneously an enzymic mixture of 50 µg lactoperoxidase (Calbiochem, Los Angeles, Calif.), and 1.25 units of glucose oxidase (Worthington Biochemical Corp., Freehold, N.H.), and 200 µCi sodium iodide ^{125}I-carrier-free for protein iodination (New England Nuclear, Boston, Mass.). After a 10 min iodination, cells were washed in PBI-G, which was identical in composition to the PBS-G, except that sodium iodide was substituted for sodium chloride to stop iodination. After 3 washed in PBI-G, cells were collected by scraping in PBI-G containing 2 mM FMSF (phenyl methyl sulfonyl fluoride) to prevent proteolytic degradation, for subsequent harvesting by centrifugation at 500 rpm for 10 min.

Immune precipitation. The serum used was goat antiserum 1S-167 to purified Tween- ether-disrupted murine leukemia virus and control goat serum. The goat antiserum showed precipitin lines by immunodiffusion with Moloney leukemia virus being nega- tive with fetal calf serum, NIH mouse spleen cells and early passages of normal rat kidney cells exhibiting density-dependent inhibition. By counterelectrophoresis, the antiserum showed 3 bands with Moloney leukemia virus, 3 bands with Rauscher mu- rine leukemia virus, and no bands with simian sarcoma virus, gibbon ape lymphoma virus, fetal calf serum, and 3T3 cells. The control goat serum exhibited no reac- tivity with murine leukemia virus by immunodiffusion. The immune sera were gener- ously provided by Dr. Jack Gruber, National Cancer Institute, Program Resources and Logistics, Bethesda, Md.

Electrophoretic Analyses. Extracts were prepared by freezing and thawing 3X in 5 M Urea, 1% Triton-X-100, 0.000 M FMSF 0.05 M Tris-HCl pH 7.5. After removal of in- soluble aggregates, the supernatants were preabsorbed with preimmune rabbit serum for 1 hour at 37° and further 16 hours at 4°. After centrifugation at 12,500 x g for 20 min, the supernatants were reacted with 0.02 ml of immune serum for collection as indicated for the preimmune precipitates. Samples for electrophoretic analysis were made 2% in sodium dodecyl sulfate (SDS); 0.002 M FMSF; 0.1 M β-mercaptoethanol; 0.1 M Tris-HCl, pH 6.8 and heated for 3 min to 90°.

Electrophoresis was carried out in 3-15% gradient gels by the high resolution pro- cedure of Laemmli (7) followed by fluorographic analysis (2). Approximate molecu- lar weights were estimated by the use of known protein standards exposed to parallel electrophoresis under identical conditions to those used for samples.

RESULTS

Restriction of the Transformation Phenotype at Low Serum Levels Affects the Expression of the gp100 Antigenically Related to Oncornavirus Proteins. As an extension of our studies on transformation-associated glycoproteins recognized by anti MLV serum, we have now investigated cell cycle fluctuations in the levels of oncornavirus-related gp 100 in non producer ts-NT$_3$-KR cells (12). Such cells can be arrested in the G_0-G_1 stage in low serum and reveal a normal morphology (Fig. 1) when grown at the restrictive temperature for the expression of transformation, as compared with the same cells which continue to grow at the same serum levels when kept at the temperature that permits the expression of the transformation phenotype (Fig. 2).

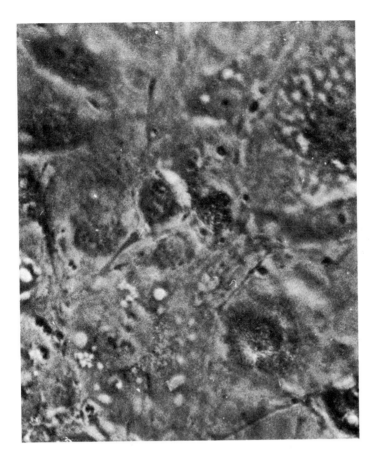

Fig. 1. Flat morphology of ts-NT$_3$-KR "normal" cells grown at the restrictive temperature for the expression of the transformed phenotype.

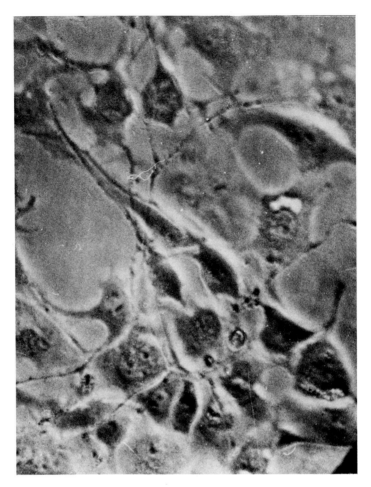

Fig. 2. Superimposed pattern of growth shown by
ts-NT$_3$-KR cells grown at the permissive temperature
for the expression of the transformed phenotype.

We have previously reported that proliferating populations of such cells express
comparable levels of the gp 100 both at the non permissive temperature of 37° and
at 33° which is the permissive temperature for the expression of transformation
(11, 12). Hence, it seemed necessary to investigate now, whether such cells limited of serum for 72 hours and labelled with ^{3}H -glucosamine during the last 16
hours of serum limitation differed in their relative concentration of oncornavirus-
related gp 100. A reaction was carried out by adjusting the relative cpm/mg cells
to equal levels prior absorption of serum-starved cells grown at 37° and 33° with
preimmune serum and subsequent reaction with anti-Moloney leukemia virus serum.

Analysis of the immune precipitates is presented in Figure 3, which reveals a relative decrease in the amount of reactive gp 100 and a corresponding increase in a
slower migrating region in serum-starved cells grown at the restrictive temperature
for the expression of transformation in contrast with the opposite result in cells
grown under permissive conditions which reveal a greater proportion of label in the
gp 100 region.

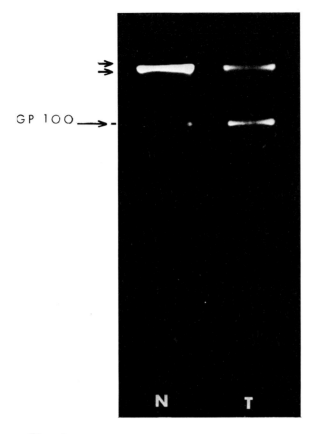

Fig. 3.
Effect of Serum Limitation on the Expression of
Cellular Glycoproteins Reactive with Anti-Murine
Leukemia Virus.
N. Immune precipitate from "normal" cells grown
for 3 days at 37° in 0.5% serum.
T. Immune precipitate from transformed cells grown
for 3 days at 33° in 0.5% serum.

The detection of components of low electrophoretic mobility observed in Fig. 3 and
the temperature-dependent decrease in the gp 100 was not apparent in ^3H -glucosa-
mine labelled extracts from serum-stimulated cultures blocked by hydroxyurea (1 mM)
in the G_1/S part of the cell cycle (not shown). This suggests that the decrease in
the gp 100 described in Fig. 3 is not associated with inhibition of DNA synthesis
but with the differential ability of "normal" ts-NT$_3$-KR to enter a resting Go state
by serum limitation, (4) depending on whether the transformed phenotype is restricted or not by the experimental temperatures used.

Transformation-Associated Surface Difference in Exposure of the Glycoproteins Antigenically related to Murine Leukemia Virus. Surface radioiodination was carried out
to determine whether the accumulation of slow-migrating components in metabolically
labelled serum-starved ts-NT$_3$-KR cells grown at 37° was also manifested by external
labelling. Figure 4 confirmed that serum-starved cells kept at 37° also manifest
an increased proportion in a 200,000 dalton surface component not detectable in

cultures maintained at the same serum levels at 33°. In contrast, identical cpm/m
of the latter cultures revealed a clearly increased proportion of label recognized
by anti-MLV serum in the molecular weight regions of 100,000 dalton and 65,000
dalton.

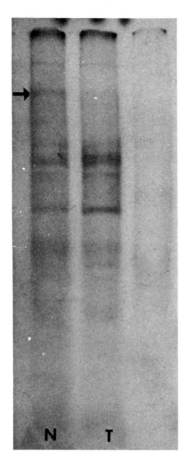

Fig. 4. Effect of Serum Limitation on the Transformation-Associated Expression of Surface Proteins
Reactive with Anti-Murine Leukemia Virus Serum.
N. Immune precipitates from surface-iodinated cells
grown at 37° for 3 days in 0.5% serum prior labelling.
T. Immune precipitates from surface-iodinated cells
grown at 33° for 3 days in 0.5% serum prior labelling.

An additional indication of a different surface exposure of components reactive with
anti-MLV serum was observed when subconfluent cultures of ts-NT$_3$-KR were washed and
incubated in situ with medium containing anti-MLV serum. Whereas anti-MLV serum
heated for 60 min to 56° did not affect the viability of the cultures, nevertheless
it became clearly apparent that the immune serum but not preimmune serum lead to a
significant agglutination of cultures grown at 33° but not at 37°, suggestive of a
surface interaction with such cells (not shown).

DISCUSSION

Our previous results by metabolic labelling with ^{3}H- glucosamine revealed on oncornavirus-related 100,000 dalton glycoprotein (gp 100) in transformed cells but not in normal and virus-infected untransformed cells (11, 12). We have now shown that cells that express conditionally transformed properties can exhibit an alteration in the proportion of the gp 100, as revealed both by metabolic labelling and by surface radioiodination. The present data indicating that cells that manifest transformed properties exhibit an increased proportion of virus-related non virion components in the 100,000 dalton region and in the 60,000 dalton region, resemble reports in avian cells in which a 100,000 dalton transformation specific surface antigen (13) and a 60,000 dalton transformation-specific sarcoma gene product (3) have been found.

More relevant to the present findings are some recent observations on Moloney leukemia virus-induced cell surface antigens. In the latter study, it has been found that such antigenic activity also appears associated with three iodinatable components in the molecular weight regions of 52,000, 92,000 and 192,000 dalton. A possible implication from our results and those related to the Moloney virus-induced cell surface antigen may be that "transformation" associated receptors exist even in "normal" cells in antigenically related forms of different molecular weight, whose interconversion may be important to the transformation process. Knowledge of the parameters that control the expression of such surface components should be useful to the understanding of growth control.

REFERENCES

1) Ali, I., Mautner, V., Lanza, R. and Hynes, R. O. (1977). Restoration of normal morphology, adhesion and cytoskeleton in transformed cells by addition of a transformation-sensitive protein. Cell 11, 115-126.
2) Bonner, W. M. and Laskey, R. A. (1974). A film detection method for tritium-labelled proteins and nucleic acids. European J. Biochem., 46, 83-88.
3) Brugge, J.S. and Erikson, R. L. (1977). Identification of a transformation-specific antigen induced by an avian sarcoma virus. Nature, 269, 346-348.
4) Burk, R. R. (1970). One-step growth cycle for BHK 21/C13 hamster fibroblasts. Exptl. Cell Res., 63, 309-316.
5) Hynes, R. O. (1976). Cell surface proteins and malignant transformation. Biochem. Biophys. Acta, 458, 73-107.
6) Hogg, N. M. (1974). A comparison of membrane proteins of normal and transformed cells by lactoperoxidase labelling. Proc. Nat. Acad. Sci. U.S.A., 71, 489-492.
7) Laemmli, U. K. (1970). Cleavage of structural proteins during the assembly of the head of bacteriophate T4. Nature, 277, 680-685.
8) Rieber, M. and Irwin, J. C. (1974). The possible correlation of growth rate and expression of transformation with temperature-dependent modification in high-molecular weight membrane glycoproteins in mammalian cells transformed by a wild-type and by a thermosensitive mutant of avian sarcoma virus. Cancer Res., 34, 3469-3473.
9) Rieber, M., Bacalao, J. and Alonso, G. (1975). Turnover of high molecular weight cell surface proteins during growth and expression of malignant transformation. Cancer Res., 35, 2104-2108.
10) Rieber, M. and Bacalao, J. (1976). A cyclic adenosine 3':5-monophosphate-mediated effect of cholera toxin on high-molecular-weight glycoprotein species of malignant cells. Cancer Res., 36, 3178-3184.
11) Rieber, M., Bacalao, J., Rieber, M. S. and Alonso, G. (1977). Demonstration of different glycosylated antigens in C-type virus-transformed and infected cells by antiserum to murine leukemia virus. Cancer Res., 37, 1165-1169.

12) Rieber, M., Bacalao, J. and Rieber, M. S. (1977). Continued presence of simi-
    lar transformation-associated antigens related to murine oncornavirus
    proteins in transformed cells, morphological revertants and cells re-
    stricted in the expression of transformation. Cancer Res., 37, 1170-1174.
13) Rohrschneider, L. R., Kurth, R. and Bauer, H. (1975). Biochemical character-
    ization of rumor-specific cell surface antigens on avian oncornavirus
    transformed cells. Virology, 66, 481-491.
14) Troy, F. A., Fenyo, E. M. and Klein, G. (1977). Moloney leukemia virus-induced
    cell surface antigen: detection and characterization in sodium dodecyl
    sulfate gels. Proc. Natl. Acad. Sci. U.S.A. 74, 5270-5274.
15) Yamada, K., Yamada, S. S. and Pastan, I. (1976). Cell surface protein partially
    restored morphology, adhesiveness and contact inhibition of movement to
    transformed fibroblasts. Proc. Natl. Acad. Sci. U.S.A. 73, 1217-1221.

Closing Remarks: Symposium 4

Eugenia Sacerdote de Lustig

*Research Department, Instituto de Oncologia Angel H. Roffo,
Avenida San Martin 5481, Buenos Aires*

Today, at the symposium of cell biology, we have been
privileged to hear a remarkable series of papers which,
although heterogeneous, show the common aim of
establishing, at a molecular level, the differences
between normal and cancer cells. A large variety of
biological systems have been used, from the simplest to
the most sophisticated as the mink cells which Aaronson
infected with feline leukemia virus. An analysis
followed on the mechanisms controlling the malignization
and the factors responsible for the redifferentiation of
transformed cells.

The symposium has contributed to the study of the
processes which stimulate DNA synthesis in tumour cells.
However, the analysis of the factors responsible for the
malignant expression in different systems leads us to the
understanding of the spontaneous transformation. It is
worth noting that in some biological systems (neuroblastoma, leukemic cells) the malignancy could be controlled: the differentiation of leukemic cells provides
clues to the mechanism of in vivo maturation arrest
characteristic of many human acute blastic leukemias, and
concluding the cancer phenotype is the result of viral,
celular and environmental factors.

We believe that the progress achieved in this symposium
is not restricted to the field of molecular biology, but
it will have an impact for the future clinical diagnosis
and treatment of cancer, enabling us to make use of
revertant cells as strong antigens, and to make use of
fetal nuclear antigens in cancer diagnosis and prognosis.

Cell Membrane and Cancer

Cell-to-Cell Communication and Growth Control

W. R. Loewenstein

*Department of Physiology & Biophysics, University of Miami School of Medicine,
P.O. Box 016430, Miami, Florida 33101, U.S.A.*

ABSTRACT

The hypothesis that the channels in permeable cell junctions are con-
duits for the cell-to-cell transmission of growth controlling molecules predicts that tissue cells of normal growth (growth-control competent) be capable of cell-to-cell transmission (channel-competent);
and that channel-incompetent dividing tissue cells be growth-control
incompetent. A survey of cells of normally growing organs and tissues and of deviant incompetent cells bears this prediction out.
Fusion of channel-competent human cells with channel-incompetent
mouse cells produces channel-competent and growth-control competent
hybrids so long as they have the sufficient chromosome complement of
the human parent cell. Upon loss of human chromosomes - in one hybrid
system, human chromosome 11, the hybrids become channel-incompetent
and growth-control incompetent. Channel competence and growth control
competence behave as genetically insegregable traits, as does the
pair of the opposite phenotype.

Cells of organized tissues have channels in their junctions that provide a path for direct flow of hydrophilic molecules between cell
interiors (Loewenstein 1966, 1975). These channels appeared early in
phylogenetic development; they are present in primitive sponges and
throughout the phylogenetic scale up to man. As a general rule, a
given cell in a tissue interconnects via such channels with many
neighbors. Thus, all cells in a salivary gland or in a thyroid acynus
are interconnected, or cells in liver and skin are widely interconnected forming continuous systems from within (Loewenstein, 1979).

From experiments in which the channels are probed with molecular yard-
stick of known dimensions, it is known that the channel bore is at
least 14 Å, wide enough to permit the passage of peptide molecules of
up to about 1000 dalton (Simpson, Rose & Loewenstein, 1977). The
aqueous bore of the channel is electrostatistically shielded; the
channel in mammalian cells discriminates against negatively charged
molecules in the 700-1000 dalton range. But for the molecules up to

500 daltons, there is not too much electrostatic hindrance (Flagg-Newton, Simpson, Loewenstein, 1978). Given these properties, the cell-to-cell channel is expected to permit the transmission of a broad range of cellular molecules: inorganic ions, metabolites, small hormones, high-energy phosphates, vitamins, nucleotides, cyclic nucleotides, and so on. It would not be too surprising, therefore, if such an ubiquitous and ancient hole between cells has adapted to many cellular functions.

I discuss here the possibility of a function in growth control. Our hypothesis is that *the cell-to-cell channel is a conduit for the cell -to-cell transmission of molecules necessary for growth control.* The *a priori* arguments and the models for growth self-regulation are given elsewhere (Loewenstein, 1968a, 1968b, 1979). Here I restate only the corollary of the hypothesis that bears directly on the cancer problem: obstruction or absence of the channels (in dividing cell populations) result in disturbance of cellular growth. And so the hypothesis makes two testable predictions: *(i) a dividing cell population competent in regulating its growth is channel-competent; and (ii) a dividing cell population which is channel-incompetent is growth-regulation incompetent, that is, it is potentially cancerous.* (The obverse, of course, does not follow from the hypothesis; not all cancerous cells need be channel-incompetent.) While I focus here on intracellular molecules of control, there is no reason to exclude additional controls by extracellular signals. In fact, there is no dearth of information for such controls by hormones, nutrients, growth factors, etc.,.

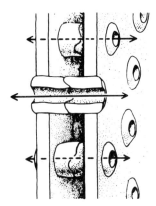

Fig. 1.   The cell-to-cell channel. Schematic diagram of a cell membrane junction, showing the cell-cell channel made of two protochannels, one from each membrane, forming a continuous leakproof tunnel through the cell membrane through which hydrophilic molecules can flow directly from one cell interior to another. (Reproduced with permission from Loewenstein 1974.)

The first prediction was born out by the work of the past ten years. All cells of organized tissues examined, capable of dividing, were found to be channel-competent. The examination covered a wide variety of tissues, including tissues in conditions where cell division is fast and generalized, such as during regeneration (liver) or wound healing (skin) (Loewenstein, 1979). The only normal tissue cells known to be channel-incompetent are (adult) skeletal muscle fibers and nerve fibers. But these cells--and nicely fitting the hypothesis--are also no longer capable of dividing. While they are capable of dividing, in the embryonic state, they are also channel-competent (Potter, Furshpan, Lennox, 1966; Sheridan, 1968).

The testing of the second prediction took longer. Our strategy here was first to search for the rare deviant cell type that is channel-incompetent and to see whether it is also growth control-incompetent; and, then, in a next step, to try to trace the incompetencies to a common genetic defect. A straightforward approach would have been to use one-step mutants; but we were unable to produce these. The next best approach that occurred to us was to use segregants, as they are provided by the spontaneous loss of chromosomes in somatic cell hybrids between channel-competent and channel-incompetent cells. This approach worked, although not at the single gene level, at the chromosome level.

We obtained channel-competent cell types by x-irradiating embryonic cells, or by searching for random mutants among various cell lines in culture. So far, a total of 17 channel-incompetent cell strains have been isolated. Our primary search here was for channel-incompentence; and only after the communication defect of the clones had been established were the growth properties tested. All 17 channel-incompetent strains turned out to be growth-control incompetent; they were density-independent in their growth in vitro and highly tumorigenic when injected into appropriate animal hosts (Borek, Higashino, Loewenstein, 1969; Azarnia, Larsen, Loewenstein, 1974; Azarnia, and Loewenstein, 1977; Loewenstein 1979).

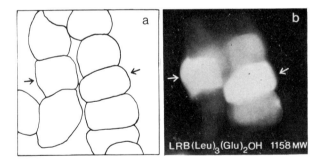

Fig. 2.   Probing the cell-cell channel with a fluorescent-tagged molecule. The linear peptide (Leu)$_3$(Glu)$_2$OH tagged with the red-fluorescent Lissamine rhodamine B is microinjected into a cell (arrow) of a salivary gland. The darkfield photomicrograph shows the cells after the tracer had passed to the adjacent cells. (Reproduced with permission from Simpson, Rose and Loewenstein 1977.)

Another approach, technically simpler, of surveying cell lines with known cancerous properties came up with 7 cancer cell types which are channel-incompetent. Among these are cells from various hepatomas (Borek, Higashino, Loewenstein, 1969; Azarnia, Loewenstein, 1971; Azarnia, Michalke, Loewenstein, 1972), neuroblastomas (Nelson, Peacoc Amano, 1971; Cox, Krauss, Balis, Dancis, 1974), and breast carcinomas (Fentiman, Taylor-Papadimitriou, Stoker, 1976; Fentiman, Taylor-Papadimitriou, 1977). All of these types seem fully channel-incompetent. Besides, 8 other cancerous cell types were found in which the channels are present but the bore or the number of the channels is abnormally small or the rate of channel formation abnormally slow (Azarnia, Loewenstein, 1976; Corsaro, Migeon, 1977).

Evidently, channel defects are not infrequent among neoplastic tissues. The latest tally, done 4 months ago, gave 32 different channel-incompetent cancer cells; there are undoubtedly more. However, the crucial question is whether the channel- and the growth defects are genetically linked. In the absence of knowledge of the identity of the growth-controlling molecules, the demonstration of such a linkage is, for the moment, the only way to obtain reasonable assurance that one is not chasing an epiphenomenon. The problem in the membrane-oriented cancer field has not been to find abnormalities; search parties for membrane defects among cancer tissues have rarely come empty-handed. The problem has been whether the defects are causally related to the cancerous state.

For an analysis of the question of a genetic linkage between the channel and growth defects, Azarnia and I made hybrids between channel competent and channel-incompetent cells. Channel-competence turned out to be a dominant trait. Thus, cell hybrids with unstable chromosome constitution, for instance, the human/mouse combination, provided a suitable tool for the analysis. In the hybrids we produced, the early generations with the nearly complete chromosome complement of both parents were channel-competent; and this correction of the communication phenotype went hand in hand with correction of the growth phenotype (Azarnia, Loewenstein, 1973, 1977). Upon chromosome loss, in unstable hybrids, many phenotypic traits segregated from each other, but channel competence never segregated from growth contro competence, nor did the opposite traits segregate from each other (Azarnia, Loewenstein, 1977).

I shall give, as an example, the results obtained with a human/mouse cell hybrid. Here the channel-competent (and growth-control competent) parent cell was a human fibroblast and the incompetent parent counterpart, a derivative (Cl-1D) of a mouse L cell. The experimental criteria for channel competence were cell-cell transmission of electrolytes (electrical coupling) and fluorescent tracer molecules, and the presence of gap-junctional intramembranous particles as seen in freeze-fracture electron microscopy. The criteria for growth control competence were density dependence of cellular growth in vitro (for the parent and all hybrid cells) and tumorigenicity in immuno-suppressed mice (parent cells and relatively stable hybrids). Both parent cells were genetically marked by enzyme defects, facilitating hybrid selection; and the rate of human chromosome loss was adequate for segregant analysis (Azarnia, Loewenstein, 1977).

The hybrid cells were channel-competent and growth-control competent so long as they had the sufficient chromosome complement of the human

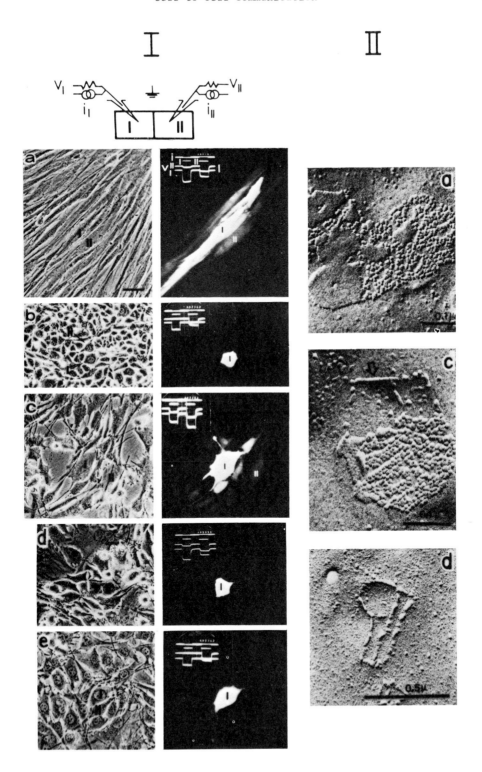

Fig. 3.　　Hybrids between a channel-competent and a channel-incompetent cell.　Column I:　Channel competence as tested by measurement of electrical coupling and fluorescein cell-cell transfer.　Top:　Electrode arrangement.　Current $(i = 2.5 \times 10^9$ A. inward) is injected into cell 1 and with a 100 msec delay, into cell II: the resulting changes in membrane potential (V) are measured in the two cells.　The microelectrodes, connected to balanced bridge circuits, pass i and record V.　Fluorescein is injected (iontophoresis) into cell I.　To left, photomicrographs of the cells in phase contrast; to right, in darkfield, showing fluorescein spread 5-10 min after injection (calibration 50 μm); insets, oscilloscope records of i and V, calibration 100 mV.　(a) The channel-competent (human) parent cell, electrical-coupling and fluorescein-transfer positive. (b) The channel-incompetent (mouse) parent cell.　(c) Early generation hybrid, channel competent.　(d) Intermediate hybrid with partial channel competence, electrical coupling positive and fluorescein transfer negative.　(e) Segregant hybrid, reverted to channel incompetence.　(Reproduced with permission from Azarnia , Loewenstein 1977.)　Column II: Junctional structure.　Freeze-fracture electronmicrographs of junction of (a) the channel-competent parent cell, showing the typical intramembranous particle aggregates of gap junction:　(c) early generation channel-competent hybrid, with gap junction and fibrillar junctional structure, of same clone as test cells in column I (c):　(d) fibrillar junctional structure, such as presented by intermediate hybrid with partial channel competence. (Reprinted with permission from Larsen, Azarnia, and Loewenstein 1977.)

parent.　As the hybrid generations lost human chromosomes, some of the hybrid clones switched to channel incompetence and this was invariably paralleled by a switch to growth control incompetence.　A total of 41 hybrid clones were analyzed (26 clones, see Azarnia, Loewenstein, 1977; plus 15 additional ones reported here).　There was segregation of several biochemical and morphological traits.　Yet in no instance did channel competence segregate from controlled growth or, in the revertants, channel incompetence from uncontrolled growth-- a nice and satisfying agreement with the hypothesis.　The analyses of two other hybrid systems gave equally good correlations.

We have now tried to identify the chromosomes that carry the genes for channel formation.　A series of 10 segregant clones from the above hybrid system, with high human chromosome complement, proved useful here.　Among these were 6 clones that had reverted to the channel-incompetent phenotype upon loss of only 3-7 identified human autosomes (identified by chromosome banding techniques).　The one autosome whose absence consistently correlated with the absence of channel-incompetence is the human chromosome 11.　This chromosome appears to carry genes necessary for the formation of the cell-to-cell channel.　However, this is not to say that it is the only carrier of such genes.　In fact, it would be surprising if all the

genes necessary for such a complex process were on the same chromosome. But it is nevertheless satisfying that the correlation between the incompetencies of channel and growth control in this hybrid
system narrows down to the level of the single chromosome.

Azarnia, R., and W.R. Loewenstein (1971). Intercellular communica-
    tion and tissue growth. V. A cancer cell strain that fails to
    make permeable membrane junctions with normal cells.
    J. Membrane Biol.,6, 368-385.
Azarnia, R., W. Michalke, and W.R. Loewenstein,   (1972). Inter-
    cellular communication and tissue growth. VI. Failure of
    exchange of endogenous molecules between cancer cells with
    defective junctions and noncancerous cells. J. Membrane Biol.,
    10, 247-258.
Azarnia, R., and W.R. Loewenstein (1973). Parallel correction of
    cancerous growth and of a genetic defect of cell-to-cell commu-
    nication. Nature, 241, 455-457.
Azarnia, R., W. Larsen, and W.R. Loewenstein (1974). The membrane
    junctions in communicating and non-communicating cells, their
    hybrids and segregants. Proc. Nat. Acad. Sci.,71, 880-884.
Azarnia, R., and W.R. Loewenstein (1976). Intercellular communica-
    tion and tissue growth. VII. A cancer cell strain with retar-
    ded formation of permeable membrane junction and reduced
    exchange of a 330-dalton molecule. J. Membrane Biol.,30, 175-
    186.
Azarnia, R., and W.R. Loewenstein (1977). Intercellular communica-
    tion and tissue growth. VIII. A genetic analysis of junction-
    al communication and cancerous growth. J. Membrane Biol.,34,
    1-37.
Borek, C., S. Higashino, and W.R. Loewenstein (1969). Intercellular
    communication and tissue growth. IV. Conductance of membrane
    junctions of normal and cancerous cells in culture. J. Membrane
    Biol., 1, 274-293.
Corsaro, C.M. and B.R. Migeon (1977). Comparison of contact-mediated
    communication in normal and transformed human cells in culture.
    Proc. Nat. Acad. Sci., 74, 4476-4480.
Cox, R.P., M.J. Krauss, M.E. Balis, and J. Dancis (1974). Metabolic
    cooperation in cell culture: Studies of the mechanism of cell
    interaction. J. Cell Physiol., 84, 237.
Fentiman, I.S., J. Taylor-Papadimitriou, and M. Stoker (1976). Selec-
    tive contact-dependent cell communication. Nature., 264, 760-
    762.
Fentiman, I.S., and J. Taylor-Papadimitriou (1977). Cultured human
    breast cancer cells lose selectivity in direct intercellular
    communication. Nature., 269, 156-157.
Flagg-Newton, J., I. Simpson, and W.R. Loewenstein (1978). The
    molecular size limit for permeation of the cell-to-cell membrane
    channels in mammalian cell junction. Science., (in press).
Loewenstein, W.R. (1966). Permeability of membrane junctions.Conf.
    on Biol. Membranes:Recent Prog. Ann. N.Y. Acad. Sci., 137, 441-
    472.
Loewenstein, W.R. (1968a). Some reflections on growth and differen-
    tiation. Perspectives in Biol. & Med. 11, 260-272.
Loewenstein, W.R. (1968b). Communication through cell junctions.
    Implications in growth control and differentiation. Devel. Biol.,
    19, (Sup. 2) 151-183.

Loewenstein, W.R. (1974). Cellular communication by permeable junctions. In Cell Membranes: Biochemistry, Cell Biology and Pathology. G. Weissmann and R. Claiborne (Eds.) H.P. Publishing Co. Inc., New York. pp. 105-114.

Loewenstein, W.R. (1975). Permeable junctions. Cold Spring Harbor Symp. Quant. Biol., 40, 49-63.

Loewenstein, W.R. (1979). Junctional intercellular communication and the control of growth. Biochim. Biophys. Acta. Reviews on Cancer., Vol. 560, 1-66.

Nelson, P.G., J.H. Peacock, and T. Amano (1971). Responses of neuroblastoma cells to iontophoretically applied acetylcholine. J. Cell Physiol., 77, 353-362.

Potter, D.D., E.J. Furshpan, and E.S. Lennox (1966). Connections between cells of the developing squid as revealed by electrophysiological methods. Proc. Nat. Acad. Sci., 55, 328.

Sheridan, J.D. (1968). Electrophysiological evidence for low-resistance intercellular junctions in the early chick embryo. J. Cell Biol., 37, 650-659.

Simpson, I., B. Rose, and W.R. Loewenstein (1977). Size limit of molecules permeating the junctional membrane channels. Science., 195, 294-296.

Specificity of Communication

M. G. P. Stoker, I. S. Fentiman and J. Taylor-Papadimitriou

Imperial Cancer Research Fund Laboratories, Lincoln's Inn Fields, London

ABSTRACT

Evidence for tissue specificity of communication came from investigations on metabolic coupling with cultured human mammary epithelial cells. From transfer of
nucleotides it was found that normal mammary epithelial cells from various sources
were able to couple freely with other mammary epithelial cells but not with mammary
fibroblasts or fibroblasts from other sources. Conversely mammary fibroblasts,
which couple with each other, did not couple with mammary epithelial cells.
Abnormal epithelial cells from all human mammary cancers examined, whether primary
cultures or cell lines, fell into two classes, non communicators which coupled with
no other cell, and non selective communicators which coupled with epithelial cells
and fibroblasts. Thus cancer may cause an alteration in the coupling specificity of
normal cells, and a change in their territorial integrity.

Cell specific communication
Coupling
Metabolic cooperation
Mammary epithelium
Mammary cancer

As already outlined in the accompanying paper (Loewenstein, 1978) direct communication between adjoining cells has been demonstrated by electrical coupling, by
transfer of dyes, and by metabolic coupling, i.e. transfer of metabolic precursors,
such as nucleotides, from cell to cell. With the exception of calcium (Rose and
Loewenstein, 1975), most molecules less than about 1,200 daltons in size can
probably travel freely from cell to cell through gap junctions. Experimental studies
with cultured cells show that the exchanges may be functional, and allow for correction of a mutant phenotype, but the natural role of such communication is unknown.

Up till recently cells examined by several methods were found to communicate freely
and reciprocally, not only with the same type, but other cell types, even from
different species (Stoker, 1967; Miehalke and Loewenstein, 1971). The only exceptions
are L cells, which lack gap junctions and are unable to couple either with other L
cells or other cell types, and cells in certain tumours *in vivo* and in culture, such
as hepatomas, which have been shown to lack electrical coupling (Gilula, Reaves and
Steinbach, 1972; Borek, Higachino and Loewenstein, 1969). On the other hand normal

and virus transformed fibroblasts, with widely differing tumourigenicity, communicate equally well (da Silva and Gilula, 1972).

Specificity of coupling was first observed in our laboratory while studying cultur
human mammary epithelial cells and stromal cells (Fentiman, Taylor-Papadimitriou a
Stoker, 1976). Concurrently Pitts and Bürk observed coupling specificity with a
hepatoma and a fibroblastic cell line (Pitts and Bürk, 1976).

Pure cultures of epithelial cells from the human mammary gland can be obtained fror
lacteal secretions, from normal breast tissue removed for cosmetic reasons, and fr
mammary tumours. Benign human tumours yield epithelium more or less indistinguishable on morphological and other grounds from normal epithelium. These apparently
normal human epithelial cells are designated Hum E cells. Malignant tumours yield
both Hum E cells and apparently abnormal poorly growing epithelium, designated
Hum E[1] cells, which may comprise the cancer cells (Hallowes, Millis, Piggott,
Shearer, Stoker and Taylor-Papadimitriou, 1977). Fibroblastic stromal cells can
also be obtained in pure culture from normal or tumour bearing breasts. The
separation and culture methods have been described elsewhere (Hallowes, Millis,
Piggott, Shearer, Stoker and Taylor-Papadimitriou, 1977).

In preliminary experiments, compact islands of Hum E cells from fibroadenomas were
grown on the surface of dishes. It is characteristic of such cells that they
remain attached to one another and do not emigrate from the edge of the islands.
Cells of a line of transformed hamster embryo fibroblasts (TG1 Cells) lacking
hypozanthine guanine phosphoribosyl transferase were added to the cultures at a
density sufficient to make contact with the epithelial cells. The TG1 cells cannot
incorporate ^{3}H hypoxanthine into nucleic acids and it was expected that this defect
would be corrected by metabolic co-operation through contact with the normal
epithelial cells and be recorded by autoradiography. Although TG1 cells show
metabolic co-operation with fibroblasts from many sources our experiments showed
no evidence of co-operation by transfer of nucleotides from the mammary epithelial
cells to the mutant fibroblasts.

In further experiments, to avoid the restriction of using mutants, we used the
method described by Pitts and Sims (1977), in which putative donor cells are exposed
to ^{3}H uridine, allowing the accumulation of labelled nucleotide pools for a period
of a few hours before incorporation into RNA. After washing to remove extracellular
nucleoside, unlabelled recipient cells were added and allowed to make contact for
periods of up to 14 hours before autoradiography. If coupling occurs under these
conditions the labelled nucleotide is transferred from the donor to adjoining
recipient cells, where it is incorporated into nucleic acid and may be detected by
autoradiography. The donors are easily identified by their heavy labelling.
Communication is demonstrated by a higher grain count in recipient cells touching a
donor compared to the more distant cells not touching a donor. Using this versatile
method we were able to test a variety of pairs of like and unlike cells. Most of
them were tested reciprocally by alternating donors and recipients, but the slow
attachment of freshly isolated epithelial cells sometimes prevented this.

Figure 1 shows the ability of human mammary epithelial cells from a fibroadenoma to
transfer nucleotide by coupling to various other cells. It will be seen that there
is no coupling to fibroblasts but there is transfer to homologous cells and to
another epithelial cell, i.e. bovine lens, and poorer transfer to an epithelial line
from liver.

Hum E cells from other sources (breast parenchyma, milk, and normal looking
epithelium from carcinomas) all failed to couple with other fibroblastic cells,
including stromal cells from the normal breast, but all coupled with lens, and in
limited tests with each other but not with Hum F cells.

Surprisingly lens epithelium which was included as an easily cultured control
behaved differently and communicated with all fibroblasts as well as all other
epithelium. The rat liver cell line in our laboratory coupled, though poorly, with
fibroblasts, but another line studied by Pitts and Bürk was reported to show selectivity and to be deficient on coupling with fibroblasts (Pitts and Bürk, 1976).

Lack of coupling might be due to failure of the cells to make contact because of a
barrier. There is in fact a strong tendency to compartmentation between epithelium
and fibroblasts (Stoker, Piggott and Riddle, 1978). Electronmicrographs (by
R. Newman) of the boundary region however show extensive regions to close contact
between epithelial cells and fibroblasts (about 10nm). Gap junctions have not so
far been found but sampling has been small. Whether the cell apposition is stable
enough for gap junctions to be formed is not known but it is clear that there is
not a continuous barrier or major gap between the fibroblasts and the epithelial
cells.

Thus the normal freshly isolated cells in culture show three classes of coupling:
1.   Selective epithelial communication;
2.   Selective fibroblast communication; and
3.   General (non-selective) communication.
The first two only communicate with their own class.

Several reviewers have discussed the possible role of cell coupling in general in
terms of transfer of signal molecules and modulation of control systems. We do not
know if the lack of communication between the cell types described here is absolute
or, as suggested by Pitts and Bürk (1976), is simply less efficient and is delayed,
though it may be noted that in our experiments with mutant fibroblasts, coupling
still failed after 24 hours in contact. Whichever is the case it indicates that
compartmentation exists between main classes of cells in the intact organism and
that direct transfer of certain molecules between these classes is forbidden, or
severely limited. This might be necessary because of incompatability of their
control systems.

Experiments with Cancer Cells

Further studies, by Fentiman and Taylor-Papadimitriou (1977), were carried out on
mammary carcinoma cells using the uridine method. First some mammary carcinoma cell
lines originally isolated from tumour metastases in various laboratories were
examined. Some, as predicted from the studies of Loewenstein, failed to couple with
any other cell tested, thus resembling L cells and hepatoma cell lines. But other
carcinoma cell lines showed an opposite pattern, and like lens cells coupled with
all others except non-communicators.

Next freshly isolated cultures of epithelium from cancers were tested. As already
indicated primary mammary cancers yield both normal looking epithelium (Hum E) and
colonies of morphologically different cells (Hum E[1]) which are more difficult to
grow and which may be the malignant cells. The Hum E cells from the carcinomas
showed selective communication like epithelium from benign tumours and normal breast
and failed to couple with fibroblasts. However the Hum E[1], putative carcinoma, cells,
like the cancer cell lines, showed a different behaviour. Some were non-
communicators, and others were general communicators like lens cells. Table 1 lists
the cell cultures tested so far and shows the type of communication which was found.
In the small series tested there was no correlation between communication pattern
and behaviour in culture, or in clinical character, or pathology of the carcinoma.

If the abnormal cells are indeed cancer cells derived from normal epithelium with
selective communication, then the neoplastic change involves a substantial alteration in ability to communicate with other cells. Lack of ability to communicate

with homologous cells could be related to abnormal behaviour through inability to receive signalling molecules, as suggested by Loewenstein (1966). On the other hand loss of coupling specificity could also result in abnormal behaviour because, in addition to normal signals from homologous cells, ectopic abnormal control signals, which are normally forbidden by the specificity of coupling, might be received from neighbouring heterologous cells. If this were so one might expect some difference in the behaviour of cancers of the two classes, and we must stress that none have so far been identified. We should also point out that non-selective communicators have only been found amongst a selected group of mammary cancers, from which cells could be cultured. More tumour types should clearly be examined, particularly by the metabolic co-operation method, which lends itself more easily to tests for coupling specificity than ionic coupling or transfer of dyes.

The molecular basis for the specificity and its loss is a matter only for speculation. Are the gap junction determinants on fibroblasts different to those on epithelial cells? Or is the interaction or lack of it due to other cell surface determinants, which affect the ability of the surfaces to approximate, thus allowing gap junctions to develop? Are non-communicating cancer cells unable to synthesise gap junction constituents or are they simply insufficiently adhesive even to homologous cells? Are the non-selective communicators (some carcinomas and lens cells) able to make both fibroblastic and epithelial type gap junctions or do they just adhere efficiently? All we can say at present is that the specificity of coupling adds another dimension to this interesting phenomenon.

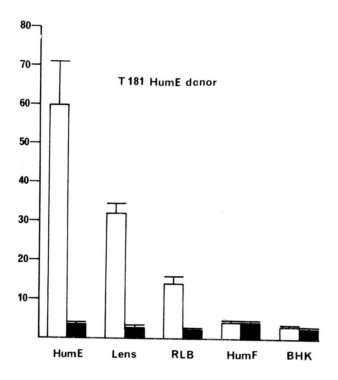

Fig. 1

Legend to Fig. 1

Metabolic co-operation between mammary epithelial cells, as donors and various recipients.

T181 Hum E: primary culture epithelial cells from fibroadenoma. Lens: bovine, primary culture. RLB: rat liver cell line. Hum F: human mammary fibroblasts, secondary culture. BHK hamster fibroblast cell line. Figures give mean grain counts with standard error per touching (open column) and non-touching (closed column) recipient cells.

Secondary cultures of epithelial cells from a fibroadenoma were prepared as previously described (Fentiman, Taylor-Papadimitriou and Stoker, 1976), 3×10^3 cells being inoculated into a 35 mm dish in medium 199 containing foetal calf serum (15%) insulin (10 µg/ml) and hydrocortisone (5 µg/ml). After incubation overnight, 2 µ£i of 5 - ^{3}H uridine (48 µCi/m mol) was added to each dish to label the donor cells. Three hours later, medium was removed and the cells washed three times before adding 2×10^5 recipient cells. The mixed cultures were fixed 3 hours later and processed for autoradiography. In each experiment 5 replicate dishes were used and experiments were repeated 3 times so that the results represented above were derived from the mean grain counts over 150 touching and 150 non-touching recipients.

TABLE 1 A Selective Communications

Primary Cultures

Hum E	Epithelium	Human breast tissue	
"	"	"	milk
"	"	"	benign breast tumour
"	"	"	(breast carcinoma)
Hum F	Fibroblast	"	breast tissue
"	"	"	benign breast tumour
"	"	"	(breast carcinoma)
"	"	"	foetal lung - passaged

Cell Lines

RL	Epithelium	Rat	liver
3T3	Fibroblast	Mouse	embryo
BHK 21	"	Hamster	kidney
Nil B	"	"	"

B Non Communicators

Primary Cultures

Hum E[1] T231	Epithelium	Human breast carcinoma	
" T595	"	"	"	"
" T629	"	"	"	"
Foam cells	Macrophages	Human milk	

Cell lines

MCF 7	Epithelium	Human breast carcinoma metastasis
Sk Br 3	"	" " " "
Cama 1	"	" " " "
Br 20	"	" " " "
L929	Fibroblasts	Mouse embryo

C General (Non Selective) Communicators

Primary Cultures

Hum E[1] T162	Epithelium	Human breast carcinoma
" T235	"	" " "
Lens	"	Bovine lens

Cell lines

HSO 578 T	"	Human breast carcinoma metastasis
MDA 157	"	" " " "
" 231	"	" " " "
Colo	"	Human skin metastasis

REFERENCES

Borek, C., S. Higachino and W.R. Loewenstein (1969). J. Membrane Biol., 1, 274-293

Fentiman, I.S., J. Taylor-Papadimitriou and M.G.P. Stoker (1976). Nature, 264, 760-762.

Fentiman, I.S. and J. Taylor-Papadimitriou (1977). Nature, 269, 156-158.

Gilula, N.B., O.R. Reeves and A. Steinbach (1972). Nature, 235, 262-265.

Hallowes, R.C., R. Millis, D. Piggott, M. Shearer, M.G.P. Stoker and J. Taylor-Papadimitriou (1977). J. Clinical Oncology, 3, 81-90.

Loewenstein, W.R. and Y. Kanno (1966). Nature, 209, 1248-1249.

Loewenstein, W.R. (1978) (accompanying paper).

Miehalke, W. and W.R. Loewenstein (1971). Nature, 232, 121-122.

Pinto da Silva, P. and N.B. Gilula (1972). Exp. Cell. Res., 71, 393-401.

Pitts, J.D. and R.R. Bürk (1976). Nature, 264, 762-764.

Pitts, J.D. and J.W. Simms (1977). Expl. Cell Res., 104, 153.

Rose, B. and W.R. Loewenstein (1975). Nature, 254, 250-252.

Stoker, M.G.P. (1967). J. Cell. Sci., 2, 293-304.

Stoker, M.G.P., D. Piggott and P. Riddle (1978). Int. J. Cancer, 21, 268-273.

The Cell Surface and Metastasis

M. M. Burger[1], J. Finne, A. Matter[2], K. Vosbeck, K. Tullberg, C. Haškovec, B. M. Jockusch and T. W. Tao

Department of Biochemistry, Biocenter, University of Basel, Klingelbergstrasse 70, 4056 Basel, Switzerland

ABSTRACT

After a brief survey of consecutive processes in metastasis, an experimental model for testing organ selectivity is discussed. Then an experimental model for testing membrane alterations in metastasis is presented: from a metastasizing mouse melanoma a variant cell line could be selected with a specific alteration in the carbohydrate structure at the cell surface. This cell line, although tumorigenic, does not metastasize. Some biological behavior, presumably relevant for metastasis and the surface biochemistry of the two related cell lines, were compared and some differences were found.

1. INTRODUCTION

The spread of tumor cells in the host is a cascading process. The transition from one site to another involves doubtlessly several different steps, the detailed numbers and the character of which are largely unknown.

While in the last few years many efforts were spent on correlating biochemical changes in the cell surface with the transformed state of the cell, almost nothing is known about the cell surface of the metastasizing cells. One of the important handicaps in the field was until recently the absence of valid experimental model systems where biochemical aspects of the cell surface for the metastasizing process could be studied. Possible consecutive stages of the metastasizing process can be analyzed as follows: (For other or similar views see Fidler, as well as Weiss in Weiss, 1976.)

1.1. Establishment of a Connection to a Disseminative Conveyer.

This includes the infiltration of surrounding tissues and penetration into vascular and lymph systems as well as body cavities. Alternatively the vascular system may enter the primary tumor (angiogenesis fac-

---

This project was supported by a grant from the Swiss National Research Foundation.

[2] F. Hoffmann-La Roche & Co., Basel, Switzerland

tor) and provide easy access to the blood system due to the lack of
a properly developed endothelium (Salsbury and others, 1974).

1.2. Release and Dissemination.

Here as well as in the foregoing process, hydrolases (Sylvén, 1968)
from proteases to mucopolysaccharidases may play an important role,
be they from necrotic or from actively growing secretory zones. Mechanical pressure, due to growth and pushing into weak tissue zones,
as well as poor cohesion among the tumor cells may facilitate their
entrance into vessels and body cavities and also the release of tumor
cells from the primary tumor. Necrotic zones may directly influence
the release of tissue fragments (Weiss, 1977).

1.3. Adhesion in the Periphery and Survival.

Despite the deformability of tumor cells (Zeidman, 1961), they can be
trapped in thin-walled veins and the capillary network. Specific adhesion may play a role in organ distribution seen for some tumor cell
but i.v. injected cells usually are arrested in the first organ where
they encounter a microcirculation bed (Roos and others, 1977,and personal observations). Thrombocytes and clotting may promote adhesion t-
endothelial cells, removing the tumor cells from the well established
killing effect of continous circulation. Platelets may even contribute growth factors, so far known to promote growth of smooth muscle
from vessel walls.

1.4. Infiltration at the Secondary Site.

Passage between or directly through endothelial cells as well as into
the surrounding tissue may not only depend on the capability of the
tumor cells to deform and to migrate, but also on the adhesiveness to
the host tissues on one hand or the secretion of lytic enzymes on the
other hand. Although cells with a high infiltrative capability may
have been selected already before they were released at the primary
site, anatomical or biochemical differences in the target organ contribute additionally to a successful infiltration and lodging of the
particular tumor cell.

1.5. Survival and Proliferation at the Secondary Site.

The distribution of tumor metastases in various organs following intra
arterial injection of the tumor cells does not follow that of blood
supply, as reflected by intra-arterial injection of radio-labelled
microspheres (personal observation). This may not only be due to differences in mechanical and adhesive properties, but also to differences in survival conditions and growth stimuli in the various organs in which the tumor cells lodge. Immunological defense, specific
or unspecific, may be expressed to a different extent in different
tissues and organs. Similarly the increasing number of growth factors
isolated recently may be produced or reach the tumor cell to a different extent in different organs.

In summary, a fine dissection of hypothetical processes and steps in
metastasis will reveal, based on the recent state of art in modern
pathology and cell biology, a multitude of interesting potential
mechanisms. We need experimental models, where pathobiological and
molecular hypotheses can be tested.

2. AN EXPERIMENTAL MODEL FOR TESTING ORGAN SELECTIVITY.

Clinically it is well known that several tumors have distinct prefe-
rences to metastasize into certain organs, which cannot be explained
by the existing knowledge of the circulatory system.

Intravenous injection of tumor cells will usually lead to lodging of
the cells, as well as the formation of tumor nodules in the lungs.
Such cells can, however, only be considered as lung-specific if the
same happens following other routes of injection, such as through
the portal system. In order to select a liver-specific tumor line we
injected melanoma cells (B16, from Dr. I. J. Fidler) into the portal
circulation system of C57/Bl-6 mice and reinjected the cells from
the tumors in the liver after passage through cell culture into the
portal system. After 8 such cycles the mother cell line, as well as
the selected cell lines, were injected i.v. The original melanoma
line gave rise almost exclusively to lung tumors and only two out of
50 animals had liver nodules, while the liver selected line produced
tumors in the liver as well as in the lungs.

A similar approach has been reported this year for a brain-colonizing
melanoma (Brunson and others, 1977).

To remove the complicating factor of "sieving" through the pulmonary
capillary network, the cells were injected through a carotid cannula
into the left ventricle. Tumors were then found in almost all the
organs except the kidneys and the spleen. In the case of the liver-
selected tumor cell line, at least 10 times more tumor nodules were
found in the liver as compared to the parent cell line.

Simultaneous intraventricular injection of isotopically labelled
(^{113}tin) Sephadex microspheres (15 μ diameter) showed that a great
number of the microspheres were found in the kidneys where, however,
no tumors could be found. Both lungs and liver had about the same
amount of microspheres, although livers had 20 to 200 times more tumor
nodules than the lungs. A careful comparison of biochemical and biological alterations between the organ selective cell line and its
parent cell line should lead to new concepts about the tendency of
malignant tumors to metastasize to specific organs.

3. AN EXPERIMENTAL MODEL FOR TESTING MEMBRANE ALTERATIONS IN METASTASIS.

Variant or mutant cell lines, which are more tumorigenic and possibly
also more metastasizing, have been selected by injecting melanoma
cells into the tail vein and passing the resulting lung tumors after
an in vitro passage back into the tail vein of the next animal
(Fidler, 1973). So far no relevant biochemical surface changes could
be found this way by Nicolson and others (1977). We decided therefore
to tackle the problem from the other side, namely by selecting cell
surface variants first (Fig.1) and then only testing the ensuing
cloned cell lines for their capability not only to give rise to
tumors by i.v. injection, but also their capability to metastasize
after i.p. administration (Tao and Burger, 1977).

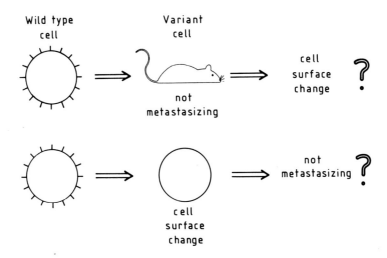

Fig. 1. Two different approaches to a search for
correlations between alterations in metastasizing
potential and cell surface alterations.

As selective agents we chose lectins, i.e. plant proteins, which are
known to bind to specific cell surface carbohydrates and were cloned
(Fig.2).

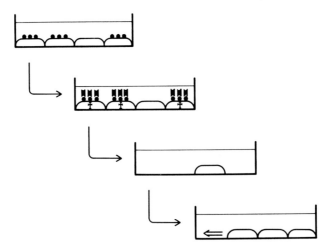

Fig.2. Approach to select a cell line with surface alterations in Petri dishes. In this case
cells were isolated which were resistant to killing by multivalent lectin.

Such a stable melanoma cell line, which was resistant to the lectin
from wheat germ (= wheat germ agglutinin, WGA) was tested for its
WGA binding capability and found to bind less of the lectin with respect to high affinity binding sites, as shown in Fig. 3.

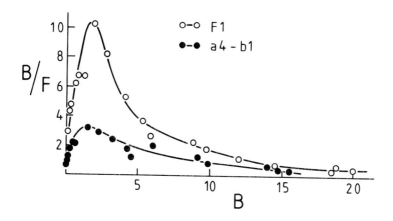

Fig.3. Binding curves (Scatchard plot) of ^{125}I-
labelled WGA to metastatic (F-1) and non-metastatic WGA-resistant daugther cells (a4-b1). On the
abscissa bound (B) and on the ordinate bound versus free (B/F) WGA are shown. In the low concentration range (high affinity sites) the metastatic
cells bind considerably more lectin. In the high
concentration range only minor differences could
be observed in the absence of serum. The increase
in B/F at the low concentrations followed by a
maximum suggests cooperative phenomena (Haškovec,
Tao and Burger, to be published).

Table 1 illustrates that the metastasizing capability of WGA resistant cells (Wa4-bl) dropped to 0 (even if longer testing times were
chosen). On the other hand the capability of these cells to give
rise to primary tumors after i.v. or i.p. administration decreased
much less. While a link between the degree of metastasizing and tumorigenicity cannot be ruled out strictly, we do not believe in a
causal coupling since i.p. injection of even large doses of the variant cells did not lead to any spread into other organs (e.g.lung).

Several other lectin resistant cells were also isolated (Table 1).
WGA-resistance (Wa4-bl) so far always led to a lower metastasizing
potential. Concanavalin A resistance (C5) so far never resulted in
lower metastasizing and Ricin (R4c-al) gave intermediate results.
Reversion of the low metastatic phenotype of WGA resistant cells
could be observed by passage in vivo (W-181) as well as by a second
round of in vitro selection with Concanavalin A (Wa4-bl-Cod).

M. M. Burger *et al.*

Table 1. Metastasizing Capacity and Tumorigenicity
of Melanoma Variants.

Cell Line	Lectin	Metastasizing Capacity	Tumorigenicity
F-1	-	$48/50$	$50/50$
Wa4-bl	WGA	$0/16$	$23/32$
W 181	WGA and then in vivo	$8/8$	$8/8$
Wa4-bl-Cod	WGA and then Con A	$8/8$	$12/12$
C5	Con A	$5/6$	$6/6$
R4c-a	Ricin	$11/26$	$7/12$

In the first column the lectins used to select the
particular cell line from the parent B16 melanoma
cell line (F-1) are indicated. W-181 was obtained
from the tumor in the animal following the injection of Wa4-bl cells.

Wa4-bl-Cod is a cell line derived from Wa4-bl after
selection for resistance to Concanavalin A in vitro.
In the second column the number of animals were scored which had tumors in mediastinal and mesenteric
lymph nodes or in other organs two to three weeks
after i.p. administration of 5×10^4 cells.

In the third column tumorigenicity is reported as
the number of animals showing tumors per total number of animals tested 2 to 3 weeks after injection
of 2×10^5 cells into the tail vein (see also Tao and
Burger, 1977).

Some properties were studied which could contribute to a lower metastasizing potential. Cell shape (Folkman and Moscona, 1978) and cell
tension (Curtis and Seehar, 1978) may not only influence growth control but also reflect or influence the deformability of a cell, a property most likely to contribute to the successful invasiveness and
implantation of a tumor cell. To what degree the extent and the structural stability of the cytoskeleton contribute to cell deformability
is not known, but we counted the cells which displayed broad cables
with monospecific anti-actin antibodies in the fluorescence microscope. Cables seem to develop primarily in cells with a decreased capability to metastasize (Table 2).

Table 2. Some Biological Properties of the Parent
Melanoma Cell Line and its Lectin Resistant
Variants and Revertants

Cell Line	Cables	Adhesion Homotypic	Adhesion Endothelial Cells	Cell Color (%Melanin) ("Release")
F-1	<7%	1	1	black (40)
Wa4-bl	>50%	1.6	1	white (78%)
W 181	<7%	-	-	black
Wa4-bl-Cod	<7%	1.1	-	black
C5	-	-	-	white
R4c-a	>40%	0.9	-	black

Under the heading "cables" the percentage of cells
is reported which had well expressed microfilament
bundles as seen in the fluorescence microscope after
staining with monospecific anti-actin antibodies
(B.M.Jockusch). Homotypic adhesion (K.Vosbeck and
J.Jenkins) as well as the preliminary results with
heterotypic endothelial adhesion (K.Tullberg) are
recorded in relative values, compared with the metastatic parent cell line (F-1). In the last column
the degree of pigmentation of the particular line
is indicated although the melanotic and amelanotic
states cannot be correlated rigorously with the degree of metastasis.

Increased adhesion of the tumor cells to themselves might decrease the
likelihood of invasiveness or release of cells into the blood stream.
For the WGA-resistant, non-metastasizing cells such an increase could
indeed be observed with the so-called single cell disappearance as
well as the monolayer adhesion assays (Table 2).

Preliminary data show that the adhesion to human umbilical cord endothelial cell monolayers did not differ significantly from the metastasizing parent cell line however (Table 2).

Rejection due to alterations in histocompatibility antigens is un-
likely since the same differences in metastasizing patterns between
F-1 cells and Wa4-bl cells were found in nude mice as in normal C57/
Bl mice.

All altered properties so far mentioned may be connected with membrane alterations including the actin cables, which are thought to be
anchored in the plasma membrane. A search for molecular alterations
in the cell surface of the WGA-resistant line was therefore initiated.
WGA-binding differences (Fig.3) were described. Labeling of the pro-

protein portions as well as labeling of sialic acid and galactose i:
cell surface glycoproteins revealed that at least 5 bands had slight
lower molecular weights and reduced labeling of the carbohydrate portion (Fig. 4).

1 2 3 4 5 6

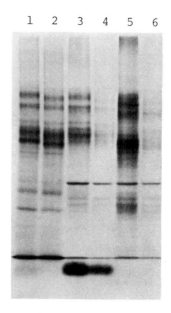

Fig.4. SDS-Polyacrylamide gel electrophoretic analysis of the surface glycoprotein alterations in
the non-metastasizing WGA-resistant cell line. Cells
for column 1 and 2 were treated with ^{125}I and lactoperoxidase, thereby labeling the protein portion
of surface glycoproteins. Cells for column 3 and 4
were treated with periodate and NaB^3H_4 (sialic acid-
labeling). Cells for column 5 and 6 were treated
with sialidase, galactose oxidase and NaB^3H_4 (ga-
lactose-labeling). Metastasizing parent cells were
used for columns 1, 3 and 5, and non-metastasizing
cells in columns 2, 4 and 6 (data from Finne, Tao
and Burger).

These results are consistent with our preliminary oligosaccharide analysis of glycoproteins which pinpoints the alteration to the loss of
only a few terminal sialic acids in some specific carbohydrate units.
The lost sialic acid residues seem to be accompanied by an increase
in fucose substituents on N-acetyl-glucosamine.

The functional significance of such a minor and very specific surface
carbohydrate change for the cell's behavior <u>in vitro</u> and particularly for the loss of metastasizing potential of this tumor cell will
have to be established and may provide us with a clue as to one of
the presumably many mechanisms for metastasis.

REFERENCES.

Brunson, K.W., G. Beattie, and G.L. Nicolson (1977). In vivo selection of malignant melanoma for organ preference of experimental metastasis. J. Cell Biol. 75, 209a.

Curtis, A.S.G., and G.M. Seehar (1978). The control of cell division by tension or diffusion. Nature, 274, 52-53.

Fidler, I.J. (1973). Selection of successive tumour lines for metastasis. Nature New Biology, 242, 148-149.

Fidler, I.J. (1976). Patterns of tumor cell arrest and development. In L. Weiss (Ed.), Fundamental Aspects of Metastasis, North Holland, Amsterdam, p.p. 275-289.

Folkman, J., and A. Moscona (1978). Role of cell shape in growth control. Nature, 273, 345-349.

Nicolson, G.L., C. R. Birdwell, K.W. Brunson, J. C. Robbins, G. Beattie and I. J. Fidler (1977). Cell interactions in the metastatic process: some cell surface properties associated with successful blood-borne tumor spread. In J. Lash and M.M.Burger (Eds.) Cell and Tissue Interactions, Raven Press, New York, p.p. 225-241.

Roos, E., K. P. Dingemans, I. V. Van der Pavert, and M. A. Van den Bergh-Weerman (1977). Invasion of lymphosarcoma cells into the perfused mouse liver. J. Nat. Cancer Inst., 58, 399-407.

Salsbury, A. J., K. Burrage, and K. Hellman (1974). Histological analysis of the antimetastatic effect of (±)-1,2-Bis(3,5-dioxopiperazin-1yl) propane. Cancer Res., 34, 843-849.

Sylvén, B. (1968). Lysosomal enzyme activity in the interstitial fluid of solid mouse tumour transplants. Eur. J. Cancer, 4, 463-474.

Weiss, L. (1976). Introduction. In L. Weiss (Ed.), Fundamental Aspects of Metastasis, North Holland, Amsterdam, p.p.1-6.

Weiss, L. (1977). Tumor necrosis and cell detachment. Int. J. Cancer 20, 87-92.

Zeidman, I. (1961). The fate of circulating tumor cells. I. Passage of cells through capillaries. Cancer Res., 21, 38-39.

The Relevance and the Effect of Cell Surface Components on Untransformed and Malignant Cells

Livio Mallucci and Valerie Wells

*Department of Microbiology, Guy's Hospital Medical School, London Bridge,
London S.E.1*

ABSTRACT. A protein component of the cell surface (F factor or F protein) is associated with the maintenance of flattened morphology. The F factor is not all immediately exposed at the cell exterior but partly masked by other macromolecular components. These may form a microenvironment where the concentration of the F protein (and other factors) is maintained and regulated during varying physiological conditions. Studies on the relevance of the F factor, which affects cell shape, to cell growth have shown the following:
1) as cells progress through the cell cycle the amount of factor exposed at the cell exterior gradually decreases; 2) untransformed cells seeded and exposed to a fraction containing the F protein are unable to progress through mitosis; 3) transformed cells, which have lower amounts of factor exposed at their surfaces, are either insensitive or sensitive to a lesser degree. A fraction containing LETS protein does not have the same effect.

In previous work we have shown that a protein component of the plasma membrane of cultured mouse embryo fibroblasts has an important function in the determination of cell form as its presence at the surface is associated with flattened cell morphology (Mallucci and Wells, 1976). This protein (M.W. $\simeq 25000$), to which we refer as F (flattening) factor, or F protein, is part of a population of macromolecules loosely bound to the cell. It can be removed from the cell surface, together with other constituents, simply by application of mild shearing forces but it is also spontaneously released into the surrounding environment (medium). Both resting cells and cells passing through S phase undergo a degree of rounding when the loosely bound macromolecular fraction is sheared away and both re-flatten when the factor is either re-synthesised or added back to the cells. In cells undergoing S phase the changes are more marked and they are similar in appearance to those naturally occurring when cells prepare for division. The development of the changes involves a transmembrane co-operation between F factor at the surface, integral macromolecular components of the cytoplasmic membrane and contractile cytoplasmic organelles (Wells and Mallucci, 1978).

We have first considered that if the F protein plays a role in the determination and modulation of cell form under physiological conditions, there should be a means of maintaining and regulating its concentration at the cell surface under varying conditions such as changes of geometry due to cellular motility and convection currents in the medium. This may be achieved by the formation of a microenvironment determined by the macromolecular components (glycoproteins) extending from the cell surface. An appreciation of these structures could be obtained observing under high resolution scanning electron microscopy cells treated with ruthenium red according to the Luft method (Luft, 1971).

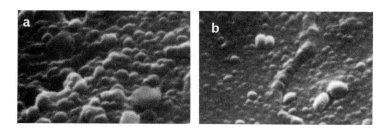

Fig. 1.   Scanning electron micrographs of tertiary mouse embryo fibroblasts after ruthenium red treatment;
a) surface of control cell; b) cell after shearing treatment x 100,000.

We interpret the "cobblestone" appearance seen in fig. 1-a as the visualization, after gold coating, of areas determined by complexes formed by sugar chains whose extension in space has been maintained by continuous bridging with ruthenium red. Figure 1-b shows loss of "cobblestones" under conditions (application of shearing forces) known to remove macromolecular constituents from the cell surface and to induce cell rounding (Mallucci and Wells, 1976). Quantitation of the F factor by means of lactoperoxidase catalyzed iodination (^{125}I), electrophoresis in acrylamide gels and band isolation under the conditions of fig. 1, show that loss of factor follows the removal of the loosely bound surface macromolecules and that an amount of factor greater than that immediately available at the surface becomes accessible to iodination after the surface fraction is sheared away (fig. 2).

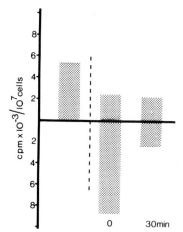

cpm x 10^{-3}/10^7 cells

0   30min

Fig. 2. Quantitation of F factor at the cell surface in band isolate. Histograms above horizontal line represent quantity before shearing (left), and amounts remaining after shearing (right). Histograms below horizontal line represent quantities detectable by labelling after removal of surface macromolecules. Notice loss of label with time.

Thus, although some factor is immediately exposed, greater quantities are hidden by structures of the microenvironment and further released while cells undergo rounding.

Quantitation of the F factor at the cell surface and in the medium (chloramine -T iodination) during and following re-flattening shows an initial accummulation of the F protein at the cell surface ensued by gradual increase in the medium as the re-flattening process undergoes completion (fig. 3). As the protein is thermolabile (half life ≃ 3h) its concentration

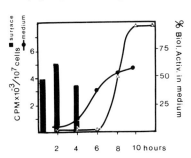

Fig. 3. Quantitation of factor at the cell surface and in the surrounding environment during the re-flattening process. Histograms represent factor at cell surface; ●———● factor in medium; △———△ biological activity.

in the medium may vary considerably during periods of different membrane turnover, and an equilibrium between concentration in the microenvironment and in the more distant environment (medium) may exist. We have found that in the medium of S phase cells concentration of the F factor is lower than in that of confluent quiescent cultures.

Changes of form are an important aspect of cellular physiology as throughout growth and division, cell movement and variations of cell morphology are continuously occurring. Variations in the constitution of the microenvironment could modulate the retention of the F protein (and any other factor) at the cell surface. We have therefore investigated the significance of the F protein in relation to cell replication. First by quantitation of the factor at the cell surface during different stages of the cell cycle, then investigating its effect, if any, on cell division. Table 1 shows progressive decrease in the amount of the factor detectable at the surface of untransformed synchronised mouse embryo fibroblasts (MEF) moving from quiescence to mitosis, while quantitation of a large M.W. protein implicated in cell adhesion (Hynes and others, 1977; Vaheri and Mosher, 1978) did not show a similarly decreasing trend. In our second approach we used a fluorescent activated cell sorter to investigate whether the F protein would affect progression through the cell cycle. When a

TABLE 1   F Factor and LETS Protein at the Cell Surface of
MEF through the Cell Cycle

Surface Protein*	G1	S 17h	22h	S-G2	M
F factor	3,577	2,940	2,472	2,250	1,825
LETS	16,000	18,000	17,500	15,000	15,000

* cpm/5 x 10^6 cells.

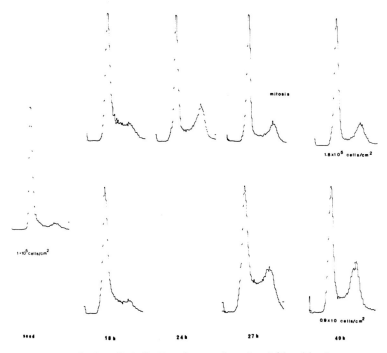

Fig. 4. Population distribution in synchronised fibroblasts progress-
ing through the cell cycle. Left, cells at seed; top, untreated cells;
bottom, cells treated with F protein preparation (fraction of components
between 10,000 and 50,000 MW shed in the absence of serum).

preparation containing the F protein was added to synchronised G-1 cells soon after plating
and at three hourly intervals the factor allowed the cells to reach the G-2 stage but it did
not allow division (fig. 4). At higher concentrations even entry into S phase was prevented.
Addition to cells already in S phase exerted no effect. An examination of cell morphology
revealed that where division had not occurred the cells had maintained a flat and well
spread shape.

TABLE 2   Oncogenic Characteristics and F Factor of Tumour Cells

Cell type	Minimum No. cells produc- ing tumours	% Tumours induced at low- est efficient dose	% Tumours induced by 10^6 cells	F Factor released	F Factor at cell surface
L-57	10^5	40	80	n. d.	12, 376
PV-TT-2	10^3	100	100	3, 000	5, 608
PV-TT-8	10^3	20	100	5, 000	3, 808
MEF	–	–	–	34, 000	15, 476

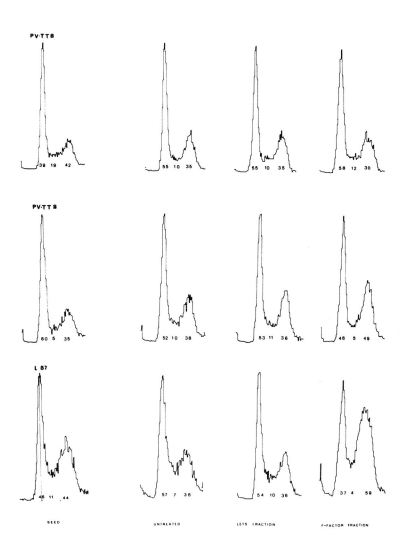

Fig. 5. Population distribution in tumour cells after two division cycles during exposure to F protein preparation (see fig. 4) and LETS preparation (fraction of components above 50,000 MW shed in absence of serum).

Our observations were then extended from untransformed cells to their transformed counterparts. We examined two highly oncogenic polyoma virus-transformed lines (PV-TT-2 and PV-TT-8) and a spontaneously transformed line (L-57) of lower oncogenicity. The data of Table 2 show that only small quantities of factor were detectable at the surface of the PV-transformed cells and that little factor was found in their medium. The value measured in the less tumourogenic line was instead closer to that of the untransformed controls. We do not know whether the low amounts represent poor synthesis or degradation by cell surface associated enzymes present in the tumour cells.

We finally investigated whether the F factor could also exert any effect on the replication of the tumour cells. These were un-synchronised populations and therefore allowed to be exposed for a period corresponding to two division cycles as only the G-1 population, as seen with the untransformed cells (fig. 4), could possibly be affected by the factor. The data of fig. 5 demonstrates that there were no significant changes in the virus-transformed lines but that a shift in the population distribution of the less oncogenic line did occur, with the G-2 peak markedly increased. Accordingly some reduction of cell number ($\approx 20\%$) after the two cycles was also observed. Figure 5 also shows that exposure of the tumour lines to the fraction containing the large M.W. protein implicated in cell adhesion exerted no effect on any of them.

The conclusion we derive from our studies is that the surface membrane of animal cells is a complex functional organelle where co-operative interaction of various components occurs. One specific peripheral protein, the F factor, affects and possibly controls processes involved in the determination of cell movement and cell form thereby having a direc relevance to cell growth and division.

Our observations also introduce the concept of a microenvironment with an operative role and the possibility that other peripheral membrane constituents may similarly have functional roles in various aspects of cell physiology.

ACKNOWLEDGEMENT

This work was supported by a grant from The Cancer Research Campaign.

REFERENCES

Hynes, R. O., A. T. Destree, V. M. Mantner and I. U. Ali (1977). Synthesis, secretion and attachment of LETS glycoprotein in normal and transformed cells. J. Supramol. Str., 7, 397-409.

Luft, J. H. (1971). Ruthenium red and violet. Chemistry, purification, methods of use for electron microscopy and mechanism of action. Anat. Record, 171, 347-368.

Mallucci, L. and V. Wells (1976). Determination of cell shape by a cell surface protein component. Nature, 262, 138-141.

Vaheri, A. and D. F. Mosher (1978). High molecular weight cell surface associated glycoprotein (fibronection) lost in malignant transformation. Biochim Biophys. Acta., 516, 1-27.

Wells, V. and L. Mallucci (1978). Determination of cell form in cultured fibroblasts. Role of surface components and cytokinetic elements. Exp. Cell Res., 116, 301-312.

Membrane Cooperative Enzymes as a Tool for the Investigation of Membrane Structure and Related Phenomena

Ricardo N. Farías

Instituto de Química Biológica, Facultad de Bioquímica,
Química y Farmacia, Universidad Nacional de Tucumán,
San M. de Tucumán, Republic Argentina

ABSTRACT

The use of membrane-bound cooperative enzymes from mammalian and bacterial system as a tool for the evaluation of membrane conformational changes is illustrated in the case of membrane-hormone interaction. The actions of insulin and L-triiodothyronine, as well as the molecular specificity for the last hormone are shown.

INTRODUCTION

Increasing and conclusive evidences have been gathered showing that allosteric transitions of the activity of a given enzyme could be correlated with changes in the "conformation" or "state" of the protein involved. The determination of this kinetic parameter in membrane-associated enzymes might give some clues as to how these enzymes are regulated by the membrane. On the other hand, that information may also indicate if some changes in membrane structure take place under a special situation, i.e., when the lipid composition of the membrane changes (Farías and co-workes, 1975). Two conditions must be fulfilled by the enzyme in order to be a suitable probe in a particular membrane: a) It must show a cooperative characteristic, b) the interactions membrane-enzyme should fall in the range of variation of the Hill coefficient for the particular system. Changes in lipid membrane-enzyme interactions of considerable low magnitude (about 0.7 - 0.8 kcal/mol) could be detected by changes in the allosteric properties of an enzyme (Siñeriz, Farías and Trucco 1975). The extent of the interaction at a given temperature can be ascerteined are since the experiments are perfomed under isothermic conditions.

It is the purpose of this presentation to discuss the potential methodological importance of the measurements of cooperative transitions of membrane bound enzymes as natural probes of the membrane conformation. Studies on change the cooperativity of membrane-bound $(Na^+ + K^+)$-ATPase and acetylcholinesterase from rat erythrocytes as well as of membrane-bound (Ca^{2+})ATPase from <u>Escherichia coli</u> in the presence of insulin and triiodothyronine $(L-T_3)$ are shown (Massa and co-workers 1975, Moreno and Farías, 1976; de Mendoza and coleagues, 1977). In addition, the molecular specificity of L-T$_3$ effect is presented here (de Mendoza, Moreno and Farias, 1978b)

RESULTS AND DISCUSSION

Relationship between membrane lipid composition and enzyme coopera-tivity. The mixed fatty acid composition of rat membrane erythrocytes was dependent on the nature of the lipid supplement of the diet (Guar nery and Johnson, 1970). A marked distinction between the fatty acid families which were endogenously synthesized and those depending on the dietary fat supplement was observed. Although the rats were able to maintain fairly constant the proportion of unsaturated fatty acid in spite of the wide differences in unsaturation of the dietary sup-plements, they were unable to maintain a constant number of total double bonds in the membrane (Bloj, Morero and Farías, 1973). The unsaturation of the dietary fat did not influence the cholesterol and lipid phosphorous content of rat membrane erythrocytes (Bloj, Mo-rero and Farías, 1973). The Hill coefficient for the inhibition by F^- of the $(Na^+ + K^+)$ATPases and acetylcholinesterase of red cell mem-brane obtained from five groups of rats (four fed with diets supple-mented with lard, olive oil, corn oil and linseed oil, respectively, and one commercial standard diet, all fatty acids sufficients animals) was determined. In addition one group was fed a fat-free diets. In an attempt to establish a correlation between the cooperative beha-vior of the membrane-bound enzymes and the fatty acid composition of the membrane, several relationships were calculated. The possibility that the dietary lipid effect were produced through changes in the membrane fluidity was considered. Since the fluidity of a lipid may be more directly dependent on the total number of double bonds pre-sent, the double bond index/saturated fatty acid ratio was calcula-ted and plotted against the value of n for the inhibition by F^- of the enzymes (Bloj, Morero, Farías and Trucco, 1973). As can be seen in Fig. 1, in the case of animals with a higher double bond index/ saturated fatty acid ratio in the membrane, the inhibition by F^- of the $(Na^+ + K^+)$-ATPase exhibited lower values of n. This relation was inverse for acetylcholinesterase.

To determine whether the above results could be generalized for procariotic cells, studies on the effect of lipid fluidity on membra-ne-bound enzymes were performed with bacteria. For this purpose,an auxotroph from Escherichia coli K-12 strain L 010 requiring unsatura-ted fatty acid was used. This mutant incorporated into their lipids the unsaturated fatty acid supplemented in the culture medium and thus provided an approach to study the relation between lipid membra-ne composition and the behavior of the membrane-bound Ca^{2+}-ATPase which was inhibited by Na^+. Growing the bacteria in media supplemen-ted with palmitoleic, vaccenic, oleic, linoleic and linolenic acids, it was possible to obtain different values of the double bond index/ saturated fatty acid ratio for the lipid composition of the membrane. The results of these experiments are presented in Fig. 2, where the values of n for the Na^+ inhibition of the Ca^+-ATPase were plotted against double bond index/saturation ratio (Siñeriz, Bloj, Farías and Trucco, 1973). A positive relation was obtained.

These correlations suggested the active role of the fluidity of the fatty acids of the membrane phospholipids in controlling the coope-rative behavior of these membrane enzymes.

Hormonal action and membrane fluidity. The correlations showed in Fig. 1 raised the possibility of evaluating changes in the membrane

fluidity through changes in the cooperativity of these enzymatic systems. The action of a effector on membrane fluidity may involve changes in the ordering or the state of compression of the lipids. This
phenomenon, in the case of insulin or L-T$_3$, should be related to membrane lipid in general since it is reflected in the behaviour of
erythrocyte acetylcholinesterase and (Na$^+$ $\pm$ K$^+$)ATPase and (Ca^{2+})ATPa-
se of E.coli (see below).

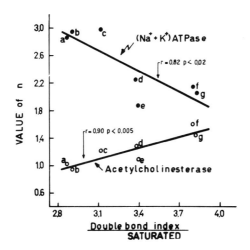

Fig. 1. Scattergram of the correlation between
        the values of n (Hill coefficient) and
        the ratio double bond index per saturated
        fatty acids from membrane erythrocytes
        lipid. The equation of the regression li-
        ne and overall correlation coefficient r
        with its significance are included. (●)
        (Na$^+$, K$^+$)-ATPase; (o) acetylcholines-
        terase; diet supplements: a, hydrogenated
        fat; b, lard; c, linseed oil; d, olive
        oil; e, fat-free; f, corn oil and g, stan
        dard diet. (Adapted from Bloj and co-wor-
        kers, 1973).

Insulin and L-T$_3$ actions: The effect of insulin and L-T$_3$ on the Hill
coefficients of acetylcholinesterase and (Na$^+$, K$^+$)-ATPase was studied in erythrocyte membranes exhibiting a high fatty acid fluidity
which were obtained from rats fed a corn oil supplemented diet, (Fig.
1, f diet). The values close to those from lard-fed (diet b of Fig.1)
rats in response to insulin 10^{-9}M. That is, the Hill coefficient for
acetylcholinesterase changed from 1.6 to 1.0 (Fig. 3A and Table 1),
whereas for (Na$^+$, K$^+$)-ATPase changes, it shifted from 2.2 to 3.0
(Table 1) (Massa and co-workers, 1975).

The presence of insulin 10^{-9}M changed the Na$^+$ inhibition curve of the
E.coli (Ca^{2+})-ATPase from a sigmoidal (n = 2.1) to hyperbolic shape (n = 1.3) (Fig. 3B and Table 1) (Moreno and Farias, 1976).

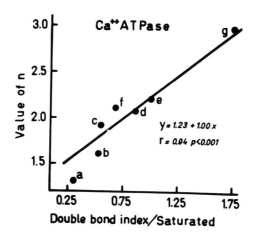

Fig. 2. Scattergram of the correlation between the
values of n (Hill coefficient) and the ratio double bond index per saturated fatty
acid from E.coli membrane lipid. The equa-
tion of the regression line and overall
correlation coefficient r with its significance are included. Cells grown at 37°
C on L broth media supplemented with unsaturated fatty acids: a, vaccenic; b, oleic
c, palmitoleic; d, linoleic, e, linolenic.
Same complex medium without glucose supplemented with unsaturated fatty acids: f,
vaccenic; g, linolenic; (From Siñeriz, F.
and coleagues, 1973).

As found with insulin, these membrane enzymes also changed in the
presence of L-T_3 10^{-9}M (Table 1) row 3) (de Mendoza and others, 1977).

The allosteric behavior of the soluble acetylcholinesterase and
(Ca^{2+})ATPase were not affected by the presence of both hormones (Massa and co-workers, 1975; Moreno and Farías, 1976 and de Mendoza and
others, 1977). The facts that:

   i) Insulin and L-T_3 action was only observed in membrane bound
      enzymes.

   ii) Insulin and L-T_3 decreases the n values of erythrocyte ace-
       tylcholinesterase and E.coli (Ca^{2+})ATPase and enhanced it
       in the erythrocyte ($Na^+ + K^+$)ATPase system.

   iii) The correlations between the membrane fluidity and the va-
        lues of n for the former enzymes were positive (Fig. 1
        and Fig. 2) whereas for the latter enzyme it was negative
        (Fig. 1).

constitute strong evidence for the hypothesis that both hormones decreases membrane fluidity.

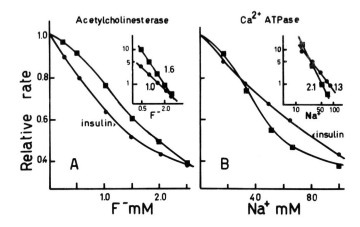

Fig. 3. Effect of the insulin on the Hill coefficient for the inhibition by F^- of rat erythrocyte acethylcholinesterase (A) and for
the inhibition by Na^+ of E.coli (Ca^{2+})ATP
ase (B). In the absence (■-■) and in the
presence (●-●) of insulin 10^{-9}M. Inset
shows Hill plots of same data. The same
membrane preparation was used for the control and hormone tests. (Adapted from Massa and co-workers, 1975 and Moreno and
Farías, 1976).

Table 1. Effect of insulin and L-T$_3$ on Hill coefficient.

Hormone (M)	n values		
	Red cell		E.coli
	Acetyl-cholinesterase	$(K^+ + Na^+)$ ATPase	(Ca^{2+}) ATPase
None	1.51 ± 0.03^a	2.30 ± 0.04^a	2.30 ± 0.05^a
Insulin 10^{-9}	1.03 ± 0.02^b	2.95 ± 0.07^b	1.14 ± 0.06^b
L-T$_3$ 10^{-9}	0.90 ± 0.10^b	3.60 ± 0.24^b	1.20 ± 0.20^b

Mean of n values of 3-5 different enzymatic preparations $\pm$
S E M; values followed by different letters were significantly different (p < 0.001) when compound by the Students
t-test. Adapted from Massa and others 1975, Moreno and Farías 1976 and de Mendoza and co-workers, 1977.

Molecular specificity of the L-T_3 action. In the second part of this presentation we will be show the use of membrane cooperative enzymes as a highly specific tool to study the action of hormones analogues.

Table 2: Effect of L-triiodothyronine analogues on n values.

Analogues (M)	n values	
	Erythrocyte Acetyl-cholinesterase	Ca^{2+} E.coli ATPase
None	1.80	1.50
L-T_3 10^{-10}	1.20	1.00
3 iodo L-tyrosine 10^{-6}	1.80	1.60
3,5 diiodo L-tyrosine 10^{-6}	1.80	1.60
D-T_3 10^{-9}	1.92	1.50
TRIAC 10^{-9}	1.83	1.55
Isopropyl L-T_2 10^{-9}	1.86	1.60
rT_3 10^{-9}	1.95	1.60
L-T_4 10^{-7}	1.80	1.60
L-T_4 10^{-4}	1.90	1.65

Analogues	3'	5'	3	5	R
L-T_3 or D-T_3	I	-	I	I	L or D-alanine
TRIAC	I	-	I	I	Acetic
Isopropyl-T_2	CH$\begin{smallmatrix}CH_3\\CH_3\end{smallmatrix}$	-	I	I	L-alanine
rT_3	I	I	I	-	L-alanine
L-T_4	I	I	I	I	L-alanine

The data are the average of a least three independent experiments which did not differ by more than 0.1 in n values.

The results of Table 1 indicated that insulin and L-T_3 behave a similar manner in the membrane cooperative enzymes systems. However, glucagon 10^{-9}M blocked the effect of insulin on these systems but not the action of L-T_3 (Melián and co-workers, 1978).

The following study was carried out with various analogues of L-T_3

(de Mendoza, Moreno and Farías, 1978).

The decrease of the values of n in the acetylcholinesterase and Ca^{2+} ATPase appear to require (Table 2):

i) the diphenyl ether structure, since 3 iodo L-thyrosine (MIT) and 3 5 diiodo L-thyrosine (DIT) are without effect (rows 3,4).

ii) L-alanine side chain, since $D-T_3$ with D-alanine side chain and TRIAC with acetic side chain have no effect (rows 5,6).

iii) iodine in the 3' position since substitution of the isopropyl group in this position yielded a compound that did not modify the n values (row 7), and

iv) 5' position iodine-free, since rT_3 and $L-T_4$ have no action (row 8-10).

The $L-T_3$ analogues, $D-T_3$, TRIAC, isopropyl-T_2 and rT_3 were used in concentrations one ten-fold higher than the $L-T_3$ concentration able to change the n values (rows 2). These experiments suggest a high specificity for $L-T_3$ to produce changes in the n values from mammalian and bacterial systems.

Liver nuclear binding sites for $L-T_3$ of high-affinity and low capacity were suggested to be involved in the iniciation of hormonal action (Oppenheimer, 1975). A reasonable agreement between relative binding affinity and thyromimetic activity for $L-T_3$ and thyroid hormones analogues was indicated (Oppenheimer, Schartz and Surks, 1973; Goslings and co-workers, 1976; De Groot and Torresani, 1975). The inhibitory effect of analogues on $L-T_3$ binding to nuclei indicated that among analogues TRIAC appears to bind with four times the affinity of $L-T_3$ and $D-T_3$ binds with equal affinity (De Groot and Torresani, 1975). By the use of "in vivo" displacements techniques, Oppenheimer and co-workers, 1973 reported similar relative displacement potencies for these compounds and isopropyl-T_2 and $L-T_3$, whereas $L-T_4$, TETRAC and rT_3 have no effect. Thus the action site is not stereospecific, does not require an L-alanine side chain and requires single bulk substitution, not necessarily iodine, in the 3' position of the phenolic ring and substituents in the 3 and 5 position of the inner ring. In the erythrocyte and E.coli systems, the iodothyronine molecules able to produce the allosteric desensitization has stereospecifity for alanine side chain and require a free 5' position (Table 2). That is, high stereospecifity molecules such as $L-T_3$ was required. Of great physiological interest is the apparent nonspecificity in the nuclear systems and the high apparent stereospecificity found in the erythrocyte and E.coli systems studied in this work. (de Mendoza, Moreno and Farías 1978b).

Speculation on the use of allosteric "Probes". Several features of the changes in the cooperative behavior of membrane enzymes in the erythrocyte membrane systems distinguish from the corresponding changes in bacterial systems, e.g. the effectors are F^- and Na^+ respectively, and enzymes and membranes differ in several aspects. The acetylcholinesterase and $(Na^+ + K^+)$ATPase from rats erythrocyte and (Ca^{2+}) ATPase from E.coli have different localization in the membrane and also have different dependence on the lipids for their enzymatic activity and differ also in their metabolic function (Farías and co-workers, 1975). Besides, the membrane from rat erythrocytes and E. coli differ largely in properties, functions and composition e.g. the

bacterial membrane does not contain sterol whereas the erythrocyte
membrane has one of the highest cholesterol/phospholipid ratios. However all the facts observed in rat erythrocyte and E.coli system
appear as a response to the general regulatory property of the membrane on cooperative enzyme. Thus, this interdependence is not confined
to one system. This suggestion may constitute the clue for general
use of a suitable "allosteric probes" to detect influence of the environment on the membrane e.g. in cancer research field. This novel
approach was illustrated in vitro and/or in vivo in the case of
cholesterol (Bloj, Morero and Farías, 1973), insulin cortisol and
progesterone (Massa and co-workers, 1975), thyroid hormones (de Mendoza and wo-workers, 1977), thyroid hormones and thyrotropin interplay (de Mendoza and Farías, 1978a), insulin, epinephrine and glucagon interplay (Melián and coleagues 1978) and organophosphorous
compounds (Domenech and others, 1977).

REFERENCES

Bloj B., R.D.Morero, R.N. Farías and R.E.Trucco (1973a). Membrane
lipid fatty acids and regulation of membrane-bound enzymes. A-
llosteric behavior of erythrocyte (Mg^{2+})ATPase $(Na^+ + K^+)$ATPase
and acetylcholinesterase from rats fed different fat-supplemen-
ted diets. Biochem.Biophys.Acta. 311, 67-79
Bloj B., R.D.Morero and R.N.Farías (1973b). Membrane fluidity, cholesterol and allosteric transitions from membrane-bound enzymes.
FEBS Letters 38, 101, 105.
De Groot L.J., and J.Torresani (1975) Triiodothyronine binding to
isolated liver cell nuclei. Endocrinology 96, 357-369.
de Mendoza D., H.Morenc, E.M.Massa, R.D.Morero and R.N.Farías (1977).
Thyroid hormone actions and membrane fluidity: Blocking action
of thyroxine on triiodothyronine effect. FEBS Letters 84, 199-
203.
de Mendoza D., and R.N.Farías (1978a). Effect of cold exposure on
rat erythrocyte membrane-bound acetylcholinesterase. Role of
thyrotropin in the thyroid hormone interplay. J.Biol.Chem. in
press.
de Mendoza, D., H.Moreno and R.N.Farías (1978b). Membrane cooperative enzymes: High molecular specificity for blocking action of
thyroxine on triiodothyronine effect in rat erythrocyte and
Escherichia coli system. J.Biol.Chem. in press
Domenech C.A., A.E.Machado de Domenech, H.Balegno, D.de Mendoza and
R.N.Farías (1977). Pesticide action and membrane fluidity: Allosteric behavior of rat erythrocytes membrane-bound acetylcholinesterase in the presence of organophosphate compounds. FEBS
Letters 74, 243-246.
Farías R.N., B.Bloj, R.D.Morero, F.Siñeriz and R.E.Trucco (1975). Regulation of allosteric membrane-bound enzymes through changes
in membrane lipid composition. Biochem.Biophys.Acta. 415, 231-
251.
Goslings B., H.L.Schwartz, W.Dillmann, M.I.Surks and J.H.Oppenheimer
(1976) Comparation of the metabolism and distribution of L-triiodothyronine and triiodothyroacetic acid in the rat: a possible explanation of differential hormonal potency. Endocrinology
98, 666-675.
Guarneri M. and R.Johnson (1970). The essential fatty acids. In R.
Paoletti and Kritchevsky D. (Ed.), Advances in Lipid Research
8, 115-174.

Massa E.M., R.D.Morero, B.Bloj and R.N.Farías (1975). Hormone action and membrane fluidity: effect of insulin and cortisol on the Hill coefficient of rat erythrocyte membrane-bound acetylcholinesterase and $(Na^+ + K^+)$ATPase. Biochem.Biophys.Res.Commun. 66, 115-122.

Melián de E.M., E.M.Massa, R.D.Morero and R.N.Farías (1978). Membrane cooperative enzymes interplay of insulin, glucagon and epinephrine on rat erythrocyte acetylcholinesterase system. FEBS Letters 92, 143-146.

Moreno H. and R.N.Farías (1976). Insulin decreased bacterial membrane fluidity. Is it a general event in its action? Biochem.Biophys. Res.Commun. 72, 74-80

Oppenheimer J.H., H.L.Schwartz and M.I.Surks (1973) Effect of thyroid hormone analogues on the displacement of ^{125}I L-triiodothyronine from hepatic and heart nuclei in vivo: possible relationship to hormonal activity. Biochem.Biophys.Res.Commun. 55, 544-550.

Oppenheimer H.J. (1975) Initiation of thyroid-hormone action. New Eng.J.Medicine 292, 1063-1068.

Siñeriz F., B.Bloj, R.N.Farías and R.E.Trucco (1973). Regulation by membrane fluidity of the allosteric behavior of the (Ca++) adenosine triphosphatase from Escherichia coli. J.Bacteriol. 115, 723-726.

Siñeriz F., R.N.Farías and R.E.Trucco (1975). The convenience of the use of allosteric "probes" for the study of lipid protein interactions in biological membranes thermodynamic consideration. J.Theor.Biol. 52, 113-120.

Surface Behaviour of Glycosphingolipids and Its Relevance to the Metabolic Changes of Gangliosides in Transformed Cells

B. Maggio and F. A. Cumar

Departamento de Química Biológica, Facultad de Ciencias Químicas,
Universidad Nacional de Córdoba, Córdoba, Argentina

ABSTRACT

The surface behaviour of glycosphingolipids reveals that the complexity of their polar head group and the presence of one or more sialosyl residues greatly influences their molecular packing and surface potential. From these studies it could be inferred that the dipolar contributions from the second and third sialosyl residues in di- and tri-sialogangliosides were of a different nature than the contributions from the first sialosyl residues and neutral carbohydrate units. The distinctive dipolar properties of the sialosyl residues in polysialogangliosides were an essential requirement for establishing particular interactions with phosphatidylcholine that were not shown by other glycosphingolipids. The intermolecular interactions shown by polysialogangliosides with phosphatidylcholine were closely correlated to the ability of these gangliosides to decrease the thermodynamic stability of the membrane and to induce the changes of permeability and morphology leading to membrane fusion both in nucleated erythrocytes and nerve endings. Since cultured cells transformed by several oncogenic agents are characterized by a lack of complex gangliosides due to enzymatic blocks in their biosynthetic pathway, this may have important consequences on the membrane organization and cellular function.

INTRODUCTION

The plasma membrane of transformed cells shows a variety of peculiar characteristics with respect to those of the corresponding control cell lines (Nicolson,1976). One of the well defined biochemical alterations at the membrane level is the decreased amounts of the more complex glycosphingolipids, particularly gangliosides (Brady and Fishman,1974; Hakomori,1975). On the other hand, the possible changes of the molecular organization of glycosphingolipids in membranes of transformed cells and the effect this may have on cellular functions has been little explored. This is probably a consequence of the lack of information on the physico-chemical surface properties of this group of lipids. In this regard, the present work will correlate the fact that the more complex gangliosides which are lacking in most transformed cell lines have a markedly different surface behaviour than simpler gangliosides or neutral glycosphingolipids.

RESULTS AND DISCUSSION

Ganglioside alterations in virus-induced transformed cell lines

Several established mouse cell lines transformed by either SV40 or polyoma virus are

141

Table 1. *Chemical structure and nomenclature of sphingolipids*

Lipid	Abbreviated nomenclature (IUPAC–IUB)*	Short symbol used in this work†
Sphingoid	Spd	Spd
N-acylsphingoid	Cer	Cer
Galβ1→1Spd	GalSpd	GalSpd
Glcβ1→1Spd	GlcSpd	GlcSpd
Galβ1→4Glcβ1→1Spd	LacSpd	LacSpd
Galβ1→1Cer	GalCer	GalCer
Glcβ1→1Cer	GlcCer	GlcCer
Galβ1→4Glcβ1→1Cer	LacCer	LacCer
GalNAcβ1→4Galβ1→4Glcβ1→1Cer	Gg$_3$Cer	Gg$_3$Cer
Galβ1→3GalNAcβ1→4Galβ1→4Glcβ1→1Cer	Gg$_4$Cer	Gg$_4$Cer
NeuGcα2→3Galβ1→4Glcβ1→1Cer	II^{3}NeuGc-LacCer	GM$_3$
NeuAcα2→8NeuAcα2→3Galβ1→4Glcβ1→1Cer	II^3(NeuAc)$_2$-LacCer	GD$_3$
GalNAcβ1→4Gal(3←2αNeuAc)β1→4Glcβ1→1Cer	II^{3}NeuAc-GgOse$_3$Cer	GM$_2$
Galβ1→3GalNAcβ1→4Gal(3←2αNeuAc)β1→4Glcβ1→1Cer	II^{3}NeuAc-GgOse$_4$Cer	GM$_1$
NeuAcα2→3Galβ1→3GalNAcβ1→4Gal(3←2αNeuAc)β1→4Glcβ1→1Cer	IV^{3}NeuAc,II^{3}NeuAc-GgOse$_4$Cer	GD$_{1a}$
NeuAcα2→3Galβ1→3GalNAcβ1→4Gal(3←2αNeuAc8←2αNeuAc)β1→4Glcβ1→1Cer	IV^{3}NeuAc,II^3(NeuAc)$_2$-GgOse$_4$Cer	GT$_1$

* IUPAC–IUB nomenclature of lipids (1976) [*Lipids* (1977) **12**, 455–468; *Biochem. J.* (1978) **171**, 21–35]. Spd and Cer are the IUPAC–IUB recommended abbreviations for sphingoid and ceramide respectively.
† For gangliosides the nomenclature of Svennerholm (1963) was used.

---

characterized by a lack of gangliosides having oligosaccharide chains longer than sialosyl-lactose (Mora and co-workers, 1969; Brady and Mora, 1970).

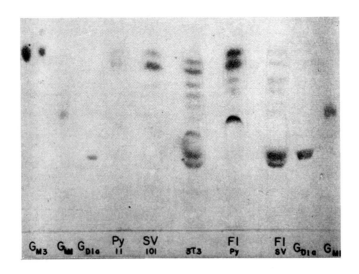

Fig. 1. Ganglioside pattern of mouse cell lines. T.l.c. of ganglioside fractions from: Py11, polyoma virus-transformed cells; SV101, SV40-transformed cells; 3T3, control cell line; Fl$_{py}$, flat revertant from polyoma virus-transformed cells; Fl$_{sv}$, flat revertant from SV40-transformed cells. GM$_3$, GM$_1$ and GD$_{1a}$ are ganglioside standards.

As illustrated in Fig. 1 the transformed cells show the presence of monosialoganglioside GM$_3$ (for abbreviations see Table 1) but almost a complete loss of the more complex monosialogangliosides GM$_2$, GM$_1$ and the disialoganglioside GD$_{1a}$ as compared with the control cell lines. The absence of complex gangliosides was found to be

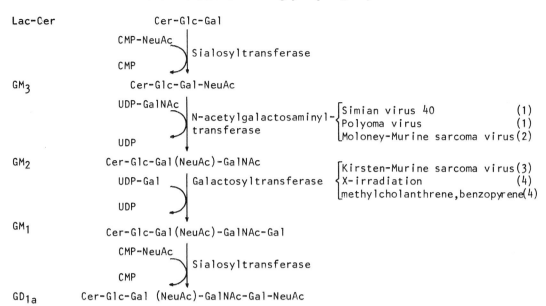

Fig. 2. Metabolic pathway of gangliosides in mouse cell lines. The step of enzymatic block is shown for cells transformed by the oncogenic agents indicated. References: (1) Cumar and co-workers, 1970; (2) Mora and co-workers, 1973; (3) Fishman and co-workers, 1974; (4) Coleman and co-workers, 1975.

the result of an enzymatic block in their biosynthesis rather than to an increase of their degradative pathway. The biosynthetic reaction affected in this case is that catalized by the enzyme UDPGalNAc:GM3 N-acetylgalactosaminyltransferase (Cumar and co-workers, 1970; Mora, Cumar and Brady, 1971), (Fig. 2 and Table 2). Similar types of enzymatic blocks leading to decreases of higher gangliosides were described in various cell lines from different animal species transformed by RNA viruses, chemical carcinogens or X-irradiation (Brady and Fishman, 1974; Hakomori, 1975), (see Fig. 2).

TABLE 2. N-Acetylgalactosaminyltransferase activity in mouse cell lines

Cell line	State	Enzyme activity (% of control)
Swiss 3T3	Normal	100
SV101	SV40-transformed	33
Py11	Polyoma-transformed	26
Fl_{sv}	Flat revertant from SV101	142
Fl_{py}	Flat revertant from Py11	46

On the other hand, in flat revertants from mouse transformed cell lines there is a tendency to normalize the ganglioside contents and enzymatic activity (Fig. 1 and Table 2) (Mora, Cumar and Brady, 1971). The fact that the transformed cells show a different ganglioside pattern may have important consequences on membrane organization and function since polysialogangliosides have remarkably different surface properties than the simpler glycosphingolipids.

Surface behaviour of gangliosides

The physico-chemical surface properties of glycosphingolipids were studied in a
model system consisting of lipid monolayers at the air-water interface (Maggio,
Cumar and Caputto, 1978a). The type and number of carbohydrate residues in the olig
saccharide chain of glycosphingolipids is a major factor conditioning their surface
properties.

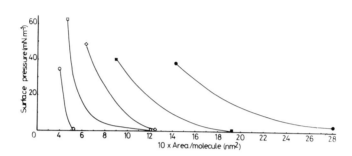

Fig. 3. Surface behaviour of glycosphingolipids. The surface pressure-area curves
were determined at 20 + 1°C on 145 mM-NaCl, pH 5.6 for: (o) Cer; (□) Gg4Cer;
(◇) GM1; (■) GD1a and (●)GT1. Other neutral glycosphingolipids, monosialoganglio
sides and disialogangliosides showed a behaviour similar to Gg4Cer, GM1 and GD1a
respectively.

The area occupied per molecule of glycosphingolipid and the liquid character of the
film was greater as the number of negatively charged sialosyl residues in the polar
head group increased (Fig. 3). From measurements of the surface potential the
resultant dipole moment of the glycosphingolipid molecule and the dipolar contributions of each carbohydrate residue of the oligosaccharide chain can be calculated
(Maggio, Cumar and Caputto, 1978a) and these results are shown in Fig. 4.

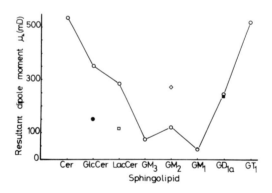

Fig. 4. Resultant dipole moment of glycosphingolipids at their limiting molecular
area. The overall resultant dipole moments on 145 mM-NaCl at pH 5.6 are shown for
the lipids indicated. Simbols outside the curve indicate: (◇) Gg4Cer, pH 5.6;
(■) GD3, pH 5.6; (●) GlcSpd, pH 10.4; (□) LacSpd, pH 10.4.

The presence of neutral carbohydrate units or a sialosyl residue attached to the

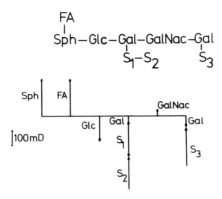

Fig. 5. Vertical dipole moment contributions from each individual carbohydrate residue of glycosphingolipids. The contributions of each residue to the overall resultant molecular dipole moment are shown for the molecule of ganglioside GT₁.

galactose proximal to the ceramide moiety causes a decrease of the overall resultant vertical dipole moment of the glycosphingolipid. Conversely, the presence of a a second or third sialosyl residue in di- and tri-sialogangliosides results in an increase of the overall molecular dipole. Fig. 5 is a diagrammatic representation

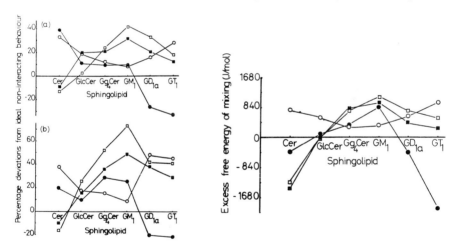

Fig. 6. Interactions of glycosphingolipids with phospholipids. Left: deviations from ideal behaviour in mean molecular area (a) and mean surface potential/molecule (b) for mixed monolayers above 30 mN.m⁻¹. Right: excess free energy of mixing for mixed monolayers up to 30 mN.m⁻¹. The curves represent the values for mixed films in molar ratio 1:1 of the sphingolipid indicated with: (●) dipalmitoylphosphatidylcholine; (○) dipalmitoylphosphatidylethanolamine; (■) phosphatidylinositol; (□) phosphatidylserine.

of the dipolar contribution of each residue in ganglioside GT₁ where it can be seen that the second and third sialosyl residues contribute with a vertical dipole moment similar in magnitude but of an opposite direction to that of the first sialosyl residue

Information on the existence and type of intermolecular interactions in lipid monolayers can be obtained by comparing properties of mixed films with those of
theoretical mixed monolayers in which no interactions are assumed (Gaines, 1966).
No interactions were found between different ganglioside species and the analysis
of the behaviour of mixed ganglioside films by the surface phase rule (cf. Gaines,
1966) indicated lack of miscibility among the ganglioside molecules. This is
probably the consequence of steric hindrance and electrostatic repulsions between
their polar head groups. These results suggested that it is unlikely that there are
regions consisting of pure or mixed gangliosides closely packed in a biological
lipid bilayer unless effects such as ganglioside-protein interactions, binding of
other ligands or ternary lipid complexes are also involved (Maggio, Cumar and
Caputto, 1978b).

By contrast, interactions involving changes in packing and surface potential were
found in mixed monolayers of gangliosides with phospholipids. Considering the
changes in mean molecular area, mean surface potential per molecule or the
spontaneity of the interaction (Fig. 6) in mixed monolayers with any of the phospholipids studied, a definite change in the trend of the interaction takes place for
di- and tri-sialogangliosides compared with monosialogangliosides and neutral
glycoshingolipids. In Fig. 6 this is evidenced by a change in the upward or downward
tendency of the curves or in the positive or negative sign of the deviations. For
mixed monolayers of phosphatidylcholine the interactions with polysialogangliosides

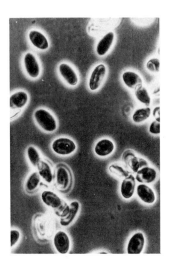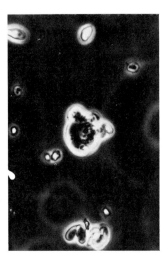

Fig. 7. Membrane fusion in chicken erythrocytes induced by polysialogangliosides.
Left: control chicken erythrocytes incubated at 37°C in the conditions described
by Maggio, Cumar and Caputto (1978c) in absence of gangliosides. Similar pictures
were obtained with erythrocytes incubated in presence of GM_1, GM_3 or neutral glycosphingolipids. Right: a multinucleated cell induced by the presence of GT_1; bi- or
multi-nucleated cells were also found after incubation with GD_{1a} or GD_3. Phase-
contrast microscopy, X 600.

were thermodinamically favoured (indicated by the negative excess free energy of
mixing, Fig. 6) and this suggests that these glycosphingolipids should be preferably
associated to phosphatidylcholine in a complex lipid interface in absence of other
constraints. As shown in Fig. 6, the interactions of di- and tri-sialogangliosides
with phosphatidylcholine were characterized by reductions of the molecular packing
and decreases of the surface potential of the mixed monolayers (Maggio, Cumar and
Caputto, 1978b).

he behaviour of polysialogangliosides in mixed monolayers with phosphatidylcholine,
articularly the modifications of the surface potential,resembled the effects on
hosphatidylcholine films of several lipidic and water-soluble compounds capable of
nducing membrane fusion (Maggio and Lucy, 1975; 1976; 1977; Maggio, Ahkong and
Lucy, 1976). On this basis it was possible to anticipate that gangliosides GD_{1a}, GD_3
and GT_1 but not GM_1, GM_3 or the neutral glycosphingolipids could induce Ca^{++} - dependent fusion of erythrocyte membranes (Fig. 7) (Maggio, Cumar and Caputto, 1978c)
and of synaptic vesicles with the plasma membrane in nerve endings (Cumar, Maggio
and Caputto, 1978).

The membrane surface potential is an important factor controlling ionic permeabilities
(Gingell, 1967; Bangham, 1968) and the reductions of the electrostatic field perpen-
dicular to the surface of a phosphatidylcholine interface together with modifications
of the membrane organization induced by polysialogangliosides may be a key event
for the initial increase of the membrane permeability to Ca^{++} (Blow, Botham and
Lucy, 1978; Ahkong and co-workers, 1973; Ahkong and co-workers, 1975; Maggio, Ahkong
and Lucy, 1976) and aggregation that leads to the fusion process (Maggio, Cumar and
Caputto, 1978c; Cumar, Maggio and Caputto, 1978).

The physico-chemical properties and function of gangliosides in membranes are still
far from being precisely understood; however, in the transformed cell lines lacking
the more complex gangliosides all of the surface properties of polysialogangliosides
described above would be presumably missing and this could undoubtedly have important
consequences on the membrane organization and cellular functions.

Acknowledgements: the research cited in this paper was supported in part by the
Organización de los Estados Americanos, National Institutes of Health, U.S.A. and
Consejo Nacional de Investigaciones Científicas y Técnicas, Argentina. We thank Dr.
R. Caputto for advice.Figs. are from references by the authors cited in the text.

REFERENCES

Ahkong, Q. F., D. Fisher, W. Tampion and J. A. Lucy (1973). The fusion of erythrocy-
    tes by fatty acids, esters, retinol and α-tocopherol. Biochem. J., 136, 147-155.
Ahkong, Q. F., W. Tampion and J. A. Lucy (1975). Promotion of cell fusion by divalent
    cation ionophores. Nature, 256, 208-209.
Bangham, A. D. (1968). Membrane models with phospholipids. Progress Biophys. Molec.
    Biol., 18, 29-95.
Blow, A. M. J., G. M. Botham and J. A. Lucy (1978). Entry of calcium into hen
    erythrocytes on treatment with fusogenic chemicals. Biochem. Soc. Trans., 6,
    284-285.
Brady, R. O. and P. T. Mora (1970) Alteration in ganglioside pattern and synthesis
    in SV40 and polyoma virus-transformed mouse cell lines. Biochim. Biophys. Acta,
    218, 308-319.
Brady, R. O. and P. H. Fishman (1974). Biosynthesis of glycolipids in virus-
    transformed cells. Biochim. Biophys. Acta, 355, 121-148.
Coleman, P. L., P. H. Fishman, R. O. Brady and G. J. Todaro (1975). Altered ganglio-
    side biosynthesis in mouse cell cultures following transformation with chemical
    carcinogens and X-irradiation. J. Biol. Chem., 250, 55-60.
Cumar, F. A., R. O. Brady, E. H. Kolodny, V. W. McFarland and P. T. Mora (1970).
    Enzymatic block in the synthesis of gangliosides in DNA virus-transformed
    tumorigenic mouse cell lines. Proc. Nat. Acad. Sci. U.S.A., 67, 757-764.
Cumar, F. A. , B. Maggio and R. Caputto (1978) Dopamine release from nerve endings
    induced by polysialogangliosides. Biochim. Biophys. Res. Comm., in press.
Fishman, P. H., R. O. Brady, R. M. Bradley, S. A. Aaronson and G. J. Todaro (1974).
    Absence of a specific ganglioside galactosyltransferase in mouse cells transfor-
    med by murine sarcoma virus. Proc. Nat. Acad. Sci. U.S.A., 71, 298-301.

Gaines, G. L. (1966) in I. Prigogine (Ed.) Interscience Monographs on Physical
    Chemistry: Insoluble Monolayers at Liquid-Gas Interfaces;Interscience.pp. 136-207-

Gingell,D(1967). Membrane surface potential in relation to a possible mechanism fc
    intercellular interactions and cellular responses: a physical basis. J. Theore
    Biol., 17, 451-482.

Hakomori,S. (1975). Structures and organization of cell surface glycolipids depend
    cy on cell growth and malignant transformation. Biochim. Biophys. Acta, 417,
    55-89.

Maggio, B. and J. A. Lucy (1975).Studies on mixed monolayers of phospholipids and
    fusogenic lipids. Biochem. J., 149, 597-608.

Maggio, B. and J. A. Lucy (1976). Polar group behaviour in mixed monolayers of
    phospholipids and fusogenic lipids. Biochem. J., 155, 353-364.

Maggio, B. and J. A. Lucy (1977). Interactions with phospholipid monolayers of
    lipids and water-soluble compounds that induce membrane fusion. In N. G. Bazán
    R. R. Brenner and N. M. Giusto (Eds.) Advances in Experimental Medicine and
    Biology, Vol. 83, Plenum Press, New York and London, pp. 225-231.

Maggio, B., Q. F. Ahkong and J. A. Lucy (1976). Poly(ethyleneglycol), surface
    potential and cell fusion. Biochem. J., 158, 647-650.

Maggio, B., F. A. Cumar and R. Caputto (1978a). Surface behaviour of gangliosides
    and related glycosphingolipids. Biochem. J., 171, 559-565.

Maggio, B., F. A. Cumar and R. Caputto (1978b). Interactions of gangliosides with
    phospholipids and glycosphingolipids in mixed monolayers. Biochem. J., in press

Maggio, B., F. A. Cumar and R. Caputto (1978c). Induction of membrane fusion by
    polysialogangliosides. FEBS Lett., 90, 149-152.

Mora, P. T., R. O. Brady, R. M. Bradley and V. W. McFarland (1969). Gangliosides in
    DNA virus-transformed and spontaneously transformed tumorigenic mouse cell line
    Proc. Nat. Acad. Sci. U.S.A., 63, 1290-1296.

Mora, P. T., F. A. Cumar and R. O. Brady (1971). A common biochemical change in
    SV40 and polyoma virus transformed mouse cells coupled to control of cell growt
    in culture. Virology, 46, 60-72.

Mora, P. T., P. H. Fishman, R. N. Bassin, R. O. Brady and V. W. McFarland (1973).
    Transformation of swiss 3T3 cells by murine sarcoma virus is followed by
    decrease in a glycolipid glycosyltransferase. Nature New Biol., 245, 226-229.

Nicolson, G. L. (1976). Transmembrane control of the receptors on normal and tumor
    cell.II. Surface changes associated with transformation and malignancy. Biochim
    Biophys. Acta, 458, 1-72.

Svennerholm, L. (1963). Chromatographic separation of human brain gangliosides.
    J. Neurochem. 10, 613-623.

Biological Markers

The Carcinoembryonic Antigen and Comparable Substances in the Diagnosis of Human Cancer*

E. D. Holyoke, T. M. Chu, J. T. Evans and A. Mittelman

*Roswell Park Memorial Institute, 666 Elm Street, Buffalo,
New York 14263, U.S.A.*

ABSTRACT

Carcinoembryonic Antigen or CEA is the best studied of a large group of tumor markers which is still increasing. CEA is discussed as a biological marker model and problems of evaluating tumor markers are discussed. The problems of initial success versus later less satisfactory results and effects of benign disease are discussed. Problems in screening are reviewed, especially the difficulties inherent in false positive results, CEA as a screening, diagnostic agent, staging assay and prognosticator is considered. Caution is recommended in declaring that a marker truly improves treatment.

INTRODUCTION

Table I presents a partial listing of a large group of biological markers discussed at the National Conference on Tumor Markers held in Washington, DC in the United States in September 1978. Since the identification of Carcino-embryonic Antigen (CEA) by Gold and Freedman (1965) in Montreal and the development of radioimmune assay for this glycoprotein (Thompson et al. 1969), a large number of new tumor associated antigens and markers have been identified and studied, and in addition, several old markers have been taken out of the closet, dusted off, and reexamined.

One reason for burgeoning interest in tumor markers has been an improved capability for measuring small quantities of material in body fluids and serum. If we consider the measurement of nanograms or 10^{-9} grams of marker per ml. as a baseline, we have increased our sensitivity of measurement of from 1,000 to 10,000 nanograms using double gel immunodiffusion or immunoelectrophoresis through 25 to 10 nanograms using counter immunoelectrophoresis or immunoradiography down to 0.25 nanogram (ng) using radioimmune assay.

CEA, partly because of its commercial availability has been the most extensively studied of these tumor markers, and during these studies, our ideas about what constitutes a viable or useful tumor marker have matured. In addition, we have

Supported in part by U.S.P.H. Grant #CA 15263-04
Contract #N01-CM-43782

learned a great deal about proper testing of clinical usefulness of tumor markers
over the last several years. As we review what we know about CEA, it is well to
keep these aspects in mind.

Table I

CARCINOEMBRYONIC ANTIGEN AND COMPARABLE SUBSTANCES
IN THE
DIAGNOSIS OF HUMAN CANCER

TUMOR MARKERS

Carcinoembryonic Antigen	CEA
Alpha Fetoprotein	AFP
Tissue Peptide Antigen	TPA
Serum Basic Fetoprotein	BFP
Serum Alpha Subunit	αCG
Serum Chorionic Gonadotrophin	CG
Serum C3 DNA-Binding Protein	C3DP
Thomsen-Friedenreich Specific Substances	T
Serum B_2-Microglobulin	
Human Sarcoma Antigen	$S_1S_2S_3$

Table II

TESTING DIFFERENT POPULATIONS

REPORT	# OF PATIENTS TESTED	PERCENT POSITIVE	DATE OF REPORT
Initial	36	97	SEPT 1969
2nd	35	91	JAN 1971
3rd	101	86	JULY 1971
4th	131	79	FEB 1972
5th	33	83	APR 1972
6th	135	72	APR 1972
7th	43	88	MAY 1972
8th	79	72	JUL 1972
9th	146	62	JUL 1972

CEA AS A BIOLOGICAL MARKER AND MODEL

Table II deserves some attention since it outlines an apparent change in CEA
sensitivity from an initial report, Thompson et al. (1969) until the Joint American
Cancer Society, National Cancer Institute of Canada Study (1972). Sensitivity of
the assay gradually fell. It is well to review this chain of events because it is
quite a general phenomenon. In the first report, only one of 36 patients with
colon cancer assayed with a false negative report. Then the reagents were passed
to other centers, the assays were conducted at other centers, and the number of

alse negative reports began to increase. We have to ask why this is the usual
tory with a new tumor marker. There are several reasons apparent at this juncture.

sually initial blood samples originating in an institution tend to be from
atients with more advanced malignancy. For present work, this has been improved
hrough early use of the Mayo Clinic-National Cancer Institute Serum Bank.
ut previously, and in many instances still, initial reports concern blood drawn
rom patients with advanced disease, particularly if coming from a university or
large cancer center where many of these patients are treated. Until more recently,
most initial reports concerned primarily the test group or well, young, healthy
individuals. Now, and properly so, most studies report early on a group of
patients with benign disease as a control group. In a search for another tumor
marker with Dr. Chu (1978) we initially tested a young healthy control group of
individuals and patients with biliary, colorectal, lung and other malignancies.
Initially, it looked as if we had a strong marker, but when we tested patients
with benign disease, it became clear that what we were measuring was non-specific.
We have also found that initial studies are usually not done properly blinded.
Before serious consideration of results some information has to be available on
properly blinded studies of a given marker.

Reagent specificity may be a problem. Recently Schuster et al. (1978) wrote
about trying to improve the specificity of our RaI assay for CEA. CEA is a glycoprotein of molecular weight of approximately 200,000. There is extensive intra
and inter molecular heterogenicity. The carbohydrate protein ratio varies from
1:1 - 6:1. The sialic acid content varies among preparations derived from
various tumor sources. There is also variation in the amino terminal end of the
polypeptide chain. Studies of different CEA standards from four different
laboratories using different antisera (Vrba 1976) have shown significant
antigenic differences between some CEA preparations. In addition, serum CEA and
the CEA obtained from a patient with hepatic metastases have been found to be
antigenically different. So that, in immune assays, which are biological assays,
reagents may vary.

Finally, as any test moves out from the laboratory towards wider use, unless it
is quite simple to perform, it will lose some sensitivity through the use of less
specialized personnel and the use of quality control rather than the type of
exactatude customary in the scientific laboratory.

THE BIOLOGICAL MARKER

The Problem

The problem we face is basically that by the time a patient becomes symptomatic
for most tumors, we are really quite far along on the growth and metastasis
curves. It is clear that the earlier we can diagnose the tumor, the more chance
by far we have for cure. A biological marker capable of detecting the presence
and growth of a malignant tumor may be useful in screening, diagnosis, staging of
disease (prognostication), monitoring disease for cure, regression or progression
in response to therapy, or it may be used to monitor progression of occult
disease and increase our clinical acumen in diagnosing clinical recurrence with
a view to earlier therapy of advancing disease.

SCREENING

The use of immunological tests for screening is probably the most difficult of
the various potential applications of any marker. For success in screening an
assay needs to be simple and practical for large scale testing. It must be
standardized and safe. A suitable high risk population should be available for
best results. The assay needs good specificity. A qualitative difference in
the marker is desirable, but not absolutely necessary.

Let us examine how a shift in sensitivity or specificity can alter our results.
If we have less than 100 percent specificity, it means that individuals without
tumor may be falsely positive. On the other hand, if we have 100 percent
specificity, but less than 100 percent sensitivity, then there are no false
positives, but only a portion of the tumors prevalent in the population are
identified. Let us think together about the consequences of lack of complete
sensitivity or specificity and how this may affect our problem of using a given
marker as a screen for malignant disease. Let us imagine that a test run is
made at a university on 100 patients, 10 with cancer. Let us assign a 90 percent
specificity to the test and a 90 percent sensitivity. We will encounter 9 of 90
patients who show a false elevated value. The sensitivity is equally good, and
we diagnose 9 of 10 patients correctly with cancer. We publish. Now let us
take the test to the community. We screen 100,000 patients looking for the
100 patients hidden in the group. We pick up 90 positives in the 100. This is
good, but we have almost 10,000 patients who are falsely positive. At this rate
still less than 1 in 100 patients who are positive will have cancer. Depending
on tumor prevalence, really very high specificity is necessary for screening.

At this Congress, Chu and Murphy (1978) reported a CEA screening study of some
3,000 older individuals over six years. Two malignancies have been found. One
an operable colon lesion, the other an inoperable lesion of the pancreas. It is
apparent that in its present form the CEA assay is not suitable for screening.

Alpha FetoProtein (AFP) has been tested as a screen in Senegal and in China
for hepatocellular cancer. The false positive rate is low, but sensitivity is
also low in these studies which did not use radioimmunoassay. Other markers
tested as screening agents are thyrocalcitonin for meduallary carcinoma of the
thyroid and possibly the use of sulfuglycoprotein in screening for gastric cancer.
The thyrocalcitonin assay with calcium or pentagastrin infusion is here to stay,
(Calmettes et al. 1977) although there are unanswered questions about its use.
The sulfoglycoprotein assay still has a problem with false positives, but its
sensitivity is good enough so that it may have a place. (Hakkinen 1976) For
many other markers, there is not enough information to determine their proper
clinical application at this time.

CEA AS A DIAGNOSTIC ADJUVANT

The first problem with the use of CEA as an adjunct to diagnosis is that it has
a rather high incidence of positivity in benign disease. At this point, we are
limiting our discussion to what CEA can accomplish as a diagnostic aid in
patients with colorectal cancer.

Table III indicates the general experience in this regard with, for example, a
CEA positivity of 31 percent in patients with ulcerative colitis. However, if
using clinical and other laboratory evaluation, known individuals with benign
disease are discounted, the false positive rate can be significantly reduced
without an adverse effect on sensitivity. This is just as well because, for

Table III

CEA IN BENIGN DISEASE

Disease	Percent Positive CEA
Emphysema	57
Alcoholics	65
Ulcerative Colitis	31
Ileitis	40
Transplants	56
Pneumonia	46
Pancreatitis	53

After Galen, Hosp, Phys. 1976

CEA and colorectal cancer, the latter is already low. Several reports and our own experience indicate that if we use the Astler-Coller modification of Dukes' Classification only 20 to 25 percent of early colon or rectal cancer victims are identified. This severely limits the use of the assay. It has been reported that the CEA assay increased the diagnostic accuracy and was additive to barium enema in a series of symptomatic patients. While we do not feel that barium enema in that study was as accurate as we have usually found it to be, we believe that the CEA assay should be included in the investigation of patients with symptoms of large bowel disease, especially those with a negative or doubtful barium enema, and that, albeit in a small group of patients, this assay may increase our diagnostic success, barium enema or colonoscopy not withstanding. Although we are impressed tht this is a very difficult aspect to quantiate.

CEA IN STAGING

Staging is an effort to describe precisely how much disease is present in a patient, but also to make a statement about prognosis. Generally staging is based on Dukes' A, B_1, or C classification in the literature. This may be modified after Astler-Coller as A1 which implies no penetration deeper than the submucosa, B1 which implies partial penetration of the bowel wall, B_2 which implies complete penetration of the bowel, C_1 which indicates lymph nodes and C_2 which generally implies both penetration of bowel wall and positive nodes. We find from our own data at Roswell Park that this approach to staging is meaningful as stage relates to prognosis.

We have used an in-house TNM class fication since 1971 when we first began to study tumor markers. It is pretty much standard with T increasing for deeper penetration, perforation, and peri-bowel wall invasion. Lymph node designation increases as nodes increase in number or are further from the primary. To assist us in staging all specimens are cleared in alcohol so that all nodes can be identified. As a result of our studies, we recommend that lymph nodes be reported on studies of colorectal cancer of prognosis or adjuvant therapy as a ratio. This should be of lymph nodes found positive over lymph nodes examined and will provide a quality control of pathology.

Our first prospective study was published several years ago. (Holyoke et al. 1972) All patients underwent curative surgery with technical removal of all tumor present. Some of the patients had recurrent disease and some local spreak in the area of the lesion, as low peritoneal seeding. As long as all visible tumor was

removed technically, the patients were included in the study. There was a
definite trend for those patients who were later to develop recurrence to have a
higher presurgical CEA with only four of twenty-three who later recurred having
a negative CEA prior to surgery.

We then undertook to conduct a very careful clinical study which has been ongoing
since 1974. We found that in order to obtain the degree of clinical precision
we needed to properly test whether or not, in our hands at least, CEA or any
other marker might be useful as a predictor or monitor, we needed to establish
a separate colon and rectum service. Forms were developed and our clinical
information for our patients is now computerized. For each visit, the research
nurse or clinician has to record if disease is present or absent according to
their best clinical judgment, progressive, regressive, or stable since the
patient's previous visit, as well as the evidence whether history, physical
finding or laboratory in which they base their decision. We find that going
back over hosital records as we used to keep them simply did not provide adequate
data. It is important that disease extent be properly staged and that progression
and regression be concisely defined.

Eighty-one patients have now been followed for five years. For Dukes B and
Cukes C patients, CEA level is significant. Dukes B patients with a CEA < 2.5 ng/m
prior to curable surgery show only 2 recurrences out of 31 after 5 years. Dukes
B patients with a CEA > 2.5 ng/ml prior to curative surgery show four recurrences
in 16 patients after 5 years. That is an increase from less than 10 percent to
25 percent. For Dukes C lesions, recurrences on a 5 year period with a pre-
surgical CEA of < 2.5 ng/ml were 6 of 18 or 33 percent. For Dukes C lesions
recurrences over a 5 year period with a pre-surgical CEA > 2.5 ng/ml in our
laboratory, were 8 of 16 or 50 percent. Based on this study, we are sure that
for our patients at least, we like to have a pre-surgical CEA to help in
estimating prognosis. For example, it would be reasonable to give a patient who
is Dukes B with a positive CEA adjuvant chemotherapy if we have such a modality.
To give it to Dukes B, CEA negative patients would be, I believe, a mistake. We
believe that CEA should be considered in stratification for treament studies to
assure no bias.

CONCLUSION

I want to leave our conclusion that the clinical study of tumor markers is a
difficult and demanding one. We believe CEA is proved prognostic and that only
very precise clinical studies can evaluate the true usefulness of a tumor marker.
It is difficult to establish that a marker is truly helpful and that its use
actually improves care and survival.

REFERENCES

. Joint National Cancer Institute of Canada/American Cancer Society Investigation.
. Collaborative Study of a Test for Carcinoembryonic Antigen (CEA) in the Sera
f Patients with Carcinoma of the Colon and Rectum. Can. Med. Assoc. J. 107,
5-33.

almettes, S.C., Moukhtar, M.S., Milhaud, G. Correlation Between Calcitonin and
arcinoembryonic Antigen Levels in Medullary Carcinoma of the Thyroid.
iomedicine (Express) 27. 52-54.

hu, T.M., Murphy, G.P. (1978). Evaluation of Carcinoembryonic Antigen as a
creening Assay in Non-cancer Clinics. Proc. U.I.C.C. XII International Con-
ress, Buenos Aires. In Press.

old, P. and Freedman, S.O. (1965) Demonstration of Tumor-Specific Antigens in
uman Colonic Carcinomata by Immunologic Tolerance and Absorption Techniques.
. Exp. Med. 121. 439-462.

akkinen, I.P. (1976). The FSA Reaction in Early Detection of Gastric Cancer.
ostrom, H. et al. Almquist and Wiksell, Stockholm, 105-117.

olyoke, E.D., Reynoso, G. and Chu, T.M. (1972). Carcinoembryonic Antigen
CEA) in Patients with Carcinoma of the Digestive Tract. Ann. Surg. 176.
59-564.

huster, J., Freedman, S.O., Gold, P. (1977) Increasing the Specificity of the
EA Radioimmunoassay. A. J. Clin. Path. 68. 679-687.

hompson, D.M.P., Krupey, J., Freedman, S.O., and Gold, P. (1969). The Radio-
mmunoassay of Circulating Carcinoembryonic Antigen of the Human Digestive
ystem. Proc. Nat. Acad. Sci. U.S.A. 64, 161-167.

rba, R., Alpert, E., Isselbacher, K.J. (Jan. 1976) Immunological Heterogenecity
f Serum Carcinoembryonic Antigen (CEA). Immunochemistry 13. 87-89.

Alpha-Fetoprotein as a Biological Marker in Cancer Diagnosis

Edward J. Sarcione

New York State Department of Health, Department of Medicine B,
Roswell Park Memorial Institute, Buffalo, NY 14263, U.S.A.

ABSTRACT

This report will review and summarize current information regarding the diagnostic significance and clinical usefulness of alpha fetoprotein measurements in patients with selected types of malignant disease. Alpha fetoprotein in a serum glycoprotein produced by the fetal liver, and found in high concentration in maternal and fetal serum. Shortly after birth, serum alpha fetoprotein levels decrease rapidly and only trace amounts are detected in normal healthy children and adults.

The diagnostic significance of alpha fetoprotein is based on observations that this fetal protein reappears in the serum of a high percentage of patients with primary hepatocellular carcinoma, germ cell tumors of the ovary and testis, and in a lower but significant percentage of some other malignant and non-malignant diseases. In cancer patients, serum alpha fetoprotein apparently originates from the tumor.

Currently available information indicates that alpha fetoprotein is the best characterized, and most specific cancer-associated biological marker for diagnosis of selected types of tumors. Quantitative measurement of this fetal serum protein is found to be clinically useful to: (a) assist in differential diagnosis of primary versus metastatic cancer, (b) follow the clinical course of disease, (c) test for completeness of resection, (d) evaluate response to therapy and (e) detect recurrence of tumor.

KEYWORDS

Alpha-fetoprotein, hepatocellular carcinoma, germ-cell tumors, chorinic gonadotropin.

INTRODUCTION

Alpha fetoprotein (AFP) is a serum glycoprotein with an electrophoretic mobility of an $alpha_1$ globulin which is found in high concentration in fetal and maternal serum, but is present in only trace amounts in normal healthy children and adults. This protein is produced by the fetal liver.

The significance of AFP to oncology is based on observations that elevated levels

159

of this fetal protein reappear in the serum of a high percentage of patients with primary hepatocellular carcinoma and germ cell tumors of the ovary and testis. In cancer patients serum, AFP originates from the tumor.

Since it is detected in both the fetus and tumor bearing hosts, it is classified as an oncofetal protein. AFP was first observed in mice with chemically induced hepatoma by Abelev and co-workers in 1963, then confirmed in humans by Tartarinov in 1964. Currently, AFP is the best characterized and most specific cancer-associated biological marker for the diagnosis and monitoring of treatment of selected types of tumors.

The objective of this report is to review and summarize current information regarding the diagnostic significance and clinical usefulness of AFP measurements in patients with malignant disease.

AFP can be detected and measured in serum by a variety of immunologic methods which vary greatly in their sensitivity. At opposite ends of the spectrum, the Ouchterlony double immunodiffusion gel precipitation technique is the least sensitive detecting approximately 1-3000 ng/ml and enzyme-linked immunoassay and radioimmunoassay are the most sensitive able to detect 1-10 ng/ml. These latter two methods are sufficiently sensitive to detect AFP in normal human serum which ranges from 10-30 ng/ml depending on the laboratory performing the assay.

AFP and Hepatocellular Carcinoma

When radioimmunoassay is used, many investigators have shown that approximately 72-93% of all patients with primary liver cancer have AFP levels elevated above the normal rnage (Abelev, 1974; Hirai and Miyaji, 1973, Masseyeff, 1974). This incidence is influenced by the age and sex of the patients, and also by the size of the tumor. Elevated AFP levels are seen more frequently in younger patients and in patients with large tumors, and is about 20% more frequent in men than in women with primary liver cancer. There also appears to be geographic and ethanic differences, but these may be explained by differences in age, sex, tumor size and detection methods used.

Extensive studies in some African countries have shown that apparently healthy individuals may have AFP levels in the range of 30-500 ng/ml, however, whether these represent high-risk subjects remains to be established (Purves and co-workers, 1973).

It should be pointed out that in all groups examined from 5-10% of histologically confirmed hepatocellular carcinomas are not accompanied by an increased AFP level. In addition, elevated AFP levels are also observed in patients with non-malignant liver disease of all types. For example, in a large series 27-36% of patients with cirrhosis, 35-53% of patients with viral and alcoholic hepatitis have elevated AFP levels (Nishi and Hirai, 1973). Furthermore, elevated AFP levels have been observed in most patients with neonatal hepatitis, childhood cirrhosis in India and hereditary tyrosinemia (Nayak and co-workers, 1972; Belanger and co-workers, 1973). These liver diseases comprise the main source of false positive results in the diagnosis of primary liver cancer. The elevated serum AFP levels found in such patients is best explained as reflecting hepatocellular damage and liver regeneration.

AFP and Other Malignant Diseases

Although an elevated AFP level is generally considered to be specific for liver

ind germ cell tumors, it should be mentioned that many investigators have observed
a lower but definite association of elevated AFP with other types of endodermally
derived tumors. For example, 19% of patients with gastric cancer and 25% with
liver metastases have elevated AFP; 13% with colon rectal cancer and 17% with
liver metastasis; 20% with pancreatic cancer and 22% with liver metastasis; (Ahai
and Kato, 1973; McIntrye and co-worker, 1975). The observation that the majority
of these patients have widely disseminated disease suggest that elevated AFP is
due to hepatic metastasis and production of AFP by damaged and regenerating hepatic cells. On the other hand, its quite possible that gastrointestinal tract
tumors can synthesize AFP, since the fetal intestine is known to synthesize this
protein.

Serial quantitative measurement of AFP can usually discriminate between most patients with primary liver cancer and those with non-malignant liver disease .

1. In general, the degree of elevation serves as an important distinction.
Most patients with non-malignant disease have serum AFP levels below 500 ng/ml
while a serum AFP concentration above this indicates the presence of primary liver
cancer 97% of the time (Ruoslahti and co-workers, 1974).

2. Furthermore, elevated serum AFP levels in non-malignant liver disease
tend to fluctuate or be transient and return to normal rapidly with remission of
disease. On the other hand, a steady or rising serum AFP level is more likely
to indicate primary liver cancer.

These observations stress the importance of performing serial quantitative
measurements of AFP rather than relying on a single measurement.

Partial Hepatectomy

The most valuable use of serum AFP measurements in hepatocellular carcinoma is to
follow the effectiveness of therapy (McIntyre and co-workers, 1976).

Following surgical removal of a primary tumor by partial hepatectomy, complete removal of tumor will produce a rapid decline of AFP to normal levels (Hirai and
co-workers, 1973). A slower rate of decrease or failure of AFP to decrease to
the normal range usually indicates residual tumor. Increasing AFP levels almost
certainly indicate recurrence of tumor.

Intra-Arterial Chemotherapy

Intra-arterial administration of methotrexate, dichloromethotrexate, 5-Fluoroura-
cil or adriamycin to patients is associated in some patients with primary liver
cancer with a marked decrease in AFP levels which parallels the clinical response,
and little or no change in other such patients. In all cases, however, there was
eventually recurrence of the tumor within 3-7 months with a return to elevated
AFP levels (Purves and co-workers, 1973). It is reasonable to assume that as more
effective chemotherapeutic agents are developed, serial measurement of AFP will be
of greater value in following the effectiveness of therapy in primary liver cancer.

AFP in Germ Cell Tumors

Elevated serum levels of AFP was also shown to be associated with teratocarcinomas
of the testis and ovary independentally by Abelev and by Masopust and their respective co-workers in 1967-68. It is now well established that approximately

69-75% of all such patients depending on the histologic type of tumor have elevated serum AFP levels when measured by radioimmunoassay. In general, both positive
incidence and serum concentrations of AFP found in patients with teratocarcinomas
is lower than in patients with primary liver cancer.

AFP and HCG

Braunstein and co-workers, 1973 and Waldmann and McIntyre, 1974 made important
contributions by demonstrating that the positive incidence of detection of these
tumors can be substantially increased by measuring both AFP and human chorinic
gonadotropin (HCG) levels in the serum. While only 16 and 14%, respectively, of
patients with teratocarcinoma of the testis had elevations of AFP and HCG, 59%
had elevations of both AFP and HCG (Waldmann and co-workers, 1977).

Teilum's Classification of Germ Cell Tumors

The relationship of elevated AFP and HCG levels in patients with germ cell tumors
is best understood when these tumors are classified histologically as advocated
by Teilum, 1965.

According to this classification, embryologically differentiated forms of the
totipotential stem cells of embryonal carcinoma are subdivided into three types
(1) endodermal sinus or yolk sac tumor, (2) choriocarcinoma and (3) teratoma.
Any combination of these and embryologically undifferentiated embryonal carcinoma
may occur.

AFP and HCG: Germ Cell Tumors

The occurence of elevated serum levels of AFP and HCG in patients with germ cell
tumors of testis and ovary, when classified histologically as advocated by
Teilum, is summarized (Norgaard-Pederson, 1976). 1) Elevations of serum AFP are
not seen in patients with pure siminomas of the testis or dysgerminomas of the
ovary, 2) In mixed germ cell tumors or embryonal cell carcinomas, elevations of
both AFP and the β chain of human chroninic gonadotropin may be seen singlally or
together. In those instances where serum AFP levels are elevated, careful histo-
pathological examination of the tumor usually reveals yolk sac elements, while
HCG elevations are associated with the presence of syncytotrophoblastic tumor
elements. 3) In pure tumors of extraembryonic origin derived from yolk sac elements (endocermal sinus tumors), AFP elevations are always present and HCG is absent. In pure choriocarcinoma the converse is true. HCG is always present and
AFP is absent. 4) In teratoblastomas, AFP and HCG are usually absent; increased
levels of either marker may, however, be present in those tumors which possess
small areas of extraembryonic tumor tissue.

AFP and HCG Levels in Treated Patients

The serial measurement of AFP and HCG is of special value in monitoring the effectiveness of therapy in patients with germ cell tumors of the testis. Perlin and
co-workers, 1976, showed that a number of different patterns were observed. In 9%
of these patients there was no clinical response to therapy and the AFP and HCG
levels increased until the patients death. In another 9% of the patients, both
markers declined to normal following surgery and chemotherapy and remained within
the normal range throughout the period of observation without recurrence of tumor.
These patients did not have recurrence of their tumor and again the AFP and HCG

levels paralelled the clinical course of the disease. In 36% of the patients, both markers declined dramatically after surgery and chemotherapy, then there were increasing levels of both markers with recurrence of the tumor. In 40% of the patients, however, following an initial decline of both markers, one marker fell to within the normal range and remained at a normal level after recurrence of the tumor. The other marker either fell transiently to the normal level after recurrence of the tumor. The other marker either fell transiently to the normal level or remained above the normal. With recurrence of the tumor this second marker returned to a very high level. This suggests that the cellular origin of these two markers is different.

SUMMARY AND CONCLUSIONS

1. Serum AFP measurement is a necessary adjunct for evaluation and management of patients with hepatocellular and germ cell malignancy.
2. When such tumors are suspected, AFP monitoring should begin before surgery:
    a) Complete removal of tumor will produce a decline of AFP equal to its 5-6 day half-life.
    b) A slower rate of decrease or failure of AFP to decrease to the normal range usually indicates residual tumor
3. In both surgically and chemotherapy treated patients, without clinical evidence of disease, AFP levels should be followed long term.
    a) Increasing AFP levels indicate recurrent tumor, unless patient developed hepatitis.
    b) Appropriate diagnostic and therapeutic measures should be instituted while the tumor mass is small and more easily eradicated.

REFERENCES

Abelev, G.I. (1974) Alpha fetoprotein as a marker of embryospecific differentiations in normal and tumor tissues. Transplant. Rev. 20, 3-37.

Abelev, G.I., Assercritova, I.V., Kraevsky, N.A., Perova, S.D. and Perevodchikova, N.I. (1967) Embryonal serum alpha-globulin in cancer patients: diagnostic value. Int. J. Cancer 2, 551-558.

Abelev, G.I., Perova, S.D., Khramkova, N.I., Postnikova, Z.A. and Irlin, I.S. (1973) Production of embryonal alpha-globulin by transplantable mouse hepatomas. Transpl. Bull. 1: 174-180.

Belanger, L., Belanger, M., Prive, L., Larochelle, J., Tremblay, M. and Auben, G. (1973) Tryosinemie hereditaire de alpha-1-fetoproteimie. Path. et Biol. 21, 449-455.

Braunstein, G.D., Vaitukaitis, J.L., Carbone, P.P. and Ross, G.T. (1973) Ectopic production of human chorionic gonadotropin by neoplasms. Ann. Intern Med. 78, 39-45.

Hirai, H. and Miyaji, T. (eds) (1973) Alpha-fetoprotein and hepatoma. Gann. Monogram Cancer Res. 14, 1-320.

Masopust, J., Jithier, K., Radl, J., Koutecky, J. and Kotal, L. (1968) Occurence of fetoprotein in patients with neoplasms and non-neoplastic diseases. Int. J. Cancer.

Masseyeff, R. (ed). (1974) Colloque, L'alpha-fetoproteine, INSERM, Paris 1-607.

McIntyre, K.R., Vogel, C.L., Primack, A., Waldmann, T.A. and Kyalwaz, S.K. (1976) Effect of surgical and chemotherapeutic treatment on alpha fetoprotein levels in patients with hepatocellular carcinoma. Cancer 37, 677-683.

McIntyre, K.R., Waldmann, T.A., Moertel, C.G. and Go, V.C.W. (1975) Serum alpha-fetoprotein in patients with neoplasm levels in people susceptible to primary liver cancer in Southern Africa. Gann Monogr. Cancer Res. 14, 51-66.

Nayak, N.C., Chawla, V., Malavivya, A.N. and Chandras, R.K. (1972) Alpha fetopro-

E. J. Sarcione

      tein in Indian childhood cirrhosis. Lancet 1, 68-72.
Nishi, S. and Hirai, H. (1973) Radioimmunoassay of alpha-fetoprotein in hepatoma,
      other liver diseases and pregnancy. Gann. Monogr. Cancer Res. 14, 79.
Norgaard-Pedersen, B. (1976) Human alpha-fetoprotein. A review of current metho-
      dological and clinical studies. Scand. J. of Immunol. 5, supp #4, 1-45.
Perlin, E., Engeler, J.E., Jr., Edson, M., Kark, D., McIntrye, K.R. and Waldemann,
      T.A. (1976). The value of serial measurement of both human choronic gonado-
      tropin and alpha fetoprotein for monitoring germinal cell tumors. Cancer
      37, 215-219.
Purves, L.R., Manso, C. and Torres, F.O. (1973) Serum alphafetoprotein levels
      in people susceptible to primary liver cancer in Southern Africa. Gann
      Monogr. Cancer Res. 14, 51-66.
Tartarinov, Y.S. (1974) Detection of embryospecific alpha-globulin in the blood
      sera of patients with primary liver tumor. Vop. Med Khim 10, 90-91.
Teilum, G. (1965) Classification of endodermal sinus tumor (mesoblastoma
      vitellinum) and so-called embryonal carcinoma of the ovary. Acta Path Micro-
      biol. Scand. 64: 407-429.
Waldmann, T.A., and McIntrye, K.R. (1974) The use of radioimmunoassay for alpha
      fetoprotein in the diagnosis of malignancy. Cancer 34, 1510-1515.

Terminal Deoxynucleotidyl Transferase as a Tumor Cell Marker in Leukemia and Lymphoma: Results from 1000 Patients

J. J. Hutton*, M. S. Coleman*, T. P. Keneklis** and F. J. Bollum**

*VA Hospital, Departments of Medicine and Biochemistry,
University of Kentucky, Lexington, Kentucky, U.S.A.
**Department of Biochemistry, Uniformed Services University of the
Health Sciences, Bethesda, Maryland, U.S.A.

ABSTRACT

Terminal deoxynucleotidyl transferase (TDT) is an unusual DNA polymerase that is normally found only in cells from thymus and bone marrow. It may, however, be present in large amounts in malignant cells from certain patients with leukemia and lymphoma. We present an assessment of the usefulness of TDT as a tumor cell marker, based upon quantitative and/or immunofluorescence measurements on tissues from over 1000 patients. TDT serves as a marker of certain classes of poorly differentiated lymphoblasts. Measurements of TDT may be of value both in the classification of hematologic neoplasms and in the detection of residual disease after treatment. The immunofluorescence assay is particularly sensitive and can be applied to fixed specimens of peripheral blood, bone marrow, lymph nodes and other tissues. Measurement of TDT activity in cells by quantitative enzymatic assay generally, but not always, correlates well with results of the immunofluorescence assay. Occasionally cells have unexpectedly high or low levels of TDT. More detailed knowledge of the biology and biochemistry of human TDT must be obtained before we can interpret some of the changes seen in human disease.

Relatively effective regimens are now available for the treatment of certain types of leukemia and lymphoma. All of these are toxic to patients and most involve complex protocols of administration of drugs and radiation. Accurate classification of leukemias and lymphomas into pathological types related to cell of origin is desirable because of differences in response to treatment. Stratification by type of disease is particularly important in clinical trials where the effectiveness of a new treatment is measured in a large number of patients. Groups of patients who respond particularly well or poorly need to be identified in a reproducible fashion. For example, most children with acute lymphoblastic leukemia of the "null" cell type do well with present treatment regimens, whereas those with T or B marked lymphoblasts do poorly and will require modified programs of therapy. The distinction between myeloid and lymphoid leukemias is difficult in a significant number of patients, yet it should be made accurately because of the different response of the two diseases to different types of drugs.

Estimation of the number of residual malignant cells during the course of treatment of a tumor is also a most important problem in oncology. Theoretically this should be relatively easy in leukemia because the blasts circulate in the peripheral blood

165

and bone marrow. Specimens of blood and marrow are readily obtained, yet there are no truly sensitive methods of detecting small numbers of malignant cells. Whether there are residual tumor cells and in what numbers are critically important questions in deciding whether chemotherapy has been effective. Physicians designing protocols for the treatment of leukemia and lymphoma debate endlessly about duration and type of chemotherapy after initial induction of remission. For example, what is the endpoint for chemotherapy in children with acute lymphoblastic leukemia?

Cytologic and cytochemical criteria have proved useful in the classification of leukemias and lymphomas. Although lymphocytes appear morphologically homogeneous, they are functionally and biochemically heterogeneous. There are several immunologic and biochemical markers of cell type and these have been applied to the classification of hematologic malignancies (Filippa and others, 1978 ; Gordon and others, 1978; Gralnick and others, 1977; Hoffbrand and others, 1977). Measurements of cell membrane receptors have been successful in acute lymphoblastic leukemia (ALL) and are of clinical relevance because of the different prognoses of null, T, and B cell disease. Quantitative measurements of the activity of terminal deoxynucleotidyl transferase (TDT) in neoplastic cells from bone marrow and peripheral blood can generally distinguish acute lymphoblastic leukemia from other types of acute leukemia (Gordon and others, 1978; Hutton and Coleman, 1976; McCaffrey and others, 1975). Measurement of TDT may also be of value in classifying non-Hodgkin's lymphomas. TDT appears to be a marker specifically related to the occurrence of certain classes of poorly differentiated lymphoblasts. Antisera to TDT have been prepared (Bollum, 1975a; Kung, Gottlieb, and Baltimore, 1976) and permit the easy cytological identification of TDT containing cells in peripheral blood, bone marrow, lymph nodes, spinal fluid, pleural effusions, and other tissues of relevance to patient management (Bollum and others, 1978; Hutton and Bollum, 1978). Detection of very small numbers of residual lymphoblasts in tissue from patients treated for leukemia or lymphoma may be possible using immunological techniques. We will discuss our initial assessment of the usefulness of TDT as a tumor cell marker, based upon quantitative and/or immunofluorescence measurements on tissues from over 1000 patients.

Terminal transferase catalyzes the addition of deoxynucleoside triphosphates to the 3´-hydroxyl ends of oligo- or polydeoxynucleotide initiators without template instruction (Bollum, 1974). This enzyme is normally present at high levels only in the thymus and low levels are found in the bone marrow. It has not been detected in cells from peripheral blood or lymph nodes (Chang, 1971; Coleman and others, 1974). Since an activity of this kind might cause modification of DNA sequence, it has been suggested that the enzyme could participate in somatic diversification of lymphoid precursors during differentiation (Baltimore, 1974; Bollum, 1975b).

In order to compare TDT activities in cells from different patients, it is essential that the conditions of extraction and assay be optimal and reproducible (Coleman, 1977a, 1977b). Clinical samples from patients with hematologic disease present special problems for the biochemist. Frequently, only small numbers of malignant cells can be obtained, so the mechanics of the assay must be tailored to meet this condition. At least 10^7 purified nucleated cells are required for a reliable TDT assay.

Terminal transferase activities in nucleated cells from the bone marrow of patients without leukemia or non-Hodgkin's lymphoma served as "controls" in our studies (Table 1). Our cytochemical criteria for the classification of adult leukemia have been described (Gordon and others, 1978). The mean TDT activity (1 unit = 1 nmole of dGTP polymerized onto poly d(pA)$_{50}$/hr) was 2.7 units/10^8 cells in 160 specimens of adult marrow. The frequency distribution of TDT activities in marrow from adult controls is illustrated in Figure 1. Statistically, activities do not follow a normal distribution, but have a distinct tailing of activities greater than the mean. The 5 patients with the highest values in marrow (14 to 27 units/10^8 cells)

Table 1. Activities of terminal deoxynucleotidyl transferase in nucleated cells from the peripheral blood and bone marrow.[1]

Type of specimen	Age Group	Bone Marrow					Peripheral Blood				
		No.	Mean	Median	Range	SD	No.	Mean	Median	Range	SD
Control	Adult	160	2.7	1.6	0-27	3.7	16	1.0	1.7	0-12	3.1
	Pediatric	198	5.9	2.6	0-219	19	51	0.5	1.0	0-3.2	0.7
Acute lymphoblastic leukemia	Adult	9	181	50	25-426	172	13	116	68	17-530	132
	Pediatric	118	85	40	0-694	122	188	70	19	0-1790	185
Acute myeloblastic leukemia	Adult	12	3.0	1.0	0.1-13	4.8	15	5.3	1.0	0-29	9.9
	Pediatric	31	8.0	1.5	0-77	19	12	2.2	1.0	0-13	3.9
Acute myelomonocytic leukemia	Adult	15	6.6	1.5	0.1-43	11.7	17	6.3	1.0	0-74	18
	Pediatric	13	33	6.1	1.2-293	79	6	4.8	3.8	0-9.9	3.6
Acute monocytic leukemia	Adult	9	1.2	0.5	0-6.0	1.9	4	0.7	1.0	0.3-1.3	0.4
	Pediatric	0									
Acute undifferentiated leukemia	Adult	15	53	19	0.2-157	53	5	8.6	4.0	0.1-30	13
	Pediatric	13	12	1.5	0-119	32	8	0.7	0.8	0-1.4	0.5
Chronic myelogenous leukemia	Adult	14	2.4	0.6	0-10.2	3.4	6	1.6	0.7	0.4-5.8	2.1
	Pediatric[2]	15	33	1.0	0-357	93	12	29	1.0	0-333	96
(blast crisis)	Adult	6	52	4.1	0.5-152	70	5	9.1	17	1.8-45	19
Chronic lymphocytic leukemia	Adult	7	0.7	0.8	0-3.4	1.3	7	1.3	0.7	0-5.1	1.8
Lymphoma (Non-Hodgkins)	Adult	14	32	4.7	0.5-127	50	11	37	1.0	0.1-275	83
	Pediatric[3]	36	11	2.6	0-63	18	16	6.8	1.0	0-42	12

[1]Specimens were assayed from patients with a variety of diseases. Control groups included marrow and peripheral blood from normal people and from those with diseases not including leukemia or non-Hodgkin's lymphoma. The numbers of specimens, each from a different patient, are listed. The mean, median, range and standard deviation of transferase activities in the specimens are recorded. Adult patients were over 15 years of age and most pediatric specimens were from children less than 15 years of age. Leukemic patients had not received chemotherapy.
[2]For children with chronic myelogenous leukemia, patients in chronic and accelerated (blastic) phase were combined.
[3]Lymphoma specimens from children included both bone marrow and cells from malignant pleural effusions.

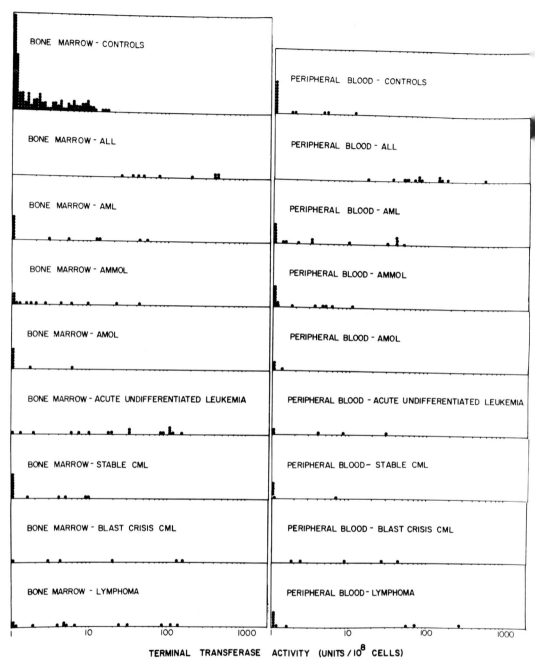

TERMINAL TRANSFERASE ACTIVITY (UNITS / 10^8 CELLS)

Figure 1.   Distribution of terminal transferase activities
in nucleated cells from the bone marrow and peripheral blood of human adults. Each point represents
one patient. None had received chemotherapy.

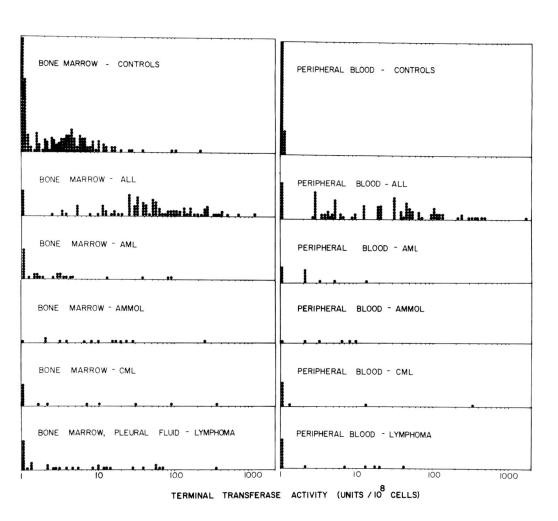

TERMINAL TRANSFERASE ACTIVITY (UNITS / 10^8 CELLS)

Figure 2.   Distribution of terminal transferase activities
in nucleated cells from the bone marrow and
peripheral blood of children. Each point
represents one patient. None had received
chemotherapy.

carried diagnoses of idiopathic thrombocytopenia (2 cases), paroxysmal nocturnal hemoglobinuria, idiopathic leukopenia, and rhabdomyosarcoma. None of these patients has developed acute leukemia or lymphoma during follow up periods of over 1 year (the patient with rhabdomyosarcoma died after several months). We have previously reported the normal activities of TDT in marrow as 2.5 ± 1.1 (SD) units/10^8 cells based on 17 morphologically normal marrows from adults without malignant disease (Hutton and Coleman, 1976). Bone marrow from 198 children without leukemia or non-Hodgkin's lymphoma contained 5.9 ± 19 (SD) units of TDT per 10^8 cells (Table 1). The median value was 2.6 units/10^8 cells, but the range was 0-219. The distribution of values is illustrated in Figure 2. Values greater than 27 units/10^8 cells were observed in 5 patients who did not develop leukemia or lymphoma during periods of 1 year or more after the high value was observed. Diagnoses were: pulmonary actinomycosis, idiopathic thrombocytopenic purpura, and neuroblastoma (3 cases). Nucleated cells from peripheral blood of adults and children usually contain 1.0 and 0.5 units of TDT activity/10^8 cells, respectively (Table 1). This activity is at the lower limits of sensitivity of the enzyme assay for TDT as we run it and may not be significantly different from zero. Higher values are occasionally observed, as in the case of an adult female with breast cancer whose peripheral blood contained 12 units TDT/10^8 cells, despite the absence of blasts.

TDT may be present in large amounts in cancer cells from certain patients with leukemia and lymphoma. Results of assay of nucleated cells from the bone marrow and peripheral blood are summarized in Table 1, Figures 1 and 2. Most patients diagnosed as having acute lymphoblastic leukemia (ALL) have markedly elevated TDT activities in cells from their bone marrow and peripheral blood. There is a significant correlation ($r = 0.73$) between TDT activity in peripheral lymphoblasts and activity in bone marrow (Greenwood and others, 1977). Blasts in ALL can be classified as null, T or B on the basis of surface membrane markers and these 3 categories of disease have distinctly different prognoses. Average TDT activity is significantly lower in T marked lymphoblasts than in null marked lymphoblasts, and is much lower in B than in either T or null lymphoblasts (Coleman and others, 1978). In 9 patients with ALL shown in Figure 2, the bone marrow contained 1 unit or less of TDT/10^8 cells. Among these we can identify two variants of ALL where TDT is usually low. In 4 patients, 50% of the blasts bore surface immunoglobulin (intense multifocal pattern with anti-IgM) so the leukemia was of B cell origin (Coleman and others, 1978). Cytologic features were indistinguishable from Burkitt's leukemia. A second group of patients diagnosed as ALL are thought to represent a "pre-B" cell neoplasm and typically have cytoplasmic IgM without surface immunoglobulin. Blasts in this variant of childhood ALL frequently contain little or no TDT activity (Vogler and others, 1978). Further definition of TDT activities in variants of ALL will require more detailed cytochemical and immunological analyses than have yet been done.

In patients with cytochemically confirmed acute myelogenous and myelomonocytic leukemia, TDT activity in bone marrow and peripheral blood is generally within the "control" range and much lower than in acute lymphoblastic leukemia (Table 1, Figures 1 and 2). In a careful study of TDT activity, membrane markers, and cytochemistry in adult acute leukemia, 3 of 27 patients with acute myeloblastic leukemia, zero of 14 with acute myelomonocytic, and zero of 7 with acute monocytic leukemia had high levels of transferase in their blasts (Gordon and others, 1978). As greater numbers of patients are studied, it appears that approximately 10% of patients with an acute myeloid or lymphoid leukemia have TDT activities in blasts that are higher or lower than expected, respectively. Whether the presence or absence of TDT is associated with a specific prognosis or response to treatment is not known.

Leukemic cells from some patients do not react positively with common cytochemical strains such as Sudan Black and periodic-acid Schiff (PAS). Such leukemias are said to be undifferentiated and cannot be classified as lymphoid or myeloid on the basis of standard morphology and cytochemistry. The activity of TDT in cells from adults and children with acute undifferentiated leukemia ranges widely in value (Table 1). High values of TDT may imply a lymphoid origin and suggest therapy appropriate for acute lymphoblastic leukemia. Certainly measurements of terminal transferase can serve as an objective marker in the classification of undifferentiated leukemias and will be particularly useful if the natural history of the diseases and/or effective therapy are related to TDT levels (Gordon and others, 1978).

Patients with chronic myelogenous leukemia in the stable phase generally have low levels of TDT in their blasts, whereas 20-30% of patients in blastic crisis have high levels of TDT. This has been observed in both children and adults (Table 1 and: Hutton and Coleman, 1976; Marks, Baltimore and McCaffrey, 1978; Sarin, Anderson and Gallo, 1976; Srivastava and others, 1977). Patients with high levels of TDT in their blasts may respond favorably, although transiently, to treatment with vincristine and prednisone.

High levels of TDT can be present in malignant cells of patients with non-Hodgkin's lymphoma. This includes cells from diverse sites such as bone marrow, peripheral blood, pleural fluid, lymph nodes and testicle. We have not observed high values in patients with Hodgkin's disease or chronic lymphocytic leukemia (Table 1). Non-Hodgkin's lymphomas with high levels of TDT are poorly differentiated and in many cases cannot be clearly distinguished from acute lymphoblastic leukemia. We evaluated cell surface markers in seven adult patients with lymphoma leukemia and found high TDT in cases that typed as null by membrane markers (Gordon and others, 1978). Other investigators have reported high levels of TDT in certain patients with undifferentiated T or null lymphoblastic lymphoma (Donlon, Jaffe and Braylon, 1977). The TDT-membrane marker relationship needs to be explored more fully in a larger series of patients.

When patients with typical null or T marked ALL relapse, TDT has been markedly elevated in all bone marrow samples examined (Greenwood and others, 1977). The mean TDT values at relapse did not differ significantly from the mean value of a comparable, but different, group of patients at initial diagnosis. These observations immediately raise the question of whether TDT can serve as a tumor cell marker.

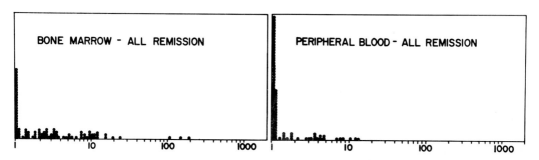

Figure 3.   Distribution of terminal transferase activities
in nucleated cells from the bone marrow and
peripheral blood of patients with acute lymphoblastic leukemia in remission.

If so, then quantitative assay of TDT in marrow and peripheral blood might be used to estimate the completeness of disease remission and to predict disease relapse. The distributions of TDT activities in nucleated cells from the peripheral blood a▪ marrow of patients with acute lymphoblastic leukemia in remission are illustrated ˙ Figure 3. The mean activity in 95 specimens of marrow was 8.4 units/10^8 cells, median 2.4, range 0-196, SD = 27.1. Corresponding values in peripheral blood were: mean 1.6, median 1.0, range 0-14, SD = 2.7. As in the case of "control" specimens shown in Figures 1 and 2, there is a tail of values greater than the mean, so it is difficult to interpret isolated high values such as 10 units of TDT/10^8 cells. Thre specimens of marrow contained greater than 100 units of TDT/10^8 cells, although morphologically the marrows appeared normal. Insufficient data are available to state whether high values of TDT can be used to predict relapse before the hematolc gist can detect relapse by morphological examination of the marrow and peripheral blood.

Most clinical reports on TDT have dealt primarily with its activity in extracts of cells from bone marrow or peripheral blood. Immunological techniques utilizing antiserum to TDT represent powerful new tools for study of the cyto- and histochem-istry of the enzyme (Barton, Goldschneider and Bollum, 1976; Bollum and others, 1978; Goldschneider and others, 1977; Gregoire and others, 1977; Hutton and Bollum, 1978). Quantitation of the number and identity of TDT containing cells is poten-tially much more informative than quantitative assay of activity in homogenates of tissues in various diseases. For example, in Figure 3 the fact that TDT activity is elevated in some patients with acute lymphoblastic leukemia in remission is interesting and suggests early relapse. However, elevated values of TDT activity can be observed in marrow from patients without malignant disease (Figures 1 and 2) High values could be due to increased numbers of normal cells containing TDT, in-creased amounts of TDT in normal cells perhaps in response to a physiologic inducer or to the presence of abnormal cells containing TDT.

Terminal transferase can be visually demonstrated in cells by the extremely sensi-tive technique of immunofluorescence (Gregoire and others, 1977; Bollum, 1978). The validity of immunological techniques is absolutely dependent on the specificity of the immunological reagents. Homogeneous, monovalent antibody to TDT has been prepared (Bollum, 1975) and used as the primary reagent for immunofluorescence studies on cells, with a secondary reagent consisting of fluorescein labeled-goat-F(ab´)2-anti-rabbit IgG. These immunospecific reagents can be applied to cells fixed with a variety of agents such as methanol. Since TDT is located within the cells and is absent from the surface membrane, immunofluorescence techniques cannot be applied to living cells. Specimens of peripheral blood and bone marrow were collected from patients with many types of diseases. The activity of TDT was quan-titatively measured in nucleated cells and the percentage of cells reacting with antiserum to TDT was determined. The correlations between TDT activity and immuno-fluorescence in 70 specimens of peripheral blood and 103 specimens of bone marrow are illustrated in Figure 4. While it is generally true that low (less than 2 units 10^8 cells) levels of TDT activity are associated with a small percentage of cells reacting with antiserum to TDT, exceptions are observed. One patient diagnosed as acute lymphoblastic leukemia in remission had 0.9 units TDT/10^8 cells in peripheral blood, but 53% of nucleated cells in the specimen reacted with antiserum to TDT. In bone marrow, 2 patients diagnosed as acute lymphoblastic leukemia had 3.4 and 8.0 units TDT/10^8 cells, but 100% and 60% of cells reacted with antiserum. One patient diagnosed as acute lymphoblastic leukemia had 176 units TDT/10^8 cells in marrow, but less than 1% of the cells reacted with antiserum. The discrepancies between the percentage of immunofluorescent cells and quantitative enzymatic acti-vity suggest heterogeneity among cells in content of TDT, as well as the possibility of antigenically reactive enzyme that is enzymatically inactive. Studies on rat thymocytes have clearly demonstrated heterogeneity among cells in level of TDT acti-vity as well as discrepancies between percentage of cells reacting with anti-TDT and enzymatic activity (Barton, Goldschneider and Bollum, 1976; Gregoire and others,

1977). In rats there are differences in the intracellular distribution of enzyme among TDT containing cells of bone marrow and thymus. TDT is located predominately in the cytoplasm of small thymocytes from adult animals, but is within the nucleus of bone marrow cells. Differences in intracellular distribution may be of biological significance and may assist in the morphological classification of cells. There is little or no information about the distribution of TDT within human cells. Such information may be of value in classifying leukemias and lymphomas, as well as in distinguishing benign from malignant cells.

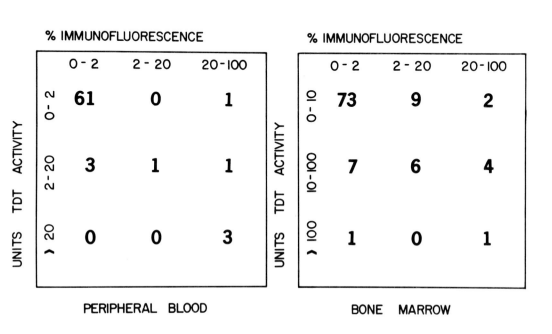

Figure 4. Specimens of peripheral blood and bone marrow were collected from patients with many types of diseases. The activity of TDT was quantitatively measured in nucleated cells and the percentage of cells reacting with antiserum to TDT was determined. The number of patients falling into each of 9 classes of TDT activity and TDT immunofluorescence is recorded in the table.

Applications of the immunofluorescence procedure to fixed specimens of peripheral blood, bone marrow, and lymph nodes opens a new dimension to the diagnosis of leukemia and lymphoma. The use of TDT immunofluorescence with standard blood and bone marrow specimens, as well as tissue sections, spinal fluid, and other effusions, provides a means of assessing the presence of certain types of malignant lymphoblasts. The results are strikingly specific and, in contrast to the quantitative assay, can be performed on ordinary clinical specimens in a short time and in an ordinary clinical laboratory. Detection and characterization of relatively small

numbers of cells containing TDT can probably be automated using fluorescence activated cell counting. This technique requires that cells be in suspension. Since
TDT is an internal rather than surface antigen, the cell membrane must be rendered
permeable to antibodies. Automated detection and characterization of cells reacting with antiserum may be particularly important in detecting small numbers of
malignant cells in patients who have been treated for leukemia or lymphoma and are
thought to be in complete clinical remission. Quantitative biochemical assays are
cumbersome and may not be sufficiently sensitive for this task. Evaluation of TDT
or any other marker as a diagnostic aid requires a large experience with readily
available materials. Immunofluorescent staining on dried specimens seems the
simplest way to gain this experience. Development of a standardized, readily
available supply of immunospecific reagents would be the most direct route to evaluation.

We conclude that TDT activity and antigen are useful objective markers of certain
types of malignant lymphoid cells and can be of value in the classification of
hematologic neoplasms. Whether measurements of TDT will be useful in predicting
the response of tumors to treatment is not known, but clinical trials to answer
this question are in progress. Development of immunofluorescence techniques for
detection of TDT in single cells makes assay of TDT more readily available. It
also greatly increases the probability that TDT can serve as a sensitive marker of
tumor cells and be used to detect residual cancer in treated patients. The biology
of TDT is poorly understood. More detailed knowledge of the normal distribution,
function, and regulation of this enzyme must be obtained before we can interpret
some of the changes in TDT activity and distribution that have been observed in
human disease.

ACKNOWLEDGMENTS

We thank the following physicians who provided many of the specimens used in this
research: Drs. M. F. Greenwood, P. Holland, B. Lampkin, C. Krill, R. Vogler, D.
Gordon, P. DeSimone, J. Gockerman and O. Nelson.

REFERENCES

Baltimore, D. (1974). Is terminal deoxynucleotidyl transferase a somatic mutagen
    in lymphocytes? *Nature*, **248**, 409-411.
Barton, R., I. Goldschneider, and F. J. Bollum. (1976). The distribution of termi-
    nal deoxynucleotidyl transferase (TdT) among subsets of thymocytes in the rat.
    J. Immunol., **116**, 462-468.
Bollum, F. J. (1974). Terminal deoxynucleotidyl transferase. In P. D. Boyer (Ed.),
    The Enzymes, Vol. 10. Academic Press, New York. pp. 145-171.
Bollum, F. J. (1975a). Antibody to terminal deoxynucleotidyl transferase. Proc.
    Natl. Acad. Sci., **72**, 4119-4122.
Bollum, F. J. (1975b). Terminal deoxynucleotidyl transferase: Source of immuno-
    logical diversity? In R. K. Zahn (Ed.), Karl-August-Forster Lectures, Vol. 14,
    Franz Steiner Verlag, Wiesbaden, W. Germany. pp. 1-47.
Bollum, F. J. (1978). Deoxynucleotide-polymerizing enzymes in mammalian cells:
    Immunofluorescence. In P. Chandra (Ed.), Antiviral Mechanisms for the Control
    of Neoplasia. North Holland Publishing Co., New York, New York.
Bollum, F. J., T. P. Keneklis, J. A. Donlon, H. R. Gralnick, and E. Jaffe. (1978).
    Immunofluorescence assay for terminal deoxynucleotidyl transferase in leukemia
    and lymphoma. Abstract XVII. International Congress of Hematology, Paris,
    France.
Chang, L. M. S. (1971). Development of terminal deoxynucleotidyl transferase
    activity in embryonic calf thymus gland. Biochem. Biophys. Res. Commun., **44**,
    124-131.

Coleman, M. S. (1977a). Terminal deoxynucleotidyl transferase: characterization of extraction and assay conditions from human and calf tissue. Arch. Biochem. Biophys., 182, 525-532.

Coleman, M. S. (1977b). A critical comparison of commonly used procedures for the assay of terminal deoxynucleotidyl transferase in crude tissue extracts. Nucleic Acids Res., 4, 4305-4312.

Coleman, M. S., M. F. Greenwood, J. J. Hutton, P. Holland, B. Lampkin, C. Krill, and J. E. Kostelic. (1978). Adenosine deaminase, terminal deoxynucleotidyl transferase, and cell surface markers in childhood acute leukemia. Blood, (in press).

Coleman, M. S., J. J. Hutton, P. DeSimone, and F. J. Bollum. (1974). Terminal deoxyribonucleotidyl transferase in human leukemia. Proc. Natl. Acad. Sci., 71, 4404-4408.

Donlon, J. A., E. S. Jaffe, and R. C. Braylon. (1977). Terminal deoxynucleotidyl transferase in malignant lymphomas. New Engl. J. Med., 297, 461-464.

Filippa, D. A., P. H. Lieberman, R. A. Erlandson, B. Koziner, F. P. Siegal, A. Turnbull, A. Zimring, and R. A. Good. (1978). A study of malignant lymphomas using light and ultramicroscopic, cytochemical and immunologic technics. Am. J. Med., 64, 259-268.

Goldschneider, I., K. E. Gregoire, R. W. Barton, and F. J. Bollum. (1977). Demonstration of terminal deoxynucleotidyl transferase in thymocytes by immunofluorescence. Proc. Natl. Acad. Sci., 74, 734-738.

Gordon, D. S., J. J. Hutton, R. V. Smalley, L. M. Meyer, and W. R. Vogler. (1978). Terminal deoxynucleotidyl transferase, cytochemistry, and membrane receptors in adult acute leukemia. Blood, (in press).

Gralnick, H. R., D. A. G. Galton, D. Catovsky, C. Sultan, and J. M. Bennett. (1977). Classification of acute leukemia. Ann. Int. Med., 87, 740-753.

Greenwood, M. F., M. S. Coleman, J. J. Hutton, B. Lampkin, K. Krill, F. J. Bollum, and P. Holland. (1977). Terminal deoxynucleotidyl transferase distribution in neoplastic and hematopoietic cells. J. Clin. Invest., 59, 889-899.

Gregoire, K. E., I. Goldschneider, R. W. Barton, and F. J. Bollum. (1977). Intracellular distribution of terminal deoxynucleotidyl transferase in rat bone marrow and thymus. Proc. Natl. Acad. Sci., 74, 3993-3996.

Hoffbrand, A. V., K. Ganeshaguru, G. Janossy, M. F. Greaves, D. Carovsky, and R. K. Woodruff. (1977). Terminal deoxynucleotidyl transferase levels and membrane phenotypes in diagnosis of acute leukemia. The Lancet, 2, 520-523.

Hutton, J. J., and F. J. Bollum. (1978). Terminal transferase and DNA polymerases in leukemia. In R. W. Ruddon (Ed.), Conference on Biological Markers of Neoplasia: Basic and Applied Aspects, Elsevier North Holland, New York.

Hutton, J. J., and M. S. Coleman. (1976). Terminal deoxynucleotidyl transferase measurements in the differential diagnosis of adult leukemias. Brit. J. Haemat., 34, 447-456.

Kung, P. C., P. D. Gottlieb, and D. Baltimore. (1976). Terminal deoxynucleotidyl transferase, serological studies and radioimmunoassay. J. Biol. Chem., 251, 2399-2404.

Marks, S. M., D. Baltimore, and R. McCaffrey. (1978). Terminal transferase as a predictor of initial responsiveness to vincristine and prednisone in blastic crisis myelogenous leukemia. New Eng. J. Med., 298, 812-814.

McCaffrey, R., T. A. Harrison, R. Parkman, and D. Baltimore. (1975). Terminal deoxynucleotidyl transferase activity in human leukemic cells and in normal thymocytes. New Eng. J. Med., 292, 775-780.

Sarin, P. S., P. N. Anderson, and R. C. Gallo. (1976). Terminal deoxynucleotidyl transferase activities in human blood leukocytes and lymphoblast cell lines: high levels in lymphoblast cell lines and in blast cells of some patients with chronic myelogenous leukemia in acute phase. Blood, 47, 11-20.

Srivastava, B. I. S., S. A. Khan, J. Minowada, G. A. Gomez, and I. Rakowski. (1977). Terminal deoxynucleotidyl transferase activity in blastic phase of chronic myelogenous leukemia. Cancer Res., 37, 3612-3618.

Vogler, L. B., W. M. Crist, D. E. Bockman, E. R. Pearl, A. R. Lawton, and M. D. Cooper. (1978). Pre-B-Leukemia. New Eng. J. Med., 298, 872-878.

Cytolysis of Cancer Cells by Antisera Against Human Tumor Markers

S. Carrel*, J.-P. Mach*, S. K. Liao** and P. Dent**

*Unit of Human Cancer Immunology, Lausanne Branch,
Ludwig Institute for Cancer Research, Epalinges s/ Lausanne, Switzerland
**Department of Pediatrics, McMaster University, Hamilton, Canada

ABSTRACT

Tumor cell lysis by antibodies against various surface membrane markers was studied using colon carcinoma and melanoma cells grown in vitro. Antisera against carcinoembryonic antigen (CEA) and normal glycoprotein crossreacting with CEA (NGP) were produced in rabbits, whereas antisera against melanoma-associated antigen(s) (MAA) were raised either in rabbits or in monkeys. All sera were rendered specific by appropriate absorption. Antibody activity was tested with two different assays, namely a complement-dependent cytotoxicity (CDC) assay and an antibody-dependent cell-mediated cytotoxicity (ADCC) assay. Lysis was assessed by short-term ^{51}Cr release from labelled target cells. Rabbit serum was used as a source of complement, whereas normal human peripheral blood lymphocytes provided the source of effector cells in the ADCC assay. Antisera directed against CEA and NGP were not cytolytic as assessed by CDC, but both sera induced significant lysis of the relevant target cells in the ADCC assay. The rabbit anti-MAA antiserum was cytolytic against 9 of 10 melanoma cell lines in both assays, while the monkey antiserum was cytolytic only in the CDC assay. As shown here, the three markers studied (CEA, NGP, MAA) not only have a selective distribution among different cell lines, but they also determine a distinct susceptibility of these cells to lysis by the corresponding antisera.

INTRODUCTION

Human tumor cells from long-term cultures are frequently used in vitro as target cells in studies searching for tumor markers or tumor-associated antigens. The assays most widely used to demonstrate the presence or absence of serologically defined membrane structures on tumor cells are based on complement-dependent cytotoxicity (CDC) (Brunner, 1968) and, more recently, antibody-dependent cell-mediated cytotoxicity (ADCC) (MacLennan, 1969 ; Perlmann, 1969). Positive results obtained with either one of the two assays indicate that the structures against which the antibodies are directed are expressed on the surface membrane of the tumor cells.

Although the end result of both assays is the same, i.e. target cell lysis, it appears that its induction requires a quite different distribution or density of

the antigens on the cell surface. The immunoglobulin class of the antibody is
also of great importance as for example only IgG antibodies can induce ADCC while
IgM and, to a lower extent, IgG antibodies are lytic in the presence of complement
Examples of such differences are given in the present study which deals with the
lytic activity of rabbit antibodies against two different markers, carcinoembryonic antigen (CEA) (Gold, 1965) and normal glycoprotein (NGP) crossreacting with
CEA (Mach, 1972 ; Von Kleist, 1972) as well as that of monkey and rabbit antibodies directed against melanoma-associated antigen(s) (MAA).

MATERIALS AND METHODS

Purification of CEA and NGP

Carcinoembryonic antigen (CEA) used for the immunization of rabbits was purified
from hepatic metastases of colon carcinoma by 0.6 M perchloric acid extraction,
followed by gel filtration as described previously (Pusztaszeri, 1973). Normal
glycoprotein (NGP) was purified from perchloric acid extracts of normal human lung
by Sephadex G-200 filtration followed by elution from an insoluble immunoadsorbent
containing anti-CEA IgG antibodies (Heumann, 1978).

Antisera

Antisera against CEA were prepared in rabbits by repeated intradermal injections
of 200 µg purified CEA with complete Freund's adjuvant. The antisera were absorbed
with perchloric acid extracts of normal lung in order to eliminate antibodies
crossreacting with NGP. Antisera against NGP were prepared in rabbits by repeated
intradermal injections of 100 µg of purified NGP with complete Freund's adjuvant.
Antisera against MAA were prepared in rabbits by repeated intradermal injections
of 1 mg crude membrane preparations in complete Freund's adjuvant. Membrane preparations from cultured melanoma cells were obtained by nitrogen cavitation as
described by Schmidt-Ulrich (1974). Monkey anti-melanoma serum was obtained by
repeated subcutaneous injections of 2×10^6 cells in complete Freund's adjuvant.
All anti-melanoma antisera were rendered specific by absorption with 6×10^8 cells/
ml from a pool of seven different lymphoid cell lines.

Cells

All target cells used in this study were obtained from long-term cultures of three
colon carcinomas (Co-115, Co-125, HT-29), seven melanomas (Mel-67, Mel-57, Mel-
2a-P, Me-43, IgR3, Me-21, SK-Mel-1), one glioblastoma (G 40), one breast carcinoma
(SK-Br-3), one cervical carcinoma (Cx-180) and one choriocarcinoma (Be-Wo). All
cells were grown in Dulbecco's modified Eagle's medium, supplemented with 10 %
heat inactivated fetal calf serum. Except for the melanoma cell line, SK-Mel-1,
which grows in suspension, all cell lines grow as monolayer cultures. They were
harvested by incubation with a mixture of 0.05 % trypsin and 0.05 % EDTA for 10
min.

Cytotoxicity assays

Target cells were labelled with ^{51}Cr by a modification of the method of Brunner
(1968) as described previously (Carrel, 1977). The CDC assay was performed as
follows. Ten thousands labelled target cells in 25 µl were distributed into
plastic tubes and incubated with 25 µl of the appropriate antiserum dilution for
30 min at 37^0 followed by 50 µl of rabbit complement diluted 1:2. After incubation
for 3 hr at 37^0, the radioactivity in the supernatant fluid was measured. Calcu-

ation of the percentage of specific lysis was done as described below for the
DCC assay, taking as control release (CR) the values obtained with target cells
incubated in the presence of complement alone. Quantitative absorption experiments
ere carried out by incubating varying numbers of cells (10^4 to 10^6 cells/50 ul)
ith 50 ul of antiserum for 1 hr at room temperature. The remaining lytic activity
as then tested as described above.

ntibody-dependent cell-mediated cytolysis (ADCC) was measured by a short-term
^{1}Cr release assay as described previously (Carrel, 1977). Briefly, 10^4 labelled
arget cells in 20 μl volumes were distributed into glass tubes and incubated
ith 20 μl of the appropriate antiserum dilution for 30 min at 37°, followed by
 x 10^5 lymphocytes in a volume of 100 μl. ^{51}Cr release in the supernatant was
letermined after incubation for 3 hr at 37°. The ratio of lymphocytes to target
:ells was 50:1 in all experiments. The percentage of specific ^{51}Cr release was
:alculated by the following formula :

$$\% \text{ specific } ^{51}\text{Cr release} = \frac{TR - CR}{MR - CR} \times 100$$

where CR, the control release, represents the values obtained by incubation of
targed cells with lymphocytes and without antiserum ; TR, the test ^{51}Cr release
of target cells incubated with lymphocytes and antiserum ; MR, the maximum ^{51}Cr
release obtained from 3 times frozen and thawed target cells in distilled water.

The specificity of the ADCC assay for CEA and NGP was demonstrated by inhibition
experiments where aliquots of the respective antisera were absorbed with increasing
amount of purified CEA or NGP and the remaining lytic activity tested as described
above.

RESULTS

Anti-CEA antibody-dependent cell-mediated cytotoxicity

In these experiments cells from three different colon carcinoma cell lines known
to express CEA on their surface were labelled with ^{51}Cr and incubated for 30 min
with various dilutions of a rabbit anti-CEA serum. Normal human peripheral blood
lymphocytes from a single donor were then added at a ratio of 50:1 lymphocytes/
tumor cell and the mixture was further incubated for 3 hr at 37°. For control
experiments three non-CEA producing cell lines, one breast carcinoma (Br-3), one glioblastoma (G 40), two melanoma (Mel-57) (Mel-67) were tested with the same antisera.

As shown in Table 1 the three CEA producing cell lines (Co-115, Co-125, HT-29) were
lysed by the rabbit anti-CEA antiserum up to a dilution of 1:800. A maximum of
about 50 % lysis was observed for each of the three colon carcinoma cell lines.
Among the 4 non-CEA producing cell lines, 2 (Br-3 and G 40) were not lysed at all,
whereas a low but detectable lysis of the 2 melanoma cell lines was also observed. These latter results are possibly due to the presence on melanoma cells
of an antigen crossreacting with CEA, different from NGP, the characterization of
which will be reported separately (Dent, in preparation).

Anti-NGP antibody-dependent cell-mediated cytotoxicity

The results obtained in ADCC with a specific rabbit anti-NGP serum are presented
in Table 2. Up to 30 % specific lysis of the three CEA producing cell lines
(Co-115, Co-125, HT-29) was observed at a serum dilution of 1:50. Significant lysis
was still obtained at a dilution of 1:200. Among the four non-CEA producing cell
lines, two of them (Br-3 and G-40) were unaffected by the same antiserum, while

TABLE   1

RABBIT ANTI-CEA

ASSAY USED	ANTISERUM DILUTION	TARGET CELLS						
		Co-115	HT-29	Co-125	G 40	Br-3	Mel-57	Mel-67
CDC	1 : 5	0[a]	0	0	0	1	1	0
	10	0	0	0	0	0	1	0
	20	0	0	0	0	0	0	0
ADCC	1 : 50	48	64	53	0	0	9	7
	100	45	52	60	0	0	8	5
	200	43	48	51	1	0	7	4
	400	41	47	44	1	0	4	2
	800	23	35	35	0	0	0	0
	1600	8	21	23	0	0	0	0

a) Values represent the percentage of specific lysis of ^{51}Cr labelled target cells.

9 % of cells from the melanoma cell lines were lysed at a serum dilution of 1:50.
Lysis of the melanoma cells did not increase at higher serum concentrations.

Complement-dependent cytotoxicity with rabbit anti-CEA and anti-NGP antibodies

In order to compare ADCC with CDC, we determined in the same experiment the degree
of lysis of colon carcinoma cells (Co-115, Co-125, HT-29) coated with either
rabbit anti-CEA or rabbit anti-NGP antiserum following incubation with either
rabbit complement or human lymphocytes. Under these conditions, the possibility
that differences in antigen expression on tumor cells related to culture conditions could interfere in the results was excluded. As shown in Tables 1 and 2, CDC
results were consistently negative, even when antisera were used at a dilution of
1:5. Control experiments showed that over 95 % of the colon carcinoma cells were
lysed by a rabbit anti-human species antiserum and complement.

Inhibition of ADCC by purified CEA and NGP

Inhibition experiments were undertaken to analyze the specificity of the ADCC
activities observed with rabbit antisera against CEA and against NGP. To this end,
500 μl of rabbit anti-CEA or anti-NGP antiserum at a dilution of 1:2 were absorbed
with increasing amounts (5,10,20,40, and 80 μg) of purified CEA or NGP, and the
residual antibody activity measured using the ADCC assay.

TABLE   2

RABBIT ANTI-NGP

ASSAY USED	ANTISERUM DILUTION	TARGET CELLS						
		Co-115	HT-29	Co-125	G 40	Br-3	Mel-57	Mel-67
CDC	1 : 5	0[a]	1	0	0	1	1	0
	10	0	0	0	0	0	1	0
	20	0	0	0	0	0	0	0
ADCC	1 : 50	37	31	43	0	1	19	17
	100	35	28	37	0	0	13	15
	200	21	20	42	0	1	8	5
	400	18	13	31	0	1	8	3
	800	2	5	27	0	0	2	1

a) Values represent the percentage of specific lysis of ^{51}Cr labelled target cells.

The results of such experiments are presented in Fig. 1. In the CEA system (Fig. 1 A), ADCC activity of the antiserum decreased progressively after absorbtion with increasing amounts of CEA. At a serum dilution of 1:1000, specific lysis dropped from 50 % for the unabsorbed antiserum to 12 % for the antiserum absorbed with 80 μg CEA. Similar results were obtained in the NGP system (Fig. 1 B). As little as 50 μg of NGP inhibited most of the lytic activity of the anti-NGP antiserum. At a serum dilution of 1:50, lysis dropped from 45 % for the unadsorbed antiserum to less than 10 % for the antiserum absorbed with 50 μg NGP. Control absorptions of the two antisera with red blood cells of different blood groups did not significantly inhibit the ADCC activity.

Complement-dependent cytotoxicity with rabbit and monkey antisera against MAA

Immunization of rabbits with membrane preparations of melanoma cells, or of monkeys with whole melanoma cells, produced antisera which, after appropriate absorption on human lymphoid cell lines, reacted only with melanoma cells. The lytic activities of a rabbit anti-melanoma serum on various human melanoma and non-melanoma cell lines as assessed in CDC assays are presented in Table 3. It can be seen that the four melanoma cell lines (Me-43, Ig-R3, Me-21, SK-Mel-1) were lysed. Maximum lysis varied from 60 to 80 %, depending on the cell line tested. Control experiments using four non-melanoma target cell lines, namely one cervical carcinoma (Cxl80), one colon carcinoma (HT-29), one choriocarcinoma (Be-Wo) and

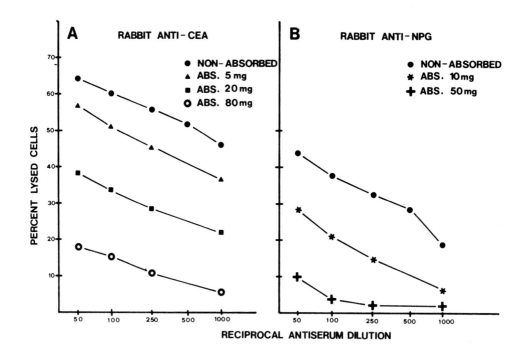

Fig. 1 A. Inhibition of the specific lysis obtained in the ADCC assay with rabbit-anti-CEA serum by absorption with increasing amounts of purified CEA.

Fig. 1 B. Inhibition of the specific lysis obtained in the ADCC assay with rabbit-anti-NGP serum by absorption with increasing amounts of purified NGP.

one breast carcinoma (Br-3), were entirely negative, thus demonstrating the melanoma specificity of the anti-melanoma serum. The CDC results obtained with a monkey anti-melanoma serum are presented in Table 4. Like the rabbit anti-MAA serum, this antiserum was cytolytic for the four melanoma cell lines tested (Mel-2aP, Mel-67, Mel-57, Me-43). Maximum lysis varied from 85 to 99 % depending on the target cell line tested. Four non-melanoma cell lines tested with the same monkey anti-melanoma serum, namely one breast (Br-3), one glioblastoma (G-40), one cervical carcinoma (Cx-180) and colon carcinoma (HT-29) were not lysed by the anti-melanoma monkey serum.

Inhibition of CDC by melanoma cells

In order to further analyze the specificity of the rabbit and monkey anti-melanoma sera, we performed absorption experiments using increasing numbers of cells from various melanoma and non-melanoma cell lines. One such absorption experiment is presented in Fig. 2. Monkey anti-melanoma serum at a dilution of 1:10 was absorbed with either one of the two melanoma cell lines (Mel 57 and Mel-67), one breast cell line (Br-3) and one colon carcinoma cell line (HT-29). While absorption with as few as 10^4 Mel-57 cells or 2.5×10^4 Mel-67 cells abolished the lytic activity of the antiserum against melanoma cells from line Me-43, no significant reduction was observed after absorption with 10^7 cells from the two non-melanoma cell lines.

TABLE 3

RABBIT ANTI-MAA

ASSAY USED	ANTISERUM DILUTION	MELANOMA TARGET CELLS				NON-MELANOMA TARGET CELLS			
		Me-43	IgR3	Me-21	SK-Mel-1	Cx-180	HT-29	BeWo	Br-3
CDC	1: 10	80[a]	77	62	76	2	4	0	0
	20	77	40	51	74	0	2	0	0
	40	67	4	23	67	0	0	0	0
	80	28	0	11	28	0	0	0	0
ADCC	1: 100	83	68	75	85	23	17	8	2
	400	65	47	63	87	4	13	0	0
	1600	41	18	41	52	0	1	0	0
	6400	13	0	11	24	0	0	0	0

a) Values represent the percentage of specific lysis of ^{51}Cr labelled target cells.

TABLE 4

MONKEY ANTI-MAA

ASSAY USED	ANTISERUM DILUTION	MELANOMA TARGET CELLS				NON-MELANOMA TARGET CELLS			
		Mel-2a-P	Me-67	Me-57	Me-43	Br-3	G-40	Cx-180	HT-29
CDC	1: 10	99[a]	99	97	85	0	0	0	0
	20	99	99	97	61	0	0	0	0
	40	97	96	68	47	0	0	0	0
	80	43	98	48	7	0	0	0	6
ADCC	1: 100	2	0	0	0	0	1	1	3
	400	2	0	1	1	0	1	0	2
	1600	1	0	0	2	0	0	0	0
	6400	0	0	0	1	0	0	0	0

a) Values represent the percentage of specific lysis of ^{51}Cr labelled target cells.

Antibody-dependent cell-mediated cytotoxicity with rabbit and monkey sera against
MAA

In parallel experiments, both anti-melanoma sera were also tested in ADCC. As show
in Table 3, 68 to 85 % of the four melanoma target cells tested (Me-43, IgR3,
Me-21, SK-Mel-1) were lysed when reacted with rabbit anti-MAA serum at a dilution
of 1:100.At a serum dilution of 1:400, significant lysis was still observed with
three of the melanoma cell lines. Two of the four non-melanoma lines, the cervical
carcinoma Cx-180 and the colon carcinoma HT-29, were partially lysed by the antiserum at a dilution of 1:100. At higher serum dilutions, however, the rabbit antiserum was not cytolytic for non-melanoma cells. The ADCC results obtained with the
monkey anti-melanoma serum are shown on Table 4. None of the four melanoma cell
lines were lysed by the antiserum. In view of these negative results, different
experimental conditions were used for the assay, such as extending the incubation
time to 24 hr and increasing the lymphocyte to target cell ratio to 100:1. In none
of the conditions used was it possible to detect any lytic activity.

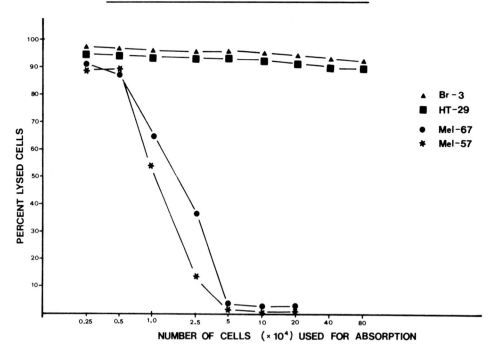

Fig. 2. Quantitative absorption of monkey anti-MAA serum. Cytotoxic assay using
^{51}Cr labelled melanoma Me-43 cells as target cells. Each point represents the cytotoxicity of the antiserum after absorption of 50 ul antiserum (1:40) with the
number of cells indicated.

DISCUSSION

In this study we demonstrated that colon carcinoma cells from long-term cultures
(HT-29, Co-115, Co-125) could be lysed by rabbit antibodies directed against CEA

nd NGP in the presence of peripheral blood effector lymphocytes. The specificity
f the lytic reactions was established by the results of absorption experiments
howing that addition of purified CEA or NGP abolished the lytic activity of the
orresponding antiserum. The specificity of the reactions was further documented
y the demonstration that target cells expressing CEA or NGP on their surface mem-
rane were lysed, while target cells not expressing these antigens were unaffected.
t is thus evident that CEA and NGP are associated with the plasma membrane in such
 way that they act as efficient target antigens for ADCC. The question whether or
ot these two antigens can be considered as integral membrane constituents is how-
ver unclear since they may be associated with the cell surface only transiently.
f interest is also the observation that only a fraction of the tumor cells were
ysed by the antisera directed against CEA and NGP. These findings may be due to an
eterogeneous expression of these two antigens. Although ADCC activity was easily
emonstrable at relatively high serum dilutions, the same antisera were totally ne-
ative in the presence of complement. These results suggest that CDC may require a
resentation or density of antigens on the target cell surface different from that
equired for ADCC killing.

When tested by CDC, the rabbit and monkey anti-melanoma sera appeared to specifi-
ally lyse melanoma target cells only. This specificity was further documented by
absorption experiments, since it was found that only cells from melanoma cell lines
were able to inhibit the cytotoxic activity of the antisera. When tested by ADCC,
the rabbit anti-melanoma serum was also specific for melanoma target cells, at
least at relatively high dilutions. Surprisingly, no lytic activity was found in
ADCC using the monkey anti-melanoma serum. We have no definitive explanation for
this observation. It is however most likely that human K cells do not recognize
the Fc portion of monkey IgG. Similar negative findings have already been observed
with goat IgG antibodies.

In conclusion, the results illustrate the importance of using different cytotoxicity methods for the identification of tumor associated antigens and/or markers. CDC
assays gave totally negative results with rabbit anti-CEA and NGP sera, whereas
the same antisera were positive on the same cell lines in ADCC. With the monkey
anti-MAA serum, the reverse observation was made, CDC assays resulting in efficient
tumor cell lysis, whereas the antiserum was totally negative in ADCC.

REFERENCES

Brunner, K.T., J. Mauel, J.-C. Cerottini, and B. Chapuis (1968). Quantitative assay
    of the lytic action of immune lymphoid cells on ^{51}Cr labeled allogeneic target
    cells in vitro; inhibition by isoantibody and by drugs. Immunol. 14:181-196.
Carrel, S., M.-C. Delisle, and J.-P. Mach (1977). Antibody-dependent cell mediated
    cytolysis of human colon carcinoma cells induced by specific antisera against
    carcinoembryonic antigen (CEA). Cancer Res. 37:2644-2650.
Gold, P., and S.O. Freedmann (1965). Specific carcinoembryonic antigens of the
    human digestive system. J. Exptl. Med. 122:467:481.
Heumann, D., Ph. Candardjis, S. Carrel, and J.-P. Mach (1978). Identification of
    the normal glycoprotein (NGP) crossreacting with CEA as a differentiation
    antigen of myeloid cells and macrophages. Proc. 6th Meeting Int. Research
    Group Carcino-Embryonic Antigen. Elsevier/North Holland Press (Ed.).
Mach, J.-P., and G. Pusztaszeri (1972). Demonstration of a partial identity bet-
    ween CEA and a normal glycoprotein. Immunochemistry 9:1031-1034.
MacLennan, I.C., G. Loewi, and A. Howard (1969). A human serum immunoglobulin with
    specificity for certain homologous target cells, which induces target cell da-
    mage by normal human lymphocytes. Immunol. 17:897-909.

Pusztaszeri, G., and J.-P. Mach (1973). Carcinoembryonic antigen (CEA) in non-
    digestive cancerous and normal tissue. Immunochemistry 10:197-204.
Perlmann, P., and G. Holm (1969). Cytotoxic effects of lymphoid cells in vitro.
    Adv. Immunol. II:117-195.
Schmidt-Ulrich, R., E. Ferber, H. Knuefermann, H. Fischer, and D.F. Hoelzl Wallach
    (1974). Analysis of the proteins in thymocyte plasma membrane and smooth endo
    plasmic reticulum by sodium dodecylsulfate-gel electrophoresis. Biochim.
    Biophys. Acta 332:175-191.
Von Kleist, S., G. Chavanel, and P. Burtin (1972). Identification of an antigen
    from normal human tissue that cross-reacts with the carcinoembryonic antigen.
    Proc. Natl. Acad. Sci. U.S. 69:2492:2494.

ACKNOWLEDGEMENTS

The authors wish to thank Dr. J.-C. Cerottini for suggestions and advice.

Membrane Changes in Malignancy: Alterations in Glycoprotein Metabolism

R. J. Bernacki, C. W. Porter, W. D. Klohs and W. Korytnyk

Department of Experimental Therapeutics, Grace Cancer Drug Center
Roswell Park Memorial Institute, Buffalo, New York 14263, U.S.A.

ABSTRACT

Increases in membrane bound sialyltransferases have been observed in human mammary tumor as compared to normal breast. These enzymes are located within the cellular Golgi membrane apparatus and on the cell's outer membrane surface from which they are presumably shed into the extracellular space. Serum sialyltransferase has been found to be elevated in rats with metastasizing mammary tumors and in women with breast cancer. We have synthesized several analogs of CMP and CMP-sialic acid and have evaluated their inhibitory activity on both tumor cell surface sialyltransferase and human serum sialyltransferase. 5'-F-CMP, ribodialdehyde CMP, and, to a lesser extent, 5'-(trans-4-N-acetylcyclo-hexyl)-CMP competetively inhibit both serum and cell surface sialyltransferase activity. Human mammary tumor cells have been observed to liberate sialyl-transferase activity into tissue culture medium. We are now studying membrane glycoconjugate turnover on such cells following plasma membrane galactoconjugate radiolabeling utilizing galactose oxidase treatement followed by $[^3H]$-NaBH$_4$ reduction. Electron microscope autoradiographs of these labeled cells confirmed that 66% of the tritium introduced by this technique was on the plasma membrane. Over a period of 20 h in culture, 70% of the label was released into the medium as low molecular weight acid soluble glycopeptides and free galactose. A small amount of membrane was released as acid insoluble material which separated into a number of high molecular weight (60,000 to 112,000) glycoproteins by SDS-polyacrylamide gel electrophoresis autofluorography. A small but significant amount of labeled membrane components was observed by electron microscope auto-radiography to be associated with lysosomal elements 20 h after radiolabeling. These studies indicate that membrane turnover is a multifaceted phenomenon encompassing both shedding and internalization. It remains to be demonstrated whether these mechanisms for membrane turnover occur in normal mammary cells and tumor cells in vivo where additional factors such as heterologous cell-to-cell contacts and circulating antibodies and complement may further modulate membrane turnover.

KEYWORDS

sialyltransferase, plasma membrane turnover, human mammary tumors, electron microscope autoradiography, cytidine analogs

INTRODUCTION

Cell surface glycoconjugates have been implicated in controlling cell division
and intercellular association in a variety of cell types. Several mitogenic
lectins have been identified and other growth factors have been postulated to
interact with cell surface glycoconjugate receptors. Therefore, alterations of
such membrane structures in malignant cells may lead to a loss of growth control
(Nicolson and Poste, 1976).

Many biochemical differences have been noted in the cell surface glycocalyx of
oncogenically transformed cells. The disappearance of a large molecular weight
glycoprotein (LETS) has been observed in a number of different transformed
tissue cultured cell lines (Hynes, 1973). Differences also have been found in
membrane enzyme activities. Increases in specific sialyltransferases have been
seen in rat (Keenan and Morré, 1973) and human (Bosmann and Hall, 1974) mammary
tumor tissue as compared to normal breast tissue. Metastasizing rat mammary
tumor SMT-2A had higher sialyltransferase levels than nonmetastasizing MT-W9B
rat mammary tumors, and serum sialyltransferase levels were elevated two-fold in
rats with SMT-2A tumors (Bernacki and Kim, 1977). These findings led to studies
of serum sialyltransferase levels in women with breast cancer. Kessel and Allen
(1975) were first to show increased sialyltransferase activity in women with
breast cancers. These findings were confirmed and extended by Ip and Dao (1978)
who observed highest serum sialyltransferase in women with metastasizing breast
cancer. This group also found 5'-nucleotidase, a plasma membrane marker, to be
elevated in serum in direct proportion with the increased levels of sialyltransferase.

These latter studies now have prompted us to look for specific inhibitors of
sialyltransferase. In this report we have examined the inhibitory action of
several newly synthesized analogs of CMP and CMP-sialic acid. These inhibitors
might enable us to study the functions of membrane and serum sialyltransferases
more fully as well as being potentially useful as chemotherapeutic agents.

Glycosyltransferases, which catalyze the addition of sugar from nucleotide-sugar
to suitable acceptors, have been localized in the Golgi apparatus and on the
cell surface of tumor cells (Porter and Bernacki, 1975; Bernacki and Porter,
1978). We have postulated that tumor cells shed surface sialyltransferase and
other membrane components and that tumor surface shedding may impair host immune
responsiveness. In the studies presented herein we provide evidence that cultured
human mammary tumor cells shed macromolecular membrane material. They also were
found to shed or secrete a soluble sialyltransferase into the culture fluid.
These findings may offer an explanation and a mechanism for the increased serum
glycosyltransferase activities that have been detected in cancer patients.
Sialyl-, galactosyl-, and fucosyltransferase activities have been found to be
elevated in the sera of cancer patients, and these enzymes can be regarded as
biological markers of malignancy (Kessel and Allen, 1975; Podolsky and Weiser,
1975; Bauer and co-workers, 1978).

MATERIALS AND METHODS

Human Mammary Tumor Cell Cultures

Human cell lines were provided by Dr. E.M. Jenson, EG & G/Mason Research Institute,
Rockville, Maryland. The two lines used in this study were an SW-613 human

mammary tumor cell line which originated from a primary adenocarcinoma of the
breast, and an MCF-7, a human mammary tumor cell line which was isolated from a
pleural effusion (Soule and co-workers, 1973). The SW-613 cell line was adapted
to grow as a monolayer culture in RPMI-1640 medium (Grand Island Biological Co.,
Buffalo, New York) supplemented with 10% fetal calf serum and 50 μg/ml neomycin,
while MCF-7 was grown in Eagle's MEM, 10% fetal calf serum, 10 μg/ml insulin,
and 50 μg/ml neomycin.

Murine Leukemia L1210

Female DBA/2J mice, weighing 20-25 g (Jackson Laboratories, Bar Harbor, Maine),
were inoculated IP with 10^5 L1210 murine leukemic cells suspended in saline.
The animals were sacrificed five to seven days later by cervical dislocation and
the ascites fluid containing the tumor cells was withdrawn and diluted with ice-
cold Dulbecco's phosphate-buffered saline (PBS). The cells were washed twice
with PBS and counted with an electronic particle counter (Coulter Electronics,
Hialeah, Florida), and the cell density was adjusted in RPMI-1640 (Grand Island
Biological Co., Buffalo, New York) containing 20 mM HEPES (Sigma, St. Louis,
Missouri) and 10 mM MOPS (Sigma), pH 7.0 (RPMI-1640 HM) (Bernacki and Porter,
1978).

Ectosialyltransferase Assay

Washed L1210 cells (5×10^7) were treated with 10 units of Vibrio cholerae
neuraminidase (VCN, Behring Diagnostic Co., Somerville, New Jersey, EC 3.2.1.18)
in 0.5 ml RPMI-1640 HM for 15 min at 37°. Following this pretreatment, VCN-
treated and untreated cells were washed three times in 5 ml RPMI-1640 HM, diluted in 1.0 ml of media, dispensed in 0.2 ml volumes (10^7 cells) in glass tubes,
and incubated for 30 min with 1 μM CMP-[^{3}H]-NANA (259 mCi/mmole, Amersham,
Chicago, Illinois, USA). The enzyme reaction was terminated by the addition of
2 ml of 1% phosphotungstic acid in 0.5 N HCl and washed twice with 2 ml of 10%
trichloroacetic acid. The final pellet was dissolved in 0.2 ml of 1 N NaOH,
neutralized, and the incorporated radioactivity determined by scintillation
counting (Bernacki and co-workers, 1978).

Serum Sialyltransferase Assay

Human blood was collected from normal individuals and allowed to clot. Serum
was obtained by centrifugation. Serum sialyltransferase assays were performed
according to procedures previously described by Bernacki and Kim (1977). A
typical assay medium consisted of 1.0 - 3.0 mg of serum protein, 3.0 mg/ml of
desialylated fetuin, 0.1 M cacodylate buffer (pH 6.5), and 9.65 μM CMP-N-acetyl-
(^{14}C)-neuraminic acid. Incubations were carried out at 37°C in a shaker bath
for 30 min. The reaction was terminated by the addition of 2.0 ml of 1% phosphotungstic acid in 0.5 N HCl and centrifuged. The pellets were washed twice in
trichloroacetic acid and once in 95% ethanol:ether (2:1, v/v) and counted in a
Packard Tri-Carb-β-λ liquid scintillation counter. Counting efficiency for ^{14}C
ranged from 70-80%. Protein was determined according to the procedure described
by Lowry and co-workers (1951). Enzyme activity is calculated as the difference
between the exogenous and endogenous activity and is expressed as DPM of N-
acetyl-(^{14}C)-neuraminic acid incorporated per hour per mg of protein.

The effects of various nucleotides, nucleotide-analogs, and nucleotide-sugar
analogs were assessed on both serum sialyltransferase and ectosialyltransferase
activity. The nucleotides were purchased from Sigma, while the analogs ribodialdehyde CMP, 5'-F-CMP, 5'-(trans-4-N-acetylcyclohexyl)cytidylic acid hydrochloride, and 5'-(cis-4-N-acetylcyclohexyl)cytidylic acid hydrochloride were
synthesized as reported elsewhere (Korytnyk and co-workers, 1978).

Cell Surface Galactoconjugate Labeling

Outer plasma membrane glycoproteins and glycolipids of SW-613 human mammary
tumor cells were labeled with tritiated sodium borohydride following neuraminidase and galactose oxidase treatment according to the procedures of Gahmberg and
Hakomori (1973) as modified by Baumann and Doyle (1978). Following radiolabeling the cells were rinsed three times and either fixed in glutaraldehyde for
electron microscope autoradiography or returned to fresh medium. The medium was
removed from these cells at various times following radiolabeling and analyzed
for radioactivity. Acid precipitable radioactive glycoconjugate was analyzed on
polyacrylamide gels according to the procedures of Laemmli (1970). Fluorographic
detection of radioactivity in these gels was carried out as outlined by Bonner
and Laskey (1974). Acid soluble radioactive material found in the medium was
analyzed on paper chromatography (Bernacki, 1974).

Electron Microscope Autoradiography

Immediately following radiolabeling and 20 h later, the medium was removed from
cell cultures and the labeled cells rinsed with PBS prior to fixation for 30 min
in ice-cold 3% phosphate buffered glutaraldehyde (pH 7.0). The cell monolayers
were collected, pelleted, and fixed for another 2 h in glutaraldehyde. The cell
pellets were washed overnight in buffer, postfixed 4 h in 1% buffered osmium
tetroxide, dehydrated in a graded alcohol series, and embedded in Epon-araldite.
Ultra-microtome sections (100 nm thick) were processed for EM autoradiography as
described previously (Porter and Bernacki, 1975). Briefly, the sections were
mounted on collodionized slides, stained with 2% uranyl acetate, carbon coated,
and overlaid with a monolayer of Ilform L-4 emulsion. The preparations were
exposed 25-55 days, developed in D-19 (Kodak, Rochester, New York) for 2 min at
24°, fixed, and photographed with a Siemens Elmiskop 101. Electron micrographs
were examined and the ultrastructural locations for over 1000 grains were determined for each experiment. Only longitudinal cell profiles which contained a
nucleus and similar amounts of cytoplasm were selected for grain distribution
analysis. The percentages of the total number of grains in each cellular compartment, including plasma membrane, mitochondria, lysosomes, vacuoles, endoplasmic reticulum, cytosol, nuclear membrane, nucleolus, heterochromatin, and
euchromatin, were then calculated.

RESULTS AND DISCUSSION

Sialyltransferase Inhibitors

Following our observations that sialyltransferase is located both on the cell
surface of L1210 leukemic cells (Bernacki, 1974) and in the sera of animals
bearing mammary tumors (Bernacki and Kim, 1977), we began to search for inhibitors of this enzyme. From previous studies we knew that CMP was a competitive
inhibitor of sialyltransferase (Bernacki, 1975). This led us to synthesize
several analogs of CMP. These include 5'-F-CMP, ribodialdehyde CMP and two CMP-
sialic acid analogs: 5'-(trans-4-N-acetylcyclohexyl)-CMP and its cis counterpart. The enzyme inhibitory activity of these agents was studied with both
L1210 cell surface sialyltransferase (Table 1) and human serum sialyltransferase
(Table 2).

ABLE 1   Effects of Nucleotides and Nucleotide-Sugar Analogs on Murine L1210
Ectosialyltransferase System

Compound	Ectosialyltransferase Activity (% control)	
	0.125 mM	1.25 mM
Cytidine	125	112
CMP	82	28
5'-F-CMP	81	26
Ribodialdehyde CMP	103	54
N-Acetylneuraminic acid	100	123
5'-(Trans-4-N-acetylcyclohexyl)-CMP	138	85
5'-(Cis-4-N-acetylcyclohexyl)-CMP	94	99

L1210 cells were obtained on day 5 from the IP ascites fluid of DBA/2 mice. The cells were washed and pretreated with Vibrio cholerae neuraminidase prior to assay in RPMI-1640 HM containing 0.25 µCi [^{14}C]-CMP-NANA plus the indicated compounds. Macromolecular radioactivity was quantitated as described in the text. All experiments were performed in duplicate on at least 2 separate occasions.

TABLE 2   Effects of Inhibitors on Human Serum Sialyltransferase Activity

Compound	Concentration (mM)	Sialyltransferase Activity (% control)
N-acetylneuraminic acid	10	100
Galactose	10	100
CMP	0.05	50
5'-F-CMP	0.07	50
Ribodialdehyde CMP	1.0	50
5'-(Trans-4-N-acetylcyclohexyl)-CMP	1.0	75
5'-(Cis-4-N-acetylcyclohexyl)-CMP	1.0	83

Enzyme activity was determined as described in the text with the addition of the indicated compounds. Activity was calculated as the difference between the exogenous and endogenous activity. Results are the average of 2 experiments, each performed in triplicate.

Cytidine and N-acetylneuraminic acid had no inhibitory activity on the ectosialyl-transferase system while CMP (1.25 mM) reduced enzyme activity to 28%. 5'-F-CMP mimicked the actions of CMP and reduced activity to 26% at 1.25 mM. Ribodialde-hyde CMP also reduced activity to 54% at 1.25 mM. Nucleotide sugar analogs, such as 5'-(trans-4-N-acetylcyclohexyl)-CMP and 5'-(cis-4-N-acetylcyclohexyl)-CMP, had little effect on the enzyme system. These studies indicate that ecto-sialyltransferase can be inhibited by cytidine nucelotides or their analogs and perhaps by other compounds, such as nucleotide-sugar analogs.

These same compounds were tested as inhibitors of human serum sialyltransferase (Table 2). CMP and 5'-F-CMP were the most effective inhibitors having apparent Ki's of 50 μM and 70 μM, respectively. The monosaccharides NANA and galactose had no inhibitory effects at 10 mM, while 1 mM ribodialdehyde CMP lowered activity to 50% of control. The CMP-NANA analogs were marginally effective inhibitors at 1 mM, lowering activity to 75 and 83%. In both systems the trans CMP-NANA analog possessed more inhibitory activity than the cis analog. This is surpris-ing in view of the fact that native CMP-NANA is in a cis configuration.

Release of Sialyltransferase

Earlier studies in our laboratory have shown that animals with metastasizing mammary tumors have elevated levels of serum sialyltransferase (Bernacki and Kim, 1977). Similar studies were conducted on women with breast cancer, where the highest enzyme activity levels were found in patients with metastasis (Ip and Dao, 1978). To determine the origin of the increased serum enzyme and the mechanism of cellular release of the enzyme, we studied the release of sialyl-transferase into the cellular media from MCF-7 human mammary tumor cells main-tained in vitro (Table 3). There was no evidence of sialyltransferase in the

TABLE 3　Shedding of Sialyltransferase Activity from MCF-7 Human Mammary Tumor Cells

	Sialyltransferase Activity	
Time (h)	Cellular Homogenate (CPM/h/μg protein)	Medium (CPM/50 μl)
0	320	0
	282	0
24	326	1046
	298	1054
48	285	1532
	294	1408

MCF-7 cells were seeded into MEM medium containing 10% heat inactivated fetal calf serum. Enzyme assays were performed at the indicated time with either cells homogenized in 0.1% Triton X-100 (5:1) or aliquots of medium. Complete assay mixtures consisted of either 50 μl cell homogenate or 50 μl medium, 20 μl fetuin minus sialic acid (15 mg/ml), 10 μl 0.5 M cacodylate buffe (pH 6.5), 10 μl 0.1 M $MgCl_2$ and 10 μl [^{14}C]-CMP-NANA (0.25 μ Ci). Results are expressed as CPM/h/μg cell protein for cell homogenates and CPM/50 μl for cell media.

:ulture medium following cell seeding. Twenty-four hours later 1050 CPM/50 μl
•f enzyme activity was detectable. Forty-eight hours later enzyme activity
ιncreased to 1470 CPM/50 μl. Total cellular sialyltransferase remained the same
Iuring this period. Therefore, we conclude that human mammary tumor cells have
:he ability to secrete or shed an active sialyltransferase.

Surface Galactoconjugate Labeling

[n order to study cell surface shedding, we used a surface radiolabeling technique
which involves galactose oxidase treatment of whole cells followed by $[^3H]$-NaBH$_4$
reduction. This method specifically introduces tritium onto the C_6 of exposed
surface galactose and N-acetylgalactosamine moieties. Initial experiments with
SW-613 human mammary tumor cells indicated that prior neuraminidase treatment increased incorporation four-fold when coupled with galactose oxidase/borohydride
reduction. Incorporation was negligible for cells treated only with neuraminidase but increased to 654 x 10^3 DPM/mg for cells treated with galactose oxidase
alone. When cells were treated with both enzymes, incorporation increased to
2363 x 10^3 DPM/mg. These labeled cells were processed for electron microscope
autoradiography or returned to culture for up to 20 h. Cellular and shed radio-
activity·were monitored during this 20 h period by polyacrylamide gel electrophoresis and paper chromatography.

Loss of Cell Surface Galactoconjugates

The disappearance of cell surface radioactivity was monitored for up to 20 h.
Cellular medium was precipitated with trichloroacetic acid and both the acid
soluble and acid insoluble fraction were quantitated and characterized. The
majority of shed radioactivity was acid soluble and consisted of small molecular
weight glycopeptides and free galactose. Acid insoluble material was present in
the medium and separated into a number of high molecular weight species on
polyacrylamide gel electrophoretograms.

Total cellular radioactivity decreased about 50% during the first 4 h following
radiolabeling and by 75% within 20 h. Polyacrylamide gel electrophoretic analysis indicated that all labeled surface glycoproteins disappeared at about the
same rate. The data therefore suggests a random first order degradation mechanism for cell surface galactoconjugates.

Electron Microscope Autoradiography

Immediately following radiolabeling the majority of the grains, indicating the
location of incorporated $[^3H]$-galactose, were located over the plasma membrane
of SW-613 cells (Fig. 1). Areas of plasma membrane rich in microvilli had an
increased grain density. Approximately 66% of the total grains was located over
the plasma membrane (Table 4) with the remaining grains scattered throughout the
cytoplasm and nuclei. Twenty hours later this grain distribution shifted so
that fewer grains were localized over the cell surface (59%) and significantly
more grains were observed in the lysosomes (from less than 1% to 4%). A cell
undergoing mitosis and having a very high density of labeled material in its
lysosomes is shown in Fig. 2. These autoradiographic results illustrate that
some membrane galactoconjugate becomes interiorized via endocytotic processes
and is presumably degraded within the lysosomes.

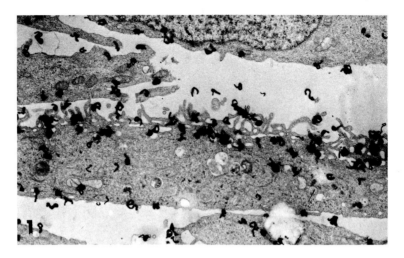

Fig. 1. Electron microscope autoradiograph of malignant
SW-613 human mammary cells fixed immediately after
the galactose oxidase [^{3}H]-NaBH$_4$ labeling sequence.
The bulk of the silver grains and, hence, the bound
radioactivity is associated with the plasma membrane
and especially with the microvilli (x 9,250).

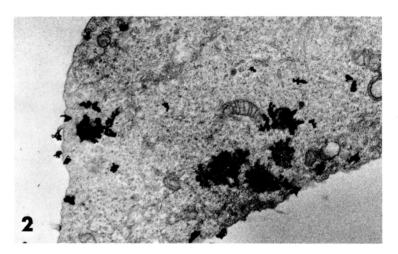

Fig. 2. Autoradiograph of cytoplasmic labeling of lysosomal
structures in SW-613 cells 20 h following the radiolabeling sequence. Two moderately labeled lysosomes
are apparent in a cell undergoing mitosis (x 8,075).

TABLE 4 Electron Microscope Autoradiographic Analysis of [3H]-Galactose
Distribution in SW-613 Human Mammary Tumor Cells

| | SW-613 Cells | | | |
| | 0 Hour* | | 20 Hour** | |
Cellular Compartment	Grains	% Total	Grains	% Total
Plasma Membrane	1433	66%	1280	59%
Cytoplasm	404	19%	645	29%
Mitochondria	105	5	121	6
Lysosomes	8	<1	91	4
Vacuoles	39	2	61	3
Endoplasmic reticulum	66	3	98	4
Golgi	5	<1	30	1
Cytosol	186	9	244	11
Nucleus	315	15%	263	12%
Membrane	187	9	155	7
Nucleolus	3	<1	0	0
Heterochromatin	5	<1	16	1
Euchromatin	120	6	92	4

 * Based on 2156 grains over 37 cells.
** Based on 1288 grains over 42 cells.

Cells were radiolabeled as described in Methods and fixed immediately in glutaraldehyde (0 hour) or allowed to incubate for 20 hours at 37°C prior to fixation and processing for electron microscope autoradiography. Grain locations were scored for each cellular compartment and the percentage distributions were calculated based on the total number of grains.

A summary of our results and current thinking on membrane turnover is illustrated in Fig. 3. Labeled cell surface galactoconjugate may be lost from the cell surface in a number of different ways. These include shedding of membrane subunits or vesicles, degradation of membrane components at the cell surface by membrane proteases (Bernacki and Bosmann, 1972) and glycosidases (Bosmann, 1971), and finally by interiorization via endocytosis followed by degradation within the lysosomes. Certain internalized membrane components may avoid degradation and may recycle back to the cell surface still intact. Membrane components, degraded intracellularly or extracellularly, are subject to reutilization at the endoplasmic reticulum and Golgi apparatus.

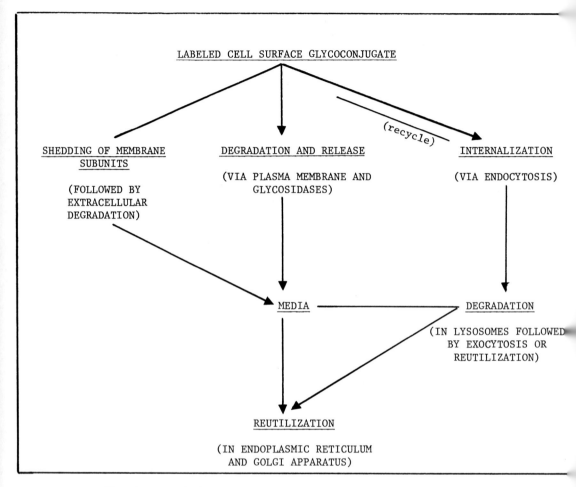

Fig. 3.   Metabolic fate of plasma membrane glycoconjugate of
          human mammary tumor.

Membrane enzymes such as sialyltransferase may be shed from tumor cell surfaces
in increased amounts as a result of cell surface turnover. We have shown that
human mammary tumor cells do secrete an active sialyltransferase in vitro. This
may be the source for the serum enzyme elevated in women with metastatic breast
cancer. Its potential as a diagnostic or prognostic marker is evident. We are
currently attempting to purify and characterize this serum sialyltransferase and
are actively engaged in synthesizing other potential inhibitors of sialytransfer-
ase which may be useful for enzyme characterization studies or as cancer chemotherapeutic agents.

auer, C.H., W.G. Reutter, K.P. Erhart, E.K. Köttgen, and W. Gerok (1978). Decrease of human serum fucosyltransferase as an indicator of successful tumor therapy. Science, 201, 1232-1233.

Bauman, H., and D. Doyle (1978). Turnover of plasma membrane glycoproteins and glycolipids of hepatoma tissue culture cells. J. Biol. Chem., 253, 4408-4418.

Bernacki, R.J., and H.B. Bosmann (1972). Red cell hydrolases II: Proteinase activities in human erythrocyte plasma membranes. J. Membrane Biol., 7, 1-14.

Bernacki, R.J. (1974). Membrane ectoglycosyltransferase activity of L1210 murine leukemic cells. J. Cellular Physiol., 83, 457-466.

Bernacki, R.J. (1975). Regulation of rat liver glycoprotein: N-acetylneuraminic acid transferase activity by pyrimidine nucleotides. Europ. J. Biochem., 58, 477-481.

Bernacki, R.J., and U. Kim (1977). Concomitant elevations in serum sialyltransferase activity and sialic acid content in rats with metastasizing mammary tumors. Science, 195, 577-580.

Bernacki, R.J., and C.W. Porter (1978). Biochemical and ultrastructural studies of ectoglycosyltransferase systems of murine L1210 leukemic cells. J. Supramolecular Structure, 8, 139-152.

Bernacki, R.J., C.W. Porter, W. Korytnyk, and E. Mihich (1978). Plasma membrane as a site for chemotherapeutic intervention. In G. Weber (ed.), Adv. Enzyme Reg., 16. Pergamon Press, Oxford. pp. 217-237.

Bonner, W.M., and R.A. Laskey (1974). A film detection method for tritium-labelled proteins and nucleic acids in polyacrylamide gels. Europ. J. Biochem., 46, 83-88.

Bosmann, H.B. (1971). Red cell hydrolases: Glycosidose activities in human erythrocyte plasma membranes. J. Membrane Biol., 4, 113-123.

Bosmann, H.B., and T.C. Hall (1974). Enzyme activity in invasive tumors of human breast and colon. Proc. Natl. Acad. Sci. U.S.A., 71, 1833-1837.

Gahmberg, C.G., and S.I. Hakamori (1973). External labeling of cell surface galactose and galactosamine in glycolipid and glycoprotein of human erythrocytes. J. Biol. Chem., 248, 4311-4317.

Hynes, R.O. (1973). Alteration of cell-surface proteins by viral transformation and by proteolysis. Proc. Natl. Acad. Sci. U.S.A., 70, 3170-3174.

Ip, C., and T. Dao (1978). Alterations in serum glycosyltransferases and 5'-nucleotidase in breast cancer patients. Cancer Res., 38, 723-728.

Kennan, T.W., and D.J. Morré (1973). Mammary carcinoma: Enzymatic block in disialoganglioside biosynthesis. Science, 12, 935-937.

Kessel, D., and J. Allen (1975). Elevated plasma sialyltransferase in the cancer patient. Cancer Res., 35, 670-672.

Korytnyk, W., N. Angelino, R.J. Bernacki, and W. Klohs (1978). CMP and CMP-sugar analogs as sialyltransferase inhibitors. Abstracts, 176th Meeting Am. Chem. Soc., CARB 29.

Laemmli, U.K. (1970). Cleavage of structural proteins during the assembly of the head of bacteriophage T4. Nature, 227, 680-683.

Lowry, O.H., N.J. Rosebrough, A.L. Farr, and R.J. Randall (1951). Protein measurement with the folin phenol reagent. J. Biol. Chem., 193, 265-275.

Nicolson, G.L., and G. Poste (1976). Dynamic aspects and modifications in cell-surface organization. New Engl. J. Med., 295, 197-203 and 253-258.

Podolsky, D.K., and M.M. Weiser (1975). Galactosyltransferase activities in human sera: Detection of a cancer-associated isoenzyme. Biochem. Biophys. Res. Commun., 65, 545-551.

Porter, C.W., and R.J. Bernacki (1975). Ultrastructural evidence for ectoglycosyltransferase systems. Nature (London), 256, 648-650.

Soule, H.D., J. Vazquez, A. Long, S. Albert, and M. Brennan (1973). A human cell line from a pleural effusion derived from a breast carcinoma. J. Natl. Cancer Inst., 51, 1409-1416.

ACKNOWLEDGEMENTS

We acknowledge the technical support in these studies provided by Marilyn Hillman, William Whitford, Janina Kaars, and Norman Angelino. These studies were supported by U.S. Public Health Service Grants CA-19814, CA-15757, CA-08793, GM-23233, and CA-13038 from the National Institutes of Health, DHEW.

Polysaccharide Storage During Carcinogenesis

Peter Bannasch

Abteilung für Cytopathologie, Institut für Experimentelle Pathologie
Deutsches Krebsforschungszentrum, Heidelberg, Federal Republic of Germany

ABSTRACT

The development of many tumours correlates with an accumulation of polysaccharides. The storage of glycogen during hepatocarcinogenesis has been studied most extensively. The appearance of hepatocellular carcinomas is regularly preceded by a persistent hepatocellular glycogenosis. The transformation of glycogen storage cells into hepatoma cells is usually accompanied by a gradual loss of the glycogen initially stored in excess. Frequently, hepatocellular tumours appear in patients with inborn glycogenosis. Another example of an epithelial tumour the development of which is correlated with a transient storage of glycogen is the clear cell kidney tumour. Some tumour types store glycogen without passing through a glycogenotic pre-stage. Mucopolysaccharides are accumulated during the development of different tumour types. Experimental cholangiocellular tumours, for instance, originate from cholangiofibrotic lesions which store and secrete abundant amounts of neutral and acid mucopolysaccharides. Similar changes have been found during the development of human cholangiocellular carcinomas. In early stages of morphogenesis of gliomas and perhaps also of basophilic renal adenomas acid mucopolysaccharides are stored. As a rule, the stored mucopolysaccharides gradually disappear again in later stages of tumourigenesis. In some experimental tumours, such as clear cell kidney tumours and lung adenomas, lipids, possibly glycolipids, are stored in addition to glycogen.

KEY WORDS

Glycogenosis - mucopolysaccharidosis - glycolipidosis - liver carcinogenesis - renal carcinogenesis - glioma development - leukemia

INTRODUCTION

Controversial histochemical and biochemical results have been reported on the presence of polysaccharides in tumours. Whereas such polysaccharides as glycogen or mucopolysaccharides were found in considerable amounts in some tumours, they were reduced or absent in others (Nigam and Cantero, 1972). However, more recent results of

cytochemical investigations in experimental animals and certain
data in humans provide convincing evidence that the development
of many tumours is regularly correlated with an excessive storage
of polysaccharides. The accumulation of polysaccharides may be
characteristic of the final tumour, but in most types of tumours
investigated more closely thus far the polysaccharide storage appears early during tumourigenesis and tends to disappear again in
later stages. Therefore, the investigation of the whole sequence
of cellular changes during the neoplastic transformation seems to
be a necessary prerequisite for clarifying the behaviour of polysaccharides in this process.

GLYCOGEN

The excessive storage of glycogen during hepatocarcinogenesis has
been studied most extensively (Bannasch, 1968, 1975; Farber, 1973).
The persistent accumulation of glycogen as shown by the PAS-reaction
or by Best's carmine stain seems to be the earliest specific cellular change which has so far been detected during the neoplastic
transformation of hepatocytes by cytochemical methods. The hepatocellular glycogenosis may develop within 8-14 days after administration of the respective carcinogen. Because of the elution of
glycogen many storage cells appear clear in routine hematoxylin and
eosin stained tissue sections. Frequently, the accumulation of glycogen is combined with a pronounced proliferation of the agranular
(smooth) endoplasmic reticulum. In this case the cytoplasm appears
acidophilic in H & E sections. The cytoplasmic volume of the storage
cells is considerably enlarged. In the electron microscope the
glycogen is usually found within the cytoplasmic matrix in the form
of α or β particles, but it may also be enclosed in large autophagic
vacuoles.

The rat liver treated with N-nitrosomorpholine was the first experimental model to show that both the clear and the acidophilic cells
form multiple glycogen storage foci during the preneoplastic phase
(Bannasch and Müller, 1964; Bannasch, 1968). These foci persist for
weeks and months even after withdrawal of the carcinogen. They regularly precede the development of neoplastic hepatic nodules and hepatocellular carcinomas. During the past decade putative preneoplastic
foci storing glycogen in excess have been described in different species (including monkeys) after administration of various chemical
carcinogens such as diethylnitrosamine (Schauer and Kunze, 1968;
Friedrich-Freksa et al., 1969; Sydow and Fey, 1969; Schmitz-Moormann and co-workers, 1972; Ruebner and co-workers, 1976; and others),
aflatoxin (Kalengayi and Desmet, 1975), methyl-allyl-nitrosa-
mine (Lesch and co-workers, 1968), dimethylaminoazobenzene (Forget
and Daoust, 1970), galactosamine (Lesch and co-workers, 1973) thio-
acetamide (Bannasch and co-workers, 1974 a), or 2-acetylaminofluorene
(Williams and co-workers 1976). Persistent glycogen storage foci have
also been induced by a single dose of diethylnitrosamine (Scherer and
co-workers, 1972) or nitrosomorpholine (unpublished observation).
Recently we have been able to confirm the carcinogen-induced hepatocellular glycogenosis by biochemical methods (Mayer and Bannasch,
1977). In addition, we were able to produce a focal hepatic glycogenosis and hepatocellular tumours prenatally by a single intraperito-
neal injection of ethylnitrosourea into pregnant mice (Bannasch and
co-workers, 1977).

Especially interesting in this context are the increasing reports on the appearance of hepatic tumours in humans suffering from inborn hepatic glycogenosis, mostly that of the von Gierke type (Mason and Anderson, 1955; Holling, 1963; Bauer, 1964; Christianson and co-workers, 1968; Fraumeni and co-workers, 1968; Zangeneh and co-workers, 1969; Spycher and Gitzelmann, 1971; Howell and co-workers, 1976, Levine and co-workers, 1976; Berant and co-workers, 1977; Roe and co-workers, 1978).

As shown in different animal models, the transformation of the hepatic glycogen storage foci into neoplastic nodules and hepatocellular carcinomas is morphologically characterized by pronounced cytoplasmic changes (Bannasch and Müller, 1964; Bannasch, 1968, 1976; Schauer and Kunze, 1968; Friedrich-Freksa and co-workers, 1969; Forget and Daoust, 1970; Bannasch and co-workers, 1972; Schmitz-Moormann and co-workers, 1972; Lesch and co-workers, 1973, Bannasch and co-workers, 1974; Ruebner and co-workers, 1976; Taper and Bannasch, 1976). The glycogen initially stored in excess is gradually reduced. At the same time the cytoplasmic basophilia increases due to a multiplication of the ribosomes. Recent findings suggest that the sequence of cellular changes during the development of human hepatocellular tumours is in principle identical (Bannasch and Klinge, 1971; Balász, 1976; Altmann, 1977, 1978; Cain and Kraus, 1977; Höhn and co-workers, 1977). Cytochemical investigations in rats and monkeys proved that both the early accumulation and the late reduction of the glycogen are often accompanied by a decrease or an increase of the activity of many enzymes, such as adenosinetriphosphatase, glucose-6-phosphatase, glycogen phosphorylase, glucose-6-phosphate-dehydrogenase, γ-glutamyltranspeptidase or acid nucleases (Schauer and Kunze, 1968; Friedrich-Freksa and co-workers, 1969; Sydow and Fey, 1969; Moulin and Daoust, 1971; Taper and co-workers, 1971, 1976; Schmitz-Moormann and co-workers, 1972; Bannasch and Angerer, 1974, Kalengayi and Desmet 1975; Ruebner and co-workers, 1976; Hacker and Bannasch, 1977 a and b; Kunz and co-workers, 1977, 1978). However, the significance of these enzymatic changes for the origin of the hepatocellular glycogenosis and the relation of this phenomenon to the neoplastic transformation remain to be elucidated (Bannasch, 1978).

Another type of epithelial tumour whose development is correlated with a transient storage of glycogen is the clear cell kidney tumour. In rats treated with N-nitrosomorpholine (NMOR) this renal tumour often appears in addition to liver tumours. The tumour originates from tubules storing glycogen in excess (Bannasch and Schacht, 1968; Bannasch and co-workers, 1978). In contrast to the focal glycogenosis of the liver which may appear very early under the influence of the carcinogen, the tubular glycogenosis develops in stop experiments, some weeks after cessation of the carcinogenic treatment. The lesion is easily detectable if the glycogen is preserved and is demonstrated by the PAS-reaction. After staining with H & E the typical clear cells with condensed nuclei are seen. Similar tubular alterations have also been described for the kidney of rats treated with dimethyl-nitrosamine. In accordance with our own interpretation the glycogenotic tubules were taken to be preneoplastic lesions by Ito and co-workers (1966), but Hard and Butler (1971) suggested that the clear cells represent a degenerative change which is unimportant for tumorigenesis.

TABLE 1 Glycogenotic (clear cell) tubules and tumours in the rat kidney at different stages after the application of N-nitrosomorpholine (12 mg ad 100 ml) in the drinking water for 7-14 weeks (from Bannasch and co-workers, 1978)

EXPERIMENTAL STAGE	NUMBER OF ANIMALS	ANIMALS WITH GLYCOGENOTIC	
		RENAL TUBULES	RENAL TUMORS
end of a 7-14 week treatment	30	0	0
3-5 weeks after stop	25	3	0
7-18 weeks after stop	15	2	0
22-97 weeks after stop	58	23	15

Table 1 shows the results of an experiment in which NMOR was added to the drinking water at a concentration of 12 mg per 100 ml. Tubules storing glycogen in excess were found in 3 of 25 animals 3-5 weeks after withdrawal of the carcinogen. After a lag period of 22-97 weeks nearly 50% of the experimental animals showed glycogenotic tubules - a lesion which was never seen in control rats. In addition to the glycogenotic tubules about 25% of the experimental animals developed glycogenotic (clear cell) tumours. Similar results were obtained by oral administration of NMOR in a concentration of 50 mg% for 3 weeks only.

The transformation of the tubules consisting of clear cells into tumours can be followed step by step. Initially the tubules show a cystic dilatation or they form a multilayered epithelium. The neoplastic nature of such alterations becomes obvious when the proliferation and atypical structure of the cells reaches a higher degree. At the same time many cells lose their glycogen and are transformed into acidophilic or slightly basophilic tumour cells. In the final tumours the clear cells may be restricted to small areas only. Electron microscopically the clear cells show a considerable amount of monoparticulate glycogen, but only a few mitochondria and ergastoplasmic profiles. In many cells substantial parts of the stored glycogen are enclosed in autophagic vacuoles - a phenomenon well known from type II of human glycogen storage disease.

In contrast to hepatocellular carcinomas and clear cell kidney tumours, some tumour types, e.g., murine lung adenomas (unpublished observations) or cholangiofibromas of the rat (Bannasch and Massner, 1977), store considerable amounts of glycogen without passing a glycogenotic pre-stage. However, during the preneoplastic phase of these tumors mucopolysaccharides may be stored.

MUCOPOLYSACCHARIDES

The development of cholangiocellular liver tumours is a most informative example for the storage of mucopolysaccharides during carcinogenesis. The cholangiocellular tumours occur especially in stop experiments with high doses of hepatocarcinogens (see Bannasch, 1975
for literature). After a 3 weeks' oral application of sublethal doses
of N-nitrosomorpholine, for example, cystic cholangiomas, cholangiofibromas and cholangiocarcinomas develop some weeks or even months
after cessation of the carcinogenic treatment (Bannasch and Reiss,
1971; Bannasch and Massner, 1976, 1977). From a morphologic point of
view these different types of tumours may be attributed to one sequence in which four distinct stages can be identified.

In the first stage, as an immediate consequence of toxic necrosis of
the liver parenchyma there is a vigorous proliferation of bile duct
epithelia (oval cells) and mesenchymal cells with subsequent fibrosis. During the second stage the ductular cell reaction proceeds to
a mucous cholangiofibrosis. Many ductular cells are converted into
goblet cells at this stage (Bannasch and Reiss, 1971; Chou and Gibson, 1972; Terao and Nakano, 1974). These cells store and secrete
abundant amounts of mucous substances which give a positive PAS- or
Hale reaction and are stained with alcian blue. The histochemical
reactions indicate that the mucus contains neutral and acid mucopolysaccharides. Therefore, we call this pathologic phenomen cholangiolar mucopolysaccharidosis (Bannasch and Reiss, 1971). After high doses of nitrosomorpholine the cholangiolar mucopolysaccharidosis
starts in some animals within a fortnight. It progresses even without further treatment, until (after some delay) it occupies nearly
all the cholangiofibrotic areas. The production of mucus in proli-
ferated bile ducts seems to be specific for carcinogenic liver in-
toxications (Bannasch and Reiss, 1971; Chou and Gibson, 1972). This
change has been observed after administration of various chemical
carcinogens in rats (Firminger and Mulay, 1955; see Bannasch, 1975,
for further literature) and hamsters (Reznik and Mohr, 1977). According to Chou and colleagues (1970, 1976) an accumulation of neutral
and acid mucopolysaccharides may also play an important role during
the development of human cholangiocellular tumours. In the third
stage of experimental cholangiocarcinogenesis benign cystic cholangiomas and cholangiofibromas originate from the mucous cholangiofibrosis (Bannasch and Reiss,1971; Bannasch and Massner, 1976).
In the fourth stage the cholangiofibroma may progress into a cholangiocarcinoma. Whereas the production of mucopolysaccharides persists
in the cholangiofibromas, the mucopolysaccharidosis gradually dis-
appears in cystic cholangiomas and in cholangiocarcinomas. In the
carcinomas a pronounced storage of glycogen may appear at the same
time.

Recently we investigated the development of gliomas induced in rats
by weekly intravenous injection of methylnitrosourea (Engelhardt and
Bannasch, 1978). The first alterations which we could detect in the
brain of the experimental animals were small areas with characteristic histochemical changes. In these areas, which exhibited no or only
a minimal proliferation of glial cells, acid mucopolysaccharides
could be demonstrated by the iron binding reaction or by alcian blue.
All intermediate stages lead from such areas to gliomatous micro-
tumours and fully developed gliomas which regularly give positive

reactions for acid mucopolysaccharides. An accumulation of acid muco
polysaccharides in experimental gliomas of the rat has also been
reported by Schiffer and Giordana (1974, 1975). Smith and Butler
(1973) described similar changes in human gliomas. According to our
own experience the alcianophilic material tends to disappear in
advanced stages of glioma development.

An excessive storage of acid mucopolysaccharides in renal tubular
epithelia has been suggested as an early event in the evolution of
basophilic renal adenomas (Bannasch and co-workers, 1971), but this
point needs further clarification.

GLYCOLIPIDS

The behaviour of glycolipids in tumours will be dealt with much more
competently by Dr. Hakamori in the following lecture, but I would
like to mention that some tumours investigated in our laboratory
show a considerable storage of lipids, possibly glycolipids. This is
especially true for the clear cell kidney tumour which often stores
lipids in addition to glycogen (Bannasch and co-workers, 1978).
The lipids form membrane-enclosed osmiophilic bodies which exhibit
a concentrically layered, or a parallel arranged pattern of dark and
light lines with a periodicity of 50-70 Å. Similar structures are
found in the nervous system, kidney and other tissues in association
with certain human storage diseases, such as mucopolysaccharidoses
and gangliosidosis (see O'Brian, 1973; Sandhoff and Harzer, 1973).
In this case the lamellar bodies seem to consist predominantly of
glycolipids. Another interesting observation on the putative storage
of glycolipids in tumours concerns the frequent appearance of
Gaucher-like cells in hematopoetic organs of humans suffering from
leukemia, especially chronic myelogeneous leukemia (see Takahashi
and co-workers, 1977 for literature).

CONCLUDING REMARKS

From the observations reported it is evident that the development of
many tumours is linked with a pathologic storage of polysaccharides.
At the cellular level the carcinogen-induced thesaurismoses are very
similar to the generalized alterations well known from human storage
diseases (Bannasch, 1974). At present it is not known whether the
disregulation of carbohydrate metabolism leading to a storage of
polysaccharides in preneoplastic or neoplastic cells plays an essential role during neoplastic transformation. The investigation of the
development of certain other tumours, such as hemangiosarcomas of
the liver or sarcomas of the brain, has so far failed to demonstrate
any storage phenomena. Nevertheless, the cellular storage of polysaccharides (or lipids) seems to indicate a more generalized principle involved in neoplastic cell transformation. In some experimental
models the stored substances may be looked upon as useful biological
markers for the detection and perhaps also for the isolation and biochemical investigation of preneoplastic cells.

REFERENCES

Altmann, H.W. (1977). Consideraciones sobre el significado y la nomenclatura de los tumores hepaticos en el hombre. Patologia, N° Extraordinario (II), 10, 1-16.

Altmann, H.W. (1978). Pathology of human liver tumours. In H. Remmer, H. M. Bolt and H. Popper (Eds.), Primary liver tumours, MTP Lancaster, in press.

Balász, M. (1976). Light and electron microscopic examination of a case of primary liver carcinoma in an infant. Zbl. allg. Path. 120, 3-13.

Bannasch, P. (1968). The cytoplasm of hepatocytes during carcinogenesis. Rec. Res. Cancer Res., vol. 19, Berlin-Heidelberg-New York, Springer

Bannasch, P. (1974). Carcinogen-induced cellular thesaurismoses and neoplastic cell transformation. Rec. Res. Cancer Res., vol. 44, 115-126.

Bannasch, P. (1975). Die Cytologie der Hepatocarcinogenese. In H.W. Altmann and colleagues (Eds.), Handbuch der Allgemeinen Pathologie, VI, 7, Berlin-Heidelberg-New York, Springer, pp. 123-276.

Bannasch, P. (1976). Cytology and cytogenesis of neoplastic (hyperplastic) hepatic nodules. Cancer Res., 36, 2555-2562.

Bannasch, P. (1978). Cellular and subcellular pathology of liver carcinogenesis. In H. Remmer, H.M. Bolt and H. Popper (Eds.), Primary liver tumours, MTP, Lancaster, in press.

Bannasch, P., and H. Angerer (1974). Glykogen und Glukose-6-Phosphatase während der Kanzerisierung der Rattenleber durch N-Nitrosomorpholin. Arch. Geschwulstforsch., 43, 105-114.

Bannasch, P., I. Hesse, and H. Angerer (1974). Hepatocelluläre Glykogenose und die Genese sogenannter hyperplastischer Knoten in der Thioacetamid-vergifteten Rattenleber. Virch. Arch. B Zellpath., 17, 29-50.

Bannasch, P., and O. Klinge (1971). Hepatocelluläre Glykogenose und Hepatombildung beim Menschen. Virch. Arch. A Path. Anat., 352, 157-164.

Bannasch, P., R. Krech, and H. Zerban (1978). Morphogenese und Mikromorphologie epithelialer Nierentumoren bei Nitrosomorpholin-vergifteten Ratten. II. Tubuläre Glykogenose und die Genese von klar- oder acidophilzelligen Tumoren. Z. Krebsforsch., 92, 63-86.

Bannasch, P., and B. Massner (1976). Histogenese und Cytogenese von Cholangiofibromen und Cholangiocarcinomen bei Nitrosomorpholin-vergifteten Ratten. Z. Krebsforsch., 87, 239-255.

Bannasch, P., and B. Massner (1977). Die Feinstruktur des Nitrosomorpholin-induzierten Cholangiofibroms der Ratte. Virchows. Arch. B. Cell Path., 24, 295-315.

Bannasch, P., and H.A. Müller (1964). Lichtmikroskopische Untersuchungen über die Wirkung von N-Nitrosomorpholin auf die Leber von Ratte und Maus. Arzneim. Forsch., 14, 805-814.

Bannasch, P., J. Papenburg, and W. Ross (1972). Cytomorphologische und morphometrische Studien der Hepatocarcinogenese. I. Reversible und irreversible Veränderungen am Cytoplasma der Leberparenchymzellen bei Nitrosomorpholin-vergifteten Ratten. Z. Krebsforsch., 77, 108-133.

Bannasch, P., and W. Reiss (1971). Histogenese und Cytogenese chol-
   angiocellulärer Tumoren bei Nitrosomorpholin-vergifteten Ratten.
   Zugleich ein Beitrag zur Morphogenese der Cystenleber.
   Z. Krebsforsch. 76, 193-215.
Bannasch, P., and U. Schacht (1968). Nitrosamin-induzierte tubuläre
   Glykogenspeicherung und Geschwulstbildung in der Rattenniere.
   Virch. Arch. B. Zellpath., 1, 95-97.
Bannasch, P., U. Schacht, R. Weidner, and E. Storch (1971). Morpho-
   genese und Mikromorphologie basophiler und onkocytärer Nieren-
   tumoren bei Nitrosamin-vergifteten Ratten. Verh. dtsch. Ges.
   Path., 55, 665-670.
Bannasch, P., G. Venske, and D. Mayer (1977). Prenatal induction by
   ENU of focal hepatic glycogenosis and hepatocellular tumors in
   mice. 4th meeting Europ. Ass. Cancer Res., p. 82.
Bauer, B. (1964). Über eine Sonderform der Gierkeschen Glykogenose
   mit Aktivitätssteigerung der α-Glucosidase in der Leber bei
   vollständigem Glucose-6-phosphatase-Mangel. Helv. Paediat.Acta,
   19, 13-28.
Berant, M., A. Horowitz, and J. Rotem (1977). Liver adenoma and
   glycogen storage disease. J. Israel Med. Ass., 17, 64-65.
Cain, H., and B. Kraus (1977). Entwicklungsstörungen der Leber und
   Leberkarzinom im Säuglings- und Kindesalter. Deut. Med.
   Wochenschr., 102, 505-509.
Chou, S.T., C.W. Chan, and W.L. Ng (1976). Mucin histochemistry of
   human cholangiocarcinoma. J. Path., 118, 165-170.
Chou, S.T., and J.B. Gibson (1970). The histochemistry of biliary
   mucins and the changes caused by Clonorchis sinensis.
   J. Path., 101, 185-197.
Chou, S.T., and J.B. Gibson, (1972). A comparative histochemical
   study of rat livers in alpha-naphthyl-iso-thiocyanate (ANIT)
   and DL-ethionine intoxication. J. Path., 108, 73-83.
Christianson, R.O., L. Page, and R.E. Greenberg (1968). Glycogen
   storage in a hepatoma: dephosphorylase kinase defect.
   Pediatrics, 42, 694-696.
Engelhardt, A., and P. Bannasch (1978). Histochemie saurer Mucopoly-
   saccharide während der Genese Methylnitrosoharnstoff-induzierter
   Hirntumoren der Ratte. Acta Neuropath., 42, 197-204.
Farber, E. (1973). Hyperplastic liver nodules. In H. Busch (Ed.),
   Methods in Cancer Research, vol. 7, New York-London:
   Academic Press, pp. 345-375.
Firminger, H.J., and A.S. Mulay (1952). Histochemical and morphologic
   differentiation of induced tumors of the liver in rats.
   J. Nat. Canc. Inst., 13, 19-34.
Forget, A., and R. Daoust (1970). Histochemical study on rat liver
   glycogen during DAB carcinogenesis. Int. J. Cancer, 5, 404-409.
Fraumeni, J.F., R.W. Miller, and J.A. Hill (1968). Primary carcinoma
   of the liver in childhood: an epidemiologic study.
   J. Nat. Canc. Inst., 40, 1087-1099.
Friedrich-Freksa, H., W. Gössner, and P. Börner (1969). Histochemi-
   sche Untersuchungen der Cancerogenese in der Rattenleber nach
   Dauergaben von Diäthylnitrosamin. Z. Krebsforsch., 72, 226-239.
Hacker, H.J., and P. Bannasch (1977a). Enzymehistochemical pattern
   of hepatic glycogen storage foci during NNM carcinogenesis.
   4th meeting Europ. Ass. Cancer Res. p.83.
Hacker, H.J., and P. Bannasch (1977b). Histochemische Muster einiger
   Schlüsselenzyme des Kohlenhydratstoffwechsels während der Hepatocarcinogenese. Verh. Dtsch. Ges. Path., 61, 481.

Hard, G.C., and W.H. Butler (1971). Morphogenesis of epithelial neo-
    plasms induced in the rat kidney by dimethylnitrosamine.
    Cancer Res., 311, 1496-1505.
Höhn, P., R. Wagner, and P. Gutjahr (1977). Patologia y clinica de
    los tumores epiteliales malignos hepaticos en edades infantiles.
    Patologia, N° Extraordinario (II), 10, 205-210.
Holling, H.E. (1963). Gout and glycogen storage disease.
    Ann. Int. Med., 58, 654-663.
Howell, R.R., R.E. Stevens, Y. Ben-Menachem, R. Phyliky and D.H.
    Berry (1976). Hepatic adenomata with Typ 1 glycogen storage
    disease. J. Am. Med. Ass., 236, 1481-1484.
Ito, N., J. Johno, M. Marugami, Y. Konishi, and Y. Hiasa (1966).
    Histopathological and autoradiographic studies on kidney tumors
    induced by N-Nitroso-dimethylamine in rat. Gann., 57, 595-604.
Kalengayi, M.M.R., and V.J. Desmet (1975). Sequential histological
    and histochemical study of the rat liver during Aflatoxin B_1-
    induced carcinogenesis. Cancer Res., 35, 2845-2852.
Kunz, W., K.E. Appel, R. Rickart, and G. Stöckle (1977). Quantitative
    analysis of enzyme-deficient cell areas to assess early pre-
    cancerous alterations of hepatocarcinogenic substances. 4th
    meeting Europ. Ass. Cancer Res., p. 45.
Kunz, W., K.E. Appel, R. Rickart, M. Schwarz, and G. Stöckle (1978).
    Enhancement and inhibition of carcinogenic effectiveness of
    nitrosamines. In H. Remmer, H.M. Bolt, and H. Popper (Eds.)
    Primary liver tumours, MTP, Lancaster, in press.
Lesch, R., Ch. Bauer, and W. Reutter (1973). The development of
    cholangiofibrosis and hepatomas in galactosamine induced
    cirrhotic rat livers. Virch. Arch. B Zellpath., 12,285-289.
Lesch, R., K. Meinhardt, and W. Oehlert (1968). Lichtmikroskopische
    und autoradiographische Befunde bei der Cancerisierung der
    Rattenleber mit Methyl-Allyl-Nitrosoharnstoff. Z. Krebsforsch.,
    70, 267-280.
Levine, G., G. Mierau, and B.E. Favara (1976). Hepatic glycogenosis,
    renal glomerular cysts, and hepatocarcinoma. Am. J. Path., 82,
    PPC-37.
Mason, H.H., and D.H. Anderson (1955). Glycogen disease of the liver
    (von Gierke's disease) with hepatomata: case report with meta-
    bolic studies. Pediatrics, 16, 785-799.
Mayer, D., and P. Bannasch (1977). Hepatic glycogenosis and activity
    of some related enzymes in early stages of NNM carcinogenesis.
    4th meeting Europ. Ass. Cancer Res., p. 82.
Moulin, M.-Ch., and R. Daoust (1971). Glucose-6-phosphatase activity
    in rat liver parenchyma during azo-dye carcinogenesis.
    Int. J. Cancer, 8, 81-85.
Nigam, V.N., and A. Cantero (1972). Polysaccharides in Cancer.
    Advanc. Cancer Res., 16, 1-96.
O'Brian, J.S. (1973). Tay-Sachs'disease and iuvenile GM2-gangliosi-
    dosis. In H.G. Hers and F. van Hoof (Eds.), Lysosomes and
    storage diseases, Academic Press, New York-London, pp. 323-344.
Reznik, G., and U. Mohr (1977). Colangiomas y colangiocarcinomas en
    el hamster europeo tras tratamiento con di-isopropanol-
    nitrosamina. Patologia, N° Extraordinario (II), 10, 171-204.
Roe, T., M. Kogut, B. Buckinham, J. Miller, G. Gates, and B. Landing
    (1978). Hepatic tumors in glycogen storage disease type I.
    Clinical Res., 26, A 191.

Ruebner, B.H., R. Kanayama, C. Michas, and P. Bannasch (1976).
    Sequential hepatic histologic and histochemical changes pro-
    duced by diethylnitrosamine in the Rhesus monkey.
    J. Nat. Canc. Inst., 57, 1261-1268.
Sandhoff, U., and K. Harzer (1973). Total hexosaminidase deficiency
    in Tay-Sachs' disease (variant O). In H.G. Hers and van Hoof,
    (Eds.) Lysosomes and storage diseases, Academic Press, New
    York-London, pp. 345-356.
Schauer, A., and E. Kunze (1968). Enzymhistochemische und autoradio-
    graphische Untersuchungen während der Cancerisierung der Ratten-
    leber durch Diäthylnitrosamin. Z. Krebsforsch., 70, 252-266.
Scherer, E., M. Hoffmann, P. Emmelot, and H. Friedrich-Freksa (1972).
    Quantitative study on foci of altered liver cells induced in
    the rat by a single dose of diethylnitrosamine and partial he-
    patectomy. J. Nat. Canc. Inst., 49, 93-106.
Schiffer, D., and M.T. Giordana (1974). On the occurrence and sig-
    nificance of acid mucopolysaccharides in oligodendrogliomas
    experimentally induced in the rat by nitrosourea derivates.
    In D. Schreiber and W. Jänisch (Eds.) Experimentelle Neuroonko-
    logie, Johann Ambrosius Barth, Leipzig, pp. 101-108.
Schiffer, D., and M.T. Giordana (1975). Acid mucopolysaccharides in
    experimental brain tumors. Proc. VII Intern. Congr. Neuropath.
    Budapest, Vol. I, Excerpta Medica, Amsterdam, pp. 533-540.
Schmitz-Moormann, P., P. Gedigk, and A. Dharamandhach (1972).
    Histologische und histochemische Frühveränderungen bei der
    experimentellen Erzeugung von Lebercarcinomen durch Diäthylni-
    trosamin. Z. Krebsforsch., 77, 9-16.
Smith, B., and M. Butler (1973). Acid mucopolysaccharides in tumours
    of the myelin sheath cells, the oligodendroglioma and the
    neurilemmoma. Acta neuropath. (Berl.), 23, 181-185.
Spycher, M.A., and R. Gitzelmann (1971). Glycogenosis type I (Gluco-
    se-6-phosphatase deficiency): Ultrastructural alterations of he-
    patocytes in a tumor bearing liver. Virchows Arch. B Zellpath.
    8, 133-142.
Sydow, G., and F. Fey (1969).Über die Glykogenose der Rattenleber nach
    Einwirkung von Diäthylnitrosamin.Acta biol.med.germ., 23, 9-13.
Takahashi, K., K. Terashima, M. Kojima, H. Yoshida, and H. Kimura.
    (1977). Pathological, histochemical and ultrastructural studies
    on sea-blue histiocytes and Gaucher-like cells in acquired
    lipidosis occuring in leukemia. Acta Path. Jap., 27, 775-797.
Taper, H.S., and P. Bannasch (1976). Histochemical correlation bet-
    ween glycogen, nucleic acids and nucleases in pre-neoplastic
    and neoplastic lesions of rat liver after short-term administra-
    tion of N-nitrosomorpholine. Z. Krebsforsch., 87, 53-65.
Taper, H.S., L. Fort, and J.-M. Brucher (1971). Histochemical activi-
    ty of alkaline and acid nucleases in the rat liver parenchyma
    during N-nitrosomorpholine carcinogenesis. Cancer Res., 31,
    913-916.
Terao, K., and M. Nakano (1974). Cholangiofibrosis induced by short-
    term feeding of 3'-methyl-4-(dimethylamino)azobenzene: an
    electron microscopic observation. Gann, 65, 249-260.
Williams, G.M., M. Klaiber, S.E. Parker,and E. Farber (1976). Nature
    of early appearing, carcinogen-induced liver lesions resistant
    to iron accumulation. J. Nat. Cancer Inst., 57, 157-165.
Zangeneh, F., G.A. Limbeck, B.L. Brown, J.R. Emch, M.M. Arcasoy, V.E.
    Goldenberg,and V.C. Kelley (1969).Hepatorenal glycogenosis (type
    I glycogenosis) and carcinoma of the liver.J.Pediat.,74, 73-83.

Chromosomes of Normal and Neoplastic Cells

Sonia B. de Salum

*Instituto de Investigaciones Hematológicas, Academia Nacional de Medicina,
Buenos Aires, Argentina*

ABSTRACT

The possible karyotype alterations are enumerated including the sequence of losses and gains for homologous chromosomes in neoplastic cells, in relation to the hete rochromatin, density of repitious DNA and G banding pattern in chromosome regions in the folded chromatin fiber chromosome model.

The chromosome banding patterns of 31 leukemia patients are presented. The results are discussed in comparison with those reported in other surveys of leukemia patients, from different geographic areas. Out of these, 13 were diagnosed as acute lymphoblastic leukemia (ALL), 1 as chronic lymphocytic leukemia (CLL), 10 as chronic myelogenous leukemia (CML) (5 of which were in acute phase), 3 acute and 1 subacute myelocytic leukemia (AMLL), and one case of hypereosinophilic syndrome (HES).

The Ph (22q-) chromosome was observed in all CML patients. In acute phase of CML, the karyotype presented abnormalities of several autosomes. The chromosome groups C and G being more frequently involved. A large proportion of ALL patients showed hyperdiploidy, each patient exhibiting a unique picture. Marker chromosomes and clonal evolution were detected in two of the AML patients. A high proportion of pseudodiploid cells was found in 4 out of 6 AML patients. These results show coincidence with chromosome changes that have been defined for both acute and chronic leukemias.

The analysis of 2 human lymphoplastoid cell lines derived from a lymphosarcoma lymph node biopsy (GH7) and the other from peripheral blood transformed lymphocytes (LDLT) revealed a cytogenetic pattern, with the presence of marker chromosomes, in many aspects comparable with the findings reported in established lines of Burkitt lymphoma.
Key words: cytogenetics, human, neoplastic,cells.

INTRODUCTION

In recent years a number of important developments have taken place in the field of cytogenetics. These include: 1) The visualitation of characteristic banding patterns within metaphase chromosomes by the use of various dyes and denaturating agents (Caspersson, Zech and Johansson, 1970; Summer, Evans and Buckland, 1971) and

2) the finding of highly repetitive satellite DNA in constitutive heterochromatin and its localization in metaphase chromosomes by in situ hibridization (Pardue and Gall, 1970).

In the chromosome model that takes into account the folded chromatin fiber, the G banding pattern and the localization of repetitive DNA can be combined to illustrate various structural elements of the chromosome (Du Praw, 1966); in this model mammalian chromosomes are believed to be composed of long chromatin fibers the bulk of which is arranged in packed and predominantly horizontal loops, which are generally visualized as deeply staining bands in the light of fluorescent microscope and are rich in repetitive and other nongenic DNA. The remaining DNA is made up of genic and intergenic DNA that is arranged in a looser and somewhat vertical fashion and is generally localized in the noncentromeric and lightly stained chromosomal bands. Pericentromeric and perinuclear bands are rich in highly repetitive satellite DNAs and correspond to the classic constitutive heterochromatin of interphase nuclei.

The dark bands on the chromosome arms are enriched in the intermediate repetitive DNA and correspond in part to the intercalary heterochromatin. This DNA replicates during the second half of the DNA synthetic period, is largely nontranscriptional and plays vital roles in chromosome structure and cell regulation.

Since the discovery of the new banding techniques is has been possible to observe chromosomal breaks and rearrangements involving the majority of the chromosomes of man with a propensity for chromosomal regions rich in nongenic DNA (such as centromeres and telomeres) to be preferentially involved in the chromosomal rearrangements. Neoplastic cells may show chromosomal abnormalities that can be summarized as follows: 1) Changes that affect entire chromosomes (heteroploidy) including euploid heteroploid and aneuploid conditions, 2) changes that involve additions or deletions of portions of individual chromosomes (duplications and deficiencies) and 3) rearrangements of chromosome material (inversions and translocations). One cannot exclude point mutations, gene deletions or duplications or hidden rearrangements. To evaluate chromosomal changes in human neoplasia it is important to consider: first their specificity and secondly the value for clinical diagnosis and prognosis.

The chromosomal changes in human neoplastic disorders appear to be confined to the tissue involved, all other somatic cells being diploid. The most interesting and relatively specific chromosomal change in human neoplasia described to date is the presence of a partly deleted member of group G, the Philadelphia or Ph'(22q-) chromosome (Nowell and Hungerford, 1960). This chromosomal aberration is virtually diagnostic for chronic myelogenous leukemia (CML). The closest approach to an association comparable to that between the Ph' chromosome and CML, was the finding that a G group chromosome is frequently lost, partially deleted or involved in structural rearrangement in meningioma cells (Mark, 1970). The Ph' chromosome is now known not to involve a simple deletion of the long arm of a chromosome 22, but a translocation, usually t (9q+, 22q-) (Rowley, 1973a).

Chromosome 9, which carries a secondary constriction, tends to be associated with the nucleolus and therefore may be involved in its organization. These related activities might bring these 2 chromosomes together in interphase and thus facilitate the chances of a specific translocation (Raposa, Natarajan and Granberg,1974).

In most instances, particular abnormalities are found to occur not in every case of a given tumour but with a strikingly increased frequency against a background of multiple rearrangements.

Examples include: the gain of a number 8 chromosome and reduplication of the long arm of a number 17 in the late (acute) stage of chronic myeloid leukemia (Mitel man, Branch and Levan, 1973; Rowley, 1973b) loss of a number 7 and gain of a number 9 in acute leukemia (Rowley, 1973c), loss or partial deletion of a number 22 in meningioma (Marck, 1970); an extra band on the long arm of a number 14 in lymphosarcoma and in myeloma (Zech and others, 1976), supernumerary numbers 8 and of numbers 7 and 22 in melanoma (McCulloch and others, 1976). For many other tumors the evidence for nonrandom chromosome aberrations is suggestive but as yet incomplete.

The present report deals with the cytogenetic examination of 31 leukemia patients whose karyotype was determined by G banding technique. The results are discussed in comparison with other surveys of leukemia patients, with comments on the chromo somal patterns in other hematological disorders.

MATERIAL AND METHODS

The diagnosis of leukemia in all cases had been established by peripheral blood and bone marrow examination, using standard procedures.

In addition leukemia cells were classified by cytochemical studies using PAS, peroxidase, and Sudan Blak B (Pavlovsky and others, 1973). Out of 31 patients, 13 were diagnosed as acute lymphoblastic leukemia(ALL), 1 as chronic lymphocytic (CLL) 10 as chronic myelogenous leukemia (CML), 5 of which were in the acute phase, 3 acute nonlymphoblastic (ANLL) and 1 subacute myelocytic leukemia (Sub AML). One patient with myelomonocytic leukemia (AMMol) and one case of hypereosinophilic syndrome. Bone marrow cells from 3 patients were analized prior to therapy (2 ALL, 1 LLC). Except for the 10 patients (9 ALL, 1 CML) in complete remission, all treated patients in partial remission or in relapse had a predominance of blasts in their marrow at the time of chromosome study (3 ALL in induction period, 2 ALL and 4 ANL in relapse). Of the 10 CML patients, 4 were in partial remission, 1 in complete remission and 5 in blast crisis).

The chromosome analysis was performed on standard and trypsin giemsa banding technique slides (Seabright, 1971). The chromosomes were identified according to the Paris Nomenclature and the karyotypes were expressed as recomended under this system (Paris Conference, 1972). The number of samples per patient ranged from 1 to 2. In most cases a minimum of 30 mitotic cells were counted and 10 of these were photographed and analysed in detail.

An abnormal clone is defined as two cells with the same extra chromosome or with the same structural rearrangement, or three cells with the same missing chromosome.

RESULTS IN CML AND COMMENTS

The Ph translocations t (9;22) was identified in two of the 10 CML Ph' positive patients. One of them had deletion of the long arm of one chromosome 11 as an additional abnormality. In the 5 CML patients in the acute phase, the chromosome group C, G and E were more frequently involved in all of the cases. Furthermore an additional abnormality was always associated with blast crisis, which consisted in a double Ph'. There were no cases with an iso- 17q chromosome - One patient in blast crisis had a clone with a complex karyotype 54XY, 2Ph' (+4C, +1D, -1E, +1F, +1G) trisomy of the 6, 13, 19 and 21 chromosomes and monosomy of the 18 were identified in G banded karyotype at the final stage of his disease.

In the literature, in patients, with Ph' positive CML (Rowley and De La Chapelle, 1978) the translocation t (9q+; 22q-) was found in 92% of them; of the remainder some had a two way translocation involving chromosome 22 with another chromosome, and others had three or four way translocations, all of which involved both chromosome 9 and 22 along with other chromosomes. The additional abnormalities seen in the chronic phase were mostly a double Ph' chromosome (5%) or +8 (2,4%) which were also those most frequently seen in the blast phase. The isochromosome for the long arm of 17 (i (17q)) was a reliable marker for the blast phase (Rowley, 1975).

RESULTS IN ACUTE LEUKEMIA AND COMMENTS

Among the 6 ANLL patients studied, 3 were diagnosed as acute, 1 as subacute myelo-cytic leukemia (AML), 1 as myelomonocytic leukemia (AMMol) and 1 was a hypereosino philic syndrome (HES).

Two of the patients had not received chemotherapy, whereas 4 had been treated and were in relapse at the time of the cytogenetic study. The aneuploid cells in the AMMol patients were either hypo or hyperdiploid. All stem line numbers were in the diploid region: 44, 46 or 47 chromosomes, with high proportion of pseudodiploid cells in 4 out of the 6 patients. In the hypereosinophilic syndrome patient 90% of the bone marrow metaphases were pseudodiploid and showed clonal evolution of the karyotype 46XY (+C, -E) to 46XY (+D, -2E, +G) karyotypes. All the 6ANLL patients had abnormal karyotypes, 4 of them with 100% abnormal cells (AA), and 2 had abnormal and normal cells (AN).

Three of them died a short time after the study was carried out. One of the AML patients, with 98% blasts in her marrow could never enter in remission, she was studied in the induction and relapse period and died three months after the onset of the disease. Abnormalities were found in 100% of the marrow cells in both opportunities and four related clones were encountered. There was an unidentified marker chromosome about the size of a 19 chromosome in each metaphase. An endo-duplicated metaphase was found with 92XX (-2C, +2M) of the major clone 46XX (-C, +M) with monosomy of chromosome 9. The additional M, appeared to be the first abnormality present in this patient and was present also in the development of three minor clones: 44XX (-2C, -D, +M) with monosomy for the 15 and 47XX (+1P, -C, +M) with trisomy form p arm of the chromosome 1; a third clone 46XX (-G, +M) was found with monosomy of chromosome 22, and the M, marker.

Another AML case, with diagnosis of AMMol had 70% normal (46XY) and 30% 46X0 (+D) as the only abnormality encountered in marrow cells. The absence of the Y chromo-some was found in 20% cells of another AML patient, finding 46X0 (+2C, -D) karyotypes and 46XY (-B, +C) with loss of a 5 and gain of a 9 chromosome and clonal evolution: 47XY (-B, +M1,+M2) cells with two unidentified small markers (M and M2).

Gain or loss of part or all of chromosome 1 was a frequent finding in cells of 3 out of the 6 ANLL patients.

The results obtained for ALL patients, have consisted of a diverse array of karyo typic alterations, aneuploidy was found in about half of the cases and a large proportion of patients had hyperploidy. In these cases all the chromosome groups showed numerical abnormalities, but the C, G and E group were more frequently involved.

Aneuploidy was found in about half of the cases and a large proportion of the patients had hyperploidy (Sandberg and others, 1968). Partial deletion of the

long arm of chromosome (6q) was observed in 4 out of 16 ALL patients serie (Oshimura and Sandberg, 1976).

In ANLL it is possible to detect structural rearrangements, nonrandom patterns of
chromosomal abnormalities and a third important observation was that acute leuke
mia can be considered as in the same sense as chronic myelogenous leukemia, a
clonal disease (Rowley and Potter, 1976). Chemotherapy did not appear to produce
a stable clone of aberrations. AML patients could be classified according to the
type of abnormality, specifically +8; -7; t (8q-, 21q+); t (15q+; 17q-), and t
(9q+, 22q-) and also, according to chromosome numbers as follows: less than 46,
equal and greater than 46 (Rowley and De La Chapelle, 1978). Results from differ
ent surveys (Golomb, Vardinam and Rowley, 1976; Trujillo and others, 1974) show
that karyotypic abnormalities observed at the time of initial examination are of
prognostic value.

The presence or absence of the Y chromosome in leukemic and cancerous cells has
received considerable attention, and it has been postulated that the cells in the
bone marrow with a missing Y as the sole karyotypic anomaly may not necessarily
be related to an acute leukemic process (Oshimura and others, 1976). It has been
indicated that when a missing Y does occur in cells of AML, it is invariably
accompanied by the prototypic karyotypic. This was the case in the two AML
patients of our ANLL series.

In an analysis of several major reviews of the HES (Chusid and others, 1975) only
four chromosomal abnormalities were demonstrated. They consisted in the finding
of Ph', lacking of single C group chromosome or a significant population of
aneuploid cells, but without specific abnormality, this was the case in our HES
patient with abnormal 46XY pseudodiploid karyotypes with groups C, E and G
involved and without presence of Ph' chromosome.

COMMENTS ON THE CHROMOSOMAL PATTERNS IN OTHER HEMATOLOGICAL DISORDERS

The analysis of human lymphoblastoid cell line (GH7) derived from a human lympho
sarcoma, and composed of blastomatous undifferentiated cells was carried out in
our laboratory (Suarez and others, 1969). A long, acrocentric marker chromosome
was present in 90% of the metaphases. Modal number was in the polyploid range
with scattered dispersion around the mode value. The cytogenetic pattern was in
many aspects comparable with the findings reported in established lines of Burkitt
 lymphoma (Salum, Suarez and Pavlovsky, 1971).Another cell line was established,
when tritiated DNA extracted from the GH7 cells was added to the culture of
apparently normal autologous peripheral leukocytes (Sen and others, 1969). This
line also exhibited a clear nonrandom cytogenetic pattern with D group marker
chromosomes (Salum, Sen and Pavlovsky, 1972). Secondary constitutions on the long
arms of a 10 group chromosome were found in 20% and in the short arms of a 7-8
group specimens in a 10%, in both lines. A striking chromosomal anomaly was seen
in 50% bone marrow metaphases of an AML patient of our serie of ANLL patients;
this very closely resembled the previously described lesions.

Secondary constrictions representing achromatic gaps in particular regions of
human chromosomes are sites which are occasionally affected by viral infection. It
has been reported that these specialized chromosome regions (many of them acting
as nucleolar organizer) become attenuated, broken or despiralized in cell lines
derived from patients with Burkitt lymphoma or infectious mononucleosis. Attenuated secondary constrictions of chromosome 9 in several cases of malignant lymphoma
have been reported (Miles and O'Neill, 1966). Some of the most common of such
constrictions (chromosomes 1 and 16) are associated with a heterochromatic segment.

These constrictions may be of particular interest in view of their inductibility
by virus.

Nonrandom karyotypic changes are not limited to disorders of bone marrow cells;
in many if not all cases of Burkitt lymphomas, a translocation t (8q-, 14q+) was
found (Manolov and Manolova, 1972) and in multiple myeloma (Wurster-Hill, 1973);
rearrangement involving chromosome 14 has also been observed in a number of
malignant lymphomas (Zech and others, 1976).

CONCLUSION

The fact that nonrandom chromosome changes are found in malignant cells suggests
that these changes provide the cells with a proliferative advantage over those
with a normal karyotype. Many of the affected chromosomes carry genes related to
nucleic acid biosynthesis, and the critical effect of these changes in gene
action within the mutant cell may be to keep it in the mitotic cycle and to
prevent the cell from intering the resting stage.

Chromosomes that are most commonly involved in aberrations are distributed nonran
domly over the different human chromosome types. The aberrations cluster in several
specific chromosomes, mainly 1,7,8,9,14,17,21, and 22.

Chronic myeloid leukemia is the best studied malignancy as regards chromosomes.
Most CML patients have the translocation t (9q+, 22q-); this is balanced translo
cation in that apparently no net changes in total material have ocurred. In the
blastic phase of CML, the most common changes are the addition of another 22q-
chromosome; producing imbalance, and then the addition of a chromosome 8, leading
to even more imbalance. A similar sequence of changes occurs in acute myeloid
leukemia.

Burkitt lymphoma is the best cytogenetically studied human lymphoid cancer. In
this lymphoma there is also a "balanced" translocation that involves chromosomes
8 and 14; t (8q-; 14q+). From these and similar studies in other cancers it
can be concluded that the usual sequence of chromosome changes in human neoplastic
cells appears to be: 1) chromosome breakage, 2) "balanced" translocation (primary
clone), 3) addition or subtraction of chromosomes, one at a time to produce
imbalance (secondary clone) and 4) further changes producing more imbalance
(tertiary clone).

Chromosome regions in cancer cells can be classified as 1) restricted (no changes
allowed), 2) semi-restricted "balanced" change or addition permitted and 3)
unrestricted (anything goes). These classes may correspond to the density of key
genes and inversely to the density of repetitive DNA (Hecht, Kaiser and Mc Caw,
1977).

Our results in this our first serie of 31 leukemia patients and 2 lymphoblastoid
cell lines, show coincidence with chromosome changes that have been reported in
the literature.

Cytogenetic examination of more human tumors is necessary, not only to establish
the validity of nonrandom chromosome aberrations but also for comparison of their
frequencies in different geographic areas. "It may be that different etiologic
agents predominate in different regions of the world, leading to geographic
variation in the chromosome aberrations of túmors" (Levan and Mitelman, 1977).

REFERENCES

Caspersson, T., Zech, L. and Johansson, C. (1970). Differential binding of alky lating fluorochrome in human chromosomes. Exp. Cell Res., 60, 315-319.

Chusid, M.J., Dale, C.D., West, B.C. and Wolff, S.M. (1975). The hypereosinophilic syndrome: Analysis of fourteen cases with review of the literature. Medicine 54, 1, 1-27.

Du Praw, E.J. (1966). Evidence for a "folded-fibre" organization in human chromo somes. Nature, 209, 577-581.

Fukuhara, S., Shirakawa, S. and Uchino, H. (1976). Specific marker chromosome 14 in malignant lymphomas. Nature, 259, 210-211.

Golomb, H.M., Vardiman, J. and Rowley, J.D. (1976). Acute nonlymphocytic leukemia in adults: Correlations with Q- banded chromosomes. Blood 48, 1, 9-21.

Hecht, F., Kaiser Mc Caw B. (1977). Chromosomes and genes in human cancer cells: Multitudiciplinary approaches to a unitary genodemographic hypothesis. In A. De La Chapelle and Sorsa (Ed.) Chromosomes Today, vol. 6, Elsevier North Holland Biomedical Press, Amsterdam. The Netherlands. pp. 357-362.

Manolov, G. and Manolova, Y. (1972). Marker band in one chromosome 14 from Burkitt lymphomas. Nature, 237, 33.

Mark, J. (1970). Chromosomal patterns in human meningiomas. Eur. J. Cancer, 6, 489-498.

Mc Culloch, P.B., Dent, O.B., Hayes, P.R. and Liao, S.K. (1976). Common and individually specific chromosome characteristics of cultured human melanoma. Cancer Res., 36, 398-404.

Miles, C.P. and O'Neil, F. (1966). Prominent constriction in a pseudodiploid human cell line. Cytogenetic, 5, 321-334.

Miles, C.P. (1974). Nonrandom chromosome changes in human cancer. Br. J. Cancer, 30, 73-85.

Mitelman, F., Brandt, L., and Levan, G. (1973). Identification of isochromosome 17 in acute myeloid leukemia. Lancet, II, 972.

Mitelman, F., Levan, G., Nillson, O.G. and Brandt, L. (1976). Nonrandom karyotypic evolution in chronic myeloid leukemia. Int. J. Cancer, 18, 24-30.

Nowell, P.C. and Hungerford, D.A. (1960). A minute chromosome in human chronic myelocytic leukemia. Science, 132, 1497.

Oshimura, M. and Sandberg, A.A. (1976). Chromosome 6q-. Anomaly in acute lympho-blastic leukemia. Lancet, II, 1045-1406.

Pardue, M.L. and Gall, J.G. (1970). Chromosomal localization of mouse satellite DNA. Science, 168, 1356-1358.

Paris Conference (1972). Standarization in human cytogenetics. The National fundation-March of Dimes. Cytogenetics, II, 313-362.

Pavlovsky, S., Peñalver, J., Eppinger-Helft, M., Sackmann Muriel, F., Bergna, L., Suarez, A., Vilaseca, G., and Andino Pavlovsky, A., and Pavlovsky, A. (1973). Induction and maintenance of remission in acute leukemia. Cancer, 31, 273-279.

Raposa, T., Natarajan, A.T. and Grandberg, I. (1974). Identification of Ph' chromosome and associated translocation in chronic myelogenous leukemia by Hoes chst 33258. J. Natl. Cancer Inst., 52, 1935-1938.

Rowley, J.D. (1973a). A new consistent chromosomal abnormality in chronic myelo-genous leukemia identified by quinacrine fluorescence and Giemsa banding. Nature (Lond.), 243, 290-293.

Rowley, J.D. (1973b). Deletions of chromosome 7 in hematological disorders. Lancet II, 1385-1386.

Rowley, J.D. (1973c). Chromosomal pattern in myelocytic leukemia. New Engl. J. Med. 289, 220-221.

Rowley, J.D. (1975). Nonrandom chromosomal abnormalities in hematologic disorders of man. Proc. Natl. Acad. Sci., 72, 152-156.

Rowley, J.D., Potter, D. (1976). Chromosomal banding patterns in acute nonlympho cytic leukemia. Blood 47, 5, 705-721.

Rowley, J.D. and De La Chapelle, A. (1978). General report on the First Interna tional Workshop on chromosomes in leukemia. Int. J. Cancer, 21, 307-308.

Sandberg, A.A., Takagi, N., Sofumi, T. and Crosswhite, L.H. (1968). Chromosomes and causation of human cancer and leukemia. V. Karyotypic aspects of acute leukemia. Cancer, 22, 1268-1282.

Salum, S.B. de, Suarez, H.G. and Pavlovsky, A. (1971). Chromosome serial studies of a cultured cell line. Rev. Europ. Etudes Clin. et Biol., 15, 711-714.

Salum, S.B. de, Sen, L. and Pavlovsky, A. (1972). Estudio citogenético de una línea celular derivada por transformación de linfocitos periféricos. Sangre, 4, 467-478.

Seabright, M. (1971). A rapid banding technique for human chromosomes. Lancet, II, 971-972.

Sen, L., Suarez, H.G., Salum, S.B. de, Pavlovsky, S., Pavlovsky, A. and Bachmann, A.E. (1972). In vitro transformation of peripheral human lymphocytes by autologous malignant DNA. Medicina 32, 5, 428-436.

Suarez, H.G., Salum, S.B. de, Pavlovsky, S., Ruibal, B. and Pavlovsky, A. (1969). Culture in vitro d'une ligneé cellulaire provenant d'un lymphosarcome humain. I. Cytochimie, cytogénétique et ultraestructure cellulaire. Int. J. Cancer, 4, 880-890.

Summer, A.T., Evans, H.J. and Buckland, R.A. (1971). New technique for distingui shing between human chromosomes. Nature, 232, 31-32.

Trujillo, J.M., Cork, A., Hart, J.S., George, S.L. and Freireich, E.J. (1974). Clinical implications of aneuploid cytogenetic profiles in adult acute leukemia. Cancer, 33, 824-834.

Wurster-Hill, D.H., Mc Intyre, O.R., Cornwell, G.G. and Maurer, L.H. (1973). Marker chromosome 14 in multiple myeloma and plasma-cell leukemia. Lancet, 2, 1031

Zech, L., Haglund, U., Nilsson, K. and Klein, G. (1976). Characteristic chromoso mal abnormalities in biopsies and lymphoid cell lines from patients with Burkitt and non-Burkitt lymphomas. Int. J. Cancer, 17, 47-56.

Biological Changes in
Human Cancer

Introduction

William H. Fishman

La Jolla Cancer Research Foundation, La Jolla, California, U.S.A.

Perhaps 20 years ago this Symposium would have been named "Tumor – Host Relationships." In those days it was never clear to what extent the tumor or the host response to the tumor was responsible for the many manifestations of cancer.

With the rapid advances in endocrinology and particularly with the introduction of the techniques of radioimmunoassay came the realization that tumors may be sites of ectopic hormone production. Hormones such as ACTH, HCG, calcitonin glucagon, etc., are produced in a number of tumors in such quantities that clinical symptoms appear. Oftentimes these humoral disorders are the circumstances which motivate the patient to see the doctor.

It has become clear in the last 10 years that there is a developmental history to certain of these paraneoplastic syndromes. As you will learn from Dr. Vaitukaitis, cells originating from the neuroectoderm of the neural crest in early development migrate and finally take up residence in sites like the thyroid, stomach, pancreas. This has been called the "microendocrine system." These cells still maintain a persistent embryonic gene expression – for example – the c-cells make calcitonin in the six week old embryo and continue in the adult. In neoplasia of these cells, there is an amplification of gene expression.

Tumors of the thymus and parathyroid glands arising from the bronchial cleft are to be discussed by Dr. Braumstein, syndromes of gut tumors by Dr. Tiscornia, and syndromes of tumors of reproductive tract and nephrogenic ridge by Dr. Ghirlanda. Dr. Silver, an invited discussant speaker, will deal with paraneoplastic markers of urogenital tumors.

Dr. Bugat then describes the coagulopathies in cancer, a manifestation which suggests the ectopic production of factors important in blood coagulation.

In my talk, I will be describing the expression of HCG and placental alkaline phosphatase in ovarian cancer from a developmental perspective. Finally, Dr. Baldi will report on homology between murine and human mammary tumor viruses from their potential as tumor markers.

To me, in the APUDOMAS and in germ cell tumors which produce AFP and HCG, we have been provided with uncomplicated model systems of human neoplasia. I am fascinated with the possibility that eutopic and ectopic polypeptide production reflects a widespread disorder in gene regulation, the nature of which merits active research.

Enzymatic Changes in Body Fluid Composition

William H. Fishman

La Jolla Cancer Research Foundation, La Jolla, California 92038, U.S.A.

Dr. Hall assigned me a title for my presentation which appears all-inclusive and which would require a Symposium for itself with at least seven speakers. However, I am sure his intention was for me to provide you some exposure to the subject of ectopic isoenzyme synthesis in cancer patients and to discuss the practical and theoretical significance of this subject. The reference to body fluid composition in the title was intended to draw attention to both blood serum and to neoplastic effusions which may be sampled for the detection of ectopic isoenzymes derived from tumor cells.

I have always been fascinated by the ectopic clinical syndromes, termed the paraneoplastic syndromes by Hall. Many times these syndromes, especially polypeptide hormone producers, have preceded the clinical diagnosis of cancer and surely if methods for the measurement of the paraneoplastic products had been applied, the diagnosis could have been made even earlier. It follows logically also that these products could still be measurable in individuals whose tumors produced insufficient amounts to cause clinical symptoms.

My plan today is to review for you the present status of enzyme changes in neoplasia and to share with you the manner of interpretation.

The area of my interest is oncodevelopmental enzyme gene expression. Oncodevelopmental proteins are defined as ones which appear during prenatal development but disappear in adulthood. They are reexpressed in neoplasia.

The first and most famous example of oncodevelopmental gene expression is alpha-fetoprotein (AFP). Abelev and Tatarinov discovered a protein in fetal liver which was absent in adult liver but was expressed in hepatoma. This AFP is a constituent also of the extraembryonic yolk sac in prenatal life but is reexpressed in yolk sac or endodermal sinus tumors of the testis. Measurements of AFP in patients with teratocarcinoma or hepatoma are clinically useful. Such fetal and yolk sac proteins are ectopic products as in the case of the polypeptide hormones.

In the field of isoenzymes, there are two main bodies of information. One deals with glycolytic enzymes studied in the experimental Morris hepatomas which have a wide range of growth rates and degrees of differentiation. Weinhouse (1) summarized these findings by concluding that in the case of the glucose-ATP phosphotransferases, aldolases, pyruvate kinases and glycogen phosphorylases a common pattern was observed. At one end of the hepatoma spectrum, described as "minimal deviation" tumors, the isozyme pattern is nearly identical with that of adult liver. At the other end, tumors which are rapidly growing have lost the adult liver enzyme phenotype but instead expressed isozymes of the fetal type. The characteristics of the latter correlated with the higher capacity for glycolysis which many tumors show. Significance is attached to the fact that the fetal isozymes, thus equipped for the more efficient utilization of metabolic fuel, have replaced those which are geared for tissue function and are controlled by dietary and hormone factors.

A second body of information has grown around the oncodevelopmental alkaline phosphatases. This began with the discovery in 1968 of the Regan isoenzyme (4), a term placental phenotype in the tumor tissue and serum of a patient with bronchogenic cancer. This is truely an oncodevelopmental isoenzyme as it is characteristic of the trophoblast and is not usually evident in adult tissues. Later, in Japan, the Nagao isoenzyme (5) was discovered. It resembled the rare D-variant phenotype of term placental alkaline phosphatase. Non-Regan isoenzyme is found in almost all tumor tissue. It is indistinguishable from early placental alkaline phosphatase (6) which, in turn, is completely different in its properties from term placental alkaline phosphatase. Finally, the Kasahara isoenzyme or Warnock and Reisman variant (7) was detected in hepatoma. It resembles an isozyme in FL-amnion cells and in fetal intestine. (Table 1, page 6)

Neoplastic Effusions

It was my esteemed colleague, Dr. Leo Stolbach, who advanced the idea in 1972 that it would be profitable to examine the malignant effusion fluids for the presence of oncodevelopmental proteins. Those fluids which were rich in tumor cells should be the best sources. Ovarian cancer was such a source.

Our first results are illustrated in Table II (page 7) (2).

From such studies in ovarian cancer effusions fluids of non-Regan alkaline phosphatase whose counterpart is early placental alkaline phosphatase; human chorionic gonadotrophin; histaminase and acidic isoferritins. Stolbach and others have identified antigen-antibody complexes and heptoglobins which may possibly be oncodevelopmental in nature.

Stolbach and I had the good fortune to work with Dr. Vaitukaitis in studying (3) the degree of concordance of expression of HCG and Regan isoenzyme in ovarian cancer fluids. We have reported longitudinal studies on such patients elsewhere. Two interesting examples are illustrated in the two following figures (pages 4 and 5).

These findings have prompted us to construct a developmental perspective in which to place these various isoenzymes of alkaline phosphatase and other oncodevelopmental proteins (8). In so doing we clearly have to distinguish between trophoblast, extraembryonic structures such as yolk sac, and pre-embryo, embryo and fetus. (Figure 1, page 3) From this arises the question of whether the destiny of a cell is affected by the reexpression of genes which provide them with the biological characteristics of embryonic cells.

We see that at seven days of gestation the blastocyst has an inner cell mass, the embryoblast, and an outer layer of cells which is trophoblast. The chorionic gonadotrophin, chorionic alkaline phosphatase and placental alkaline phosphatase are only expressed in the trophoblast progression, never in embryoblast. On the other hand, CEA and AFP are gene products of the embryoblast progression and not of trophoblast.

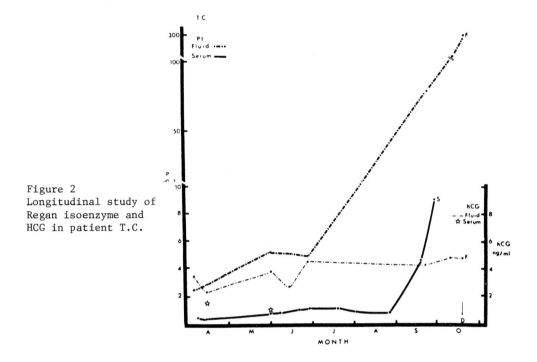

Figure 2
Longitudinal study of
Regan isoenzyme and
HCG in patient T.C.

Case 4 -- A 68-year-old female (T.C.) had an exploratory laparotomy in April 1972
that revealed papillary cystadenocarcinoma of the ovary with extensive involvement
of mesentery and omentum, as well as a pelvic mass. She required paracentesis
every 2-4 weeks during her illness. She showed slow progressive disease despite
treatment with: 1) Alkeran; 2) Cytoxan, 5-FU, and methotrexate; and 3) BCNU. She
died in October 1972; autopsy revealed extensive involvement of mesentery, serosal
surfaces, and liver.

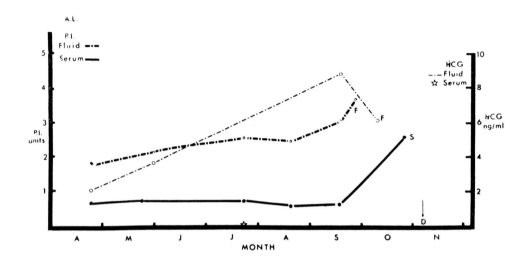

Case 1 -- A 76-year-old female (A.L.) had an exploratory laparotomy in March 1974 that revealed carcinoma of the ovary with metastases to liver, kidney, omentum, and cul-de-sac. She had massive ascites requiring paracentesis every 1-2 weeks throughout her illness. From April 1974 to September 1974 she was treated with chlorambucil. She had slow progression of disease and was switched in October 1974 to combination therapy with Cytoxan, methotrexate, and 50fluorouracil (5-FU). There was no significant response. She died on November 5, 1974, and extensive intra-abdominal involvement by metastatic tumor was found at autopsy.

TABLE I

TUMOR AND DEVELOPMENTAL PHENOTYPES OF ALKALINE PHOSPHATASE

Isoenzyme in cancer tissue	Developmental counterpart	Distinguishing biochemical characteristics					Antigenic determinants	Most frequent expression in cancer of the
		Heat stability*	Inhibition					
			5 mM L-phenyl-alanine	4 mM L-leucine	8 mM L-homoar-ginine			
Regan (1978	Term placental F. FS, S pheno-types (1973)	+	+	–	–	Term placental	Ovary, testes, pancreas
Nagao (1970)	Term placental D-phenotype (1973)	+	+	+	–	Term placental	Ovary, lung, colon
Regan variant (1969)	Amnion (FL) (1975)	+|–	+	+	–	"Intestine"	Liver
Non-Regan (1968)	Chorion (1975)	–	–	–	+	"Liver"	Lung, ovary, chorio-carcinoma

* Activity surviving 5 min. at 65°

TABLE II

| Patient | Specimen | Site of Cancer | Carcinoplacental Phenotypes | | Human Chorionic Gonadotropin Nanograms/ml | Carcinofetal Phenotypes | |
			Regan Isozyme Placental Units/100 ml Values	Ab test		Carcino-embryonic Antigen Nanograms/ml	α-Fetoprotein
P	Asc.	Ovary	0.77	+	1.46	3.6	–
C 1	Asc.	Ovary	2.8	+	2.20	2.6	–
C 2	Asc.	Ovary	304.0	+	4.70	2	–
O'C	Pl.	Ovary	239.0	+	1.24	2	–
B	Asc.	Ovary	11.5	+	1.05	14.5	–
M	Asc.	Ovary	0.74	+	0.66	2	–
Ch	Asc.	Ovary	5.33	+	0.60	30	–
K	Asc.	Ovary	2.23	+	36.6	2	–
S	Asc.	Ovary	0.06	+	1.8	30	–
M	Pl.	Lung	200.0	+	25	89	–
					Max. value non-cancer = 1 ng/ml	Max. value non-cancer = 10 ng/ml	

Comparison of 10 fluid samples from cancer patients producing various amounts of Regan isozyme with β-hcg, CEA and α-fetoprotein assays.

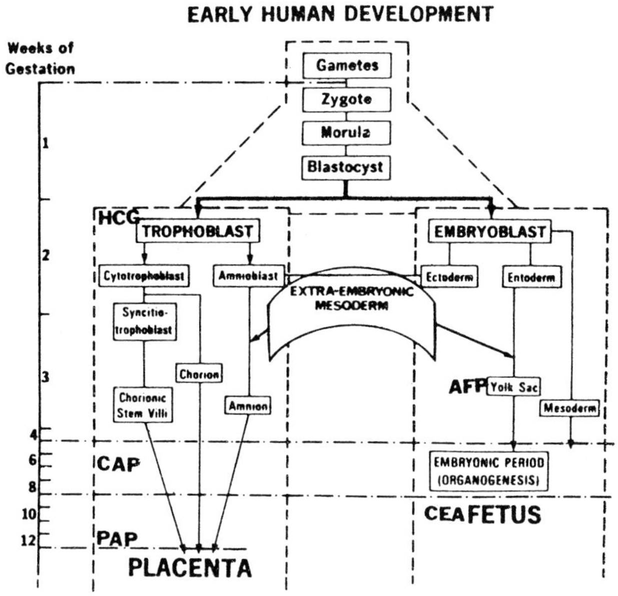

EARLY HUMAN DEVELOPMENT

Chart 1. Chronology of development of oncological gene products. *AFP*, α-fetoprotein; *CAP*, chorionic alkaline phosphatase; *PAP*, placental alkaline phosphatase.

Let us look at developmental enzyme expression as it occurs in non-neoplastic proliferative states. Here one often observes the products of late fetal stage genes which appear to be turned-off when proliferation stops. In tumor cells, since the cells continue to multiply, the retrodifferentiated state persists.

On the other hand, in retrodifferentiation, the neoplastic cells can drop back in development to the trophoblast or yolk sac stage, with the appearance of products like HCG and AFP. Is this event of any important in the behavior of such a cell with respect to its benign neighbors?

SUMMARY

The enzymatic changes in body bluid composition of interest to my laboratory are those which involve oncodevelopmental enzymes . . . that is, enzymes characteristic of a particular phase in embryonic development, absent in the adult which reappear in neoplasia.

In particular, we have focussed on three developmental isoenzymes of alkaline phosphatase which are expressed singly or in combination in a variety of human tumors. The Regan isoenzyme or term placental form is often expressed in association with HCG in the ascites fluid and serum of patients with ovarian cancer, although discondant expression occurs also.

The reexpression of developmental proteins in proliferative disorders including cancer provide an insight into the nature of cancer which is now being pursued vigorously in many countries.

SUPPORTED BY GRANTS-IN-AID (CA-21967) FROM THE NATIONAL CANCER INSTITUTE, NIH, USPHS, BETHESDA, MARYLAND, USA.

REFERENCES

1. Weinhouse, S. Glycolysis respiration and anomalous gene expression in exper-
    iment hepatomas. Cancer Res. 32: 2007, 1972.

2. Fishman, W.H. Carcinoplacental Isozymes in Isozymes III Developmental Biol-
    ogy, (C.L. Markert, ed.) Academic Press, Inc., 1975, pp. 900.

3. Fishman, W.H., Inglis, N.R., Vaitukaitis, J. and Stolbach, L.L. Regan isoen-
    zyme and human chorionic gonadotropin in ovarian cancer. National Cancer
    Institute Monograph #42, Symposium on Ovarian Carcinoma, 1974, 63.

4. Fishman, W.H., Inglis, N.R., Stolbach, L.L. and Krant, M.J. A serum alkaline
    phosphatase isoenzyme of human neoplastic cell origin. Cancer Res. 28: 150,
    1968.

5. Nakayama, T., Yoshida, M. and Kitamura, M. L-leucine sensitive, heat-stable
    alkaline phosphatase isoenzyme detected in a patient with pleuritis carcino-
    matosa. Clin. Chim. Acta 30: 546, 1970.

6. Fishman, L., Miyayama, H., Driscoll, S.G. and Fishman, W.H. Developmental
    phase-specific alkaline phosphatase isoenzymes of human placenta and their
    occurence in human cancer. Cancer Res. 36: 2268, 1976.

7. Higashino, K., Kudo, S., Ohtani, R., Yamamura, Y., Honda, T. and Sakurai, J.
    A hepatoma-associated alkaline phosphatase, the Kasahara isoenzyme, compared
    the one of the isoenzymes of FL amnion cells. Annal. N.Y. Acad. Sci. 259:
    337.

8. Fishman, W.H. and Singer, R.M. Regulatory controls of oncotrophoblast pro-
    teins and developmental alkaline phosphatases in cancer cells. Cancer Res.
    36: 4256, 1976.

Paraneoplastic Tumour Markers in Urogenital Ridge Tumours

H. K. B. Silver, F. A. Salinas and K. A. Karim

Department of Advanced Therapeutics, Cancer Control Agency of British Columbia and Department of Medicine, University of British Columbia

It is convenient to classify paraneoplastic syndromes according to whether or not they cause symptomatic disorders. In the case of tumours arising from the urogenital ridge, the symptomatic paraneoplastic syndromes have been well reviewed in this symposium and elsewhere[1]. It is the purpose of this paper to emphasize the non-symptomatic syndromes of urogenital ridge tumours and their use as tumour markers. In addition to an examination of established tumour markers, we briefly review our own data on further markers undergoing continued development.

The role of tumour markers is becoming widely accepted in the clinical management of cancer patients. It is now known that tumour markers such as carcinoembryonic antigen (CEA) and alpha$_1$-fetoprotein (AFP) may be invaluable in either detecting early recurrence, or especially in following the response to therapy[2-4]. Many of the paraneoplastic features of urogenital ridge tumours could be utilized as tumour markers. However, only a few of these features have been evaluated for this purpose, and this discussion is limited to those tumour markers with some proven clinical potential. Markers vary greatly in their specificity for the underlying histologic type of neoplasm. While it is possible to envisage a truly specific tumour antigen, in practice the clinically important tumour markers tend to be either relatively specific or relatively nonspecific. A simple classification on this basis for urogenital ridge neoplasms is shown in Table 1.

TABLE 1
Urogenital Ridge Tumour Markers

Relatively specific:

    Hormones
    Enzymes
    Tumour "specific" antigens

Relatively non-specific:

    Tumour associated antigens
    Immune complexes
    Acute phase reactants
    Sialylglycoproteins

RELATIVELY SPECIFIC TUMOUR MARKERS

Hormones

The hormone of most immediate promise is human chorionic gonadotrophin. The radio-immunoassay for the beta subunit (β-HCG) is now in common use. It is the specificity for the beta subunit that ensures measurement of HCG without contamination by luteinizing hormone[5]. Serum β-HCG elevations have been detected sporadically in association with a variety of neoplasms[6-10].

Among the utogenital ridge tumours, β-HCG is of most clinical value for patients harbouring non-seminomatous testicular neoplasms. The potential usefulness of this marker is suggested by the fact that 40-77% of patients with established disease show significant serum elevations, as is reviewed in Table 2[5,6,9,10].

TABLE 2
AFP and HCG in Non-seminomatous Testis Tumours

Investigator	AFP		HCG		AFP and/or HCG	
Silver, H.	15/18	(83%)				
Bourgeaux, C.	16/28	(57%)				
Kohn, J.	54/88	(61%)				
Grigor, K.M.	56/84	(67%)				
Wahren, B.	11/18	(61%)				
Scardino, P.T.	21/36	(58%)	28/36	(77%)	33/36	(91%)
Lange, P.H.	34/40	(81%)	24/40	(60%)	38/40	(98%)
Braunstein, G.D.			35/56	(62%)		
Cochran, J.S.			14/35	(40%)		
Total	192/294	(66%)	101/167	(60%)	71/76	(93%)

Data obtained from refs. 2, 9, 11, 22, 23, 25-28.

It is known that changes in serum β-HCG concentrations with time usually reflect changes in tumour burden. In particular, rising levels of β-HCG are almost always indicative of advancing disease and may antedate other evidence of recurrence by weeks or months[5,9,10]. The use of β-HCG as a tumour marker for ovarian carcinoma has not been as thoroughly investigated. Preliminary evidence suggests that the incidence of significant serum elevations is not as high in ovarian carcinoma as in non-seminomatous testis tumour[6-8]. However, it is possible that use of β-HCG in combination with other markers may prove more valuable[7,8]. Elevations of serum β-HCG in association with other urogenital ridge neoplasms such as prostate carcinoma or renal cell carcinoma have been observed, but the relatively infrequent occurrence of serum elevations suggests that this would not be a clinically valuable marker in these cases[1,10].

Other hormones produced by urogenital ridge tumours have not been well investigated as tumour markers. Polypeptide hormones such as parathormone and ACTH have been found elevated in some patients with urogenital ridge tumours but the relationship to tumour burden has not been well documented[1,12]. The use of erythropoetin as a marker for Wilm's tumour has been reported. Although demonstrable increases in erythropoetic activity were found, variable results and technical difficulties suggest that this would not presently be a highly valuable clinical test[13].

Enzymes

Acid phosphatase is a well known marker for prastatic carcinoma. Tradiational assays of phosphatase activity at acid Ph have been somewhat definicient in sensitivity and specificity, probably because there are several acid phosphatases[14]. More recently, the development of a radioimmunoassay (RIA) said to be specific for prastatic acid phosphatase has led to a remarkable improvement in both sensitivity and specificity[14-16]. In a study by Foti and others, improvement in detection rate in patients with relatively localised disease was striking[14]. Whereas only 3 of 24 (12%) of patients with minimal (Stage I) disease demonstrated serum acid phosphatase elevations by conventional enzyme assay, 8 of the patients (33%) demonstrated more specific RIA elevations. The improvement in sensitivity was even more striking for patients with relatively advanced diseas▲. As this radioimmunoassay requires the production of a specific antibody for prostatic acid phosphatase, it is unlikely that this test will be widely available in the near future.

There has been a developing interest in other tumour related enzyme systems. For a variety of enzymes the isoenzyme pattern normally seen in fetal life has also been detected in adult tumour disease[17]. In most cases it has yet to be demonstrated that the fetal isoenzyme pattern is apparent in readily accessible body fluids or that changes in isoenzyme concentration are related to progress of disease. The alkaline phosphatase isoenzymes have been most extensively investigated and are of most immediate clinical interest. Significant elevations of the Regan isoenzyme of alkaline phosphatase have been demonstrated in the sera of patients harbouring a variety of neoplasms[18,19]. Preliminary clinical studies of ovarian carcinoma patients suggest that Regan isoenzyme may be useful especially in conjunction with other markers such as β-HCG and CEA[20].

Tumour "Specific" Antigens

With the development of highly sensitive detection procedures the catalogue of truly specific tumour antigens will continue to diminish. However, it is important that markers such as AFP are relatively specific in comparison with other antigen markers such as CEA. AFP is a normal serum constituent in fetal life, but is only found in extremely low concentrations in the normal adult[2]. Using our RIA we have previously demonstrated that mild elevations of serum AFP may be seen in association with some non-malignant hepatic disorders[2,22-24]. However, significant elevations are almost entirely restricted to patients with primary hepatocellular carcinoma, non-seminomatous testicular tumours or endodermal sinus tumour of the ovary[2,24]. The incidence of serum AFP elevations among patients harbouring non-seminomatous testicular tumours has been examined by ourselves and others, and is reviewed in Table 2[2,10,11,21-23,25-28]. It is of interest that AFP elevations are almost never observed while disease is confined to the testicle[9,11,23,28]. As a result, AFP elevations at the time of primary diagnosis has prognostic significance, and can be used to stage patients with a probable greater accuracy than other staging techniques[10]. Elevated serum AFP is occasionally seen in association with "pure" seminoma, but this leads one to suspect that there may be unrecognised non-seminomatous elements[16].

There is, of course, great interest in the relative usefulness of AFP and β-HCG in non-seminomatous testicular tumours. The incidence of elevations of either moiety in patients with established disease is similar[9,11]. However, if both tests are used there is a clear improvement in sensitivity, as shown in Table 2[9,11]. The increase in serum concentration of either of these tumour markers is excellent evidence of advancing disease and may antedate other evidence of disease progression by weeks or months[9,11,26]. Further, a fall to normal of either marker after surgery is of definite prognostic importance[9,11,21,22,25-27]. However, problems arise in the evaluation of response to chemotherapy. It has now been shown that cancer chemotherapeutic agents may result in disappearance of some histologic elements of the tumour, leaving other usually more differentiated elements relatively intact[29] Tumour marker evaluation may not always accurately reflect this variable response to chemotherapy treatment[30]. It has further been found that in response to chemotherapy one of these tumour markers may return to normal while the other remains elevated[7,11]. As a result, a more accurate reflection of response to chemotherapy treatment can be achieved by looking at both tumour markers.

A number of laboratories, including our own, have been investigating other highly specific tumour associated antigens for possible clinical use[31,32]. Carcinoma of the ovary is one of the tumours under investigation[33,34]. However, the detection techniques used have not yet been well validated, nor are they widely available.

RELATIVELY NON-SPECIFIC TUMOUR MARKERS

Tumour Associated Antigens

Some tumour antigen markers may be detected in associated with tumours of a relatively broad variety of histologic types. Among these, CEA has been the most actively studied and widely accepted for clinical use. The urogenital ridge tumour most commonly associated with serum CEA elevations is ovarian carcinoma. Unfortunately, in this case the use of CEA may be limited to use in patients with clearly advanced disease[7,8,35-38]. In those demonstrating serum SEA elevations it would be expected that changed in serum concentration would reflect corresponding changes in tumour burden[8,38].

Acute Phase Reactants

A variety of serum constituents known as acute phase reactants (APRs) can be detected in abnormal concentration in association with a great variety of acute and chronic illnesses, including cancer. A partial list of the APRs include α_1-antitrypsin, α_1-acid glycoprotein, prealbumin, C-reactive protein, and haptoglobin[39]. Until recently the clinical value of these entirely non-specific tumour markers has been overlooked in favour of more specific tumour related substances. However, the major clinical application of tumour markers at present is not as initial diagnostic aids, but rather to detect early recurrence and monitor response to treatment. In this role the APRs may be as useful as more specific markers, and have the distinct advantage of being applicable to a broad variety of tumour types.

Used as monitors of tumour burden these serum proteins could provide valuable clinical guidance especially in assessing response to therapy. With this in mind there has been renewed interest in the role of APRs in neoplastic disease[40,41]. Clinical problems may arise in recognising sources of APRs not related to tumour burden, such as trauma, inflammation, or the administration of anticancer agents such as hormones. This may be a factor in the interpretation of results in patients with prostate cancer, for example[42]. This problem may be at least partially resolved through the use of multiple markers[41,42].

Immune Complexes

Tumour antigen, specific antibody and related immune complexes (IC) have all been detected in association with human malignancy[3,43-45]. As with the other immune ractants it appears that the circulating serum concentration of IC can be related to tumour burden. Our own investigations of IC have been based on our previous observation that complement fixing IC bind to fetal liver cells[46]. An RIA based on this finding has been developed[47]. Evaluation of malignant melanoma and ovarian carcinoma patients has demonstrated elevated serum IC concentrations and a direct relationship to tumour burden[48]. There is as yet only an incomplete understanding of how IC relate to stafe of disease and prognosis. If the circulating immune complexes have an immune blocking function, as can be demonstrated in laboratory animals[49], then it is possible that the appearance of significant circulating complexes presages a poor prognosis even before there has been a significant change of tumour burden as detected by other means. This has yet to be demonstrated. The assays for immune complexes as routinely performed are non-specific and would not distinguish many of the non-neoplastic sources of immune complexes[50]. In our own experience the assay can be rendered more specific through antigen blocking of the basic assay[48]. Clearly, further studies are necessary before the quantitation of immune complexes becomes a reliable clinical aid.

Sialylglycoproteins

Sialic acid (n-acetyl neuraminic acid) constitutes the terminal residue of the carbohydrate chains of many glycoproteins[51]. As a result, quantitation of the sialic acid hydrolyzed from the attached glycoprotein serves as an entirely non-specific measurement of underlying sialylglycoprotein concentration. Since increased sialic acid at the cell surface of malignant or transformed cells has been demonstrated, and there is a rapid turnover of these cell surface components, it would be reasonable to look for circulating sialylglycoproteins as tumour markers[34,52,53]. Preliminary clinical studies in our laboratory have shown that serum sialic acid levels can be used as a monitor of tumour burden[54-57]. At least part of the increase in serum sialic acid concentration can be explained by APRs, as these are also sialylglycoproteins. In our own examination of ovarian carcinoma patients for this tumour marker there was a clear statistically significant relationship between serum sialic acid and tumour burden, much as has already been demonstrated for malignant melanoma[54,55]. Furthermore, the measurement of serum sialic acid provided a more sensitive indicator of tumour burden than CEA[57].

CONCLUSIONS

Although the clinical significance of individual urogenital ridge tumour markers has been reviewed, general principles for clinical application have been obscured by the fragmentary development in this field. The question of most immediate clinical interest is whether or not an individual marker can be of value in primary diagnosis, staging, evaluation of prognosis, detection of early recurrence, or as a monitor of progress of established disease. A marker that is extremely valuable for one purpose may be worthless for another. For primary diagnostic use, great specificity and sensitivity are required is early detection of a given neoplasm is to be effected. Although primary diagnosis has been the prime goal of most investigation in this field, there is no single marker that clearly fulfills the ideal criteria of both sensitivity and absolute specificity. AFP and β-HCG used together in non-seminomatous testis tumours come closest to this ideal.

Tumour markers have more immediate application once primary diagnosis has been established. Some serum markers may only show significant elevation with regional or distant metastatic disease, and may then be especially useful for clinical staging. Indeed, AFP analysis may be the single most important staging technique for non-seminomatous testis tumours[10]. Similarly, there may be great prognostic value in determining tumour marker status at the time of initial treatment. This will be especially important as surgical adjuvant chemotherapy programs continue to develop. Because of toxicity the use of some adjuvant programs may only be justified where an appropriate high risk group of patients can be identified.

The most promising immediate application of tumour markers is to detect early
recurrence of neoplasms or to monitor the progress of established disease. In both
cases the marker need not be tumour specific. However, marker concentration must
be related to tumour burden, and in the case of early recurrence there must be a
high degree of sensitivity for small tumour burden. Both AFP and β-HCG have been
proven effective markers for early recurrence of non-seminomatous testic neoplasms.
The specific prostatic acid phosphatase assay for prostate carcinoma may be another
example. A variety of markers may have broad application as monitors of disease
progress. In this group could be included the less specific markers such as acute
phase reactants and sialylglycoproteins. These markers are valuable when judgement
of effectiveness of treatment, especially for the more toxic programs, must be made
in the absence of more obvious disease to follow.

Further progress can be expected in several areas. Many tumour markers have yet to
be detected, isolated or evaluated. Other potentially valuable markers, many isoenzymes and hormones for example, have yet to be clinically validated. Further
work is in progress on the advantage to be expected from use of multiple markers.
Equally important, but perhaps not as obvious, is the fact that for widespread
application, the relevant assays may need further modification and development to
ensure reliability and low cost. An expensive procedure requiring days of work, as
is true for some radioimmunoassays, is less desirable than an equally reliable,
inexpensive assay, lending itself to high output automation. It can be expected
that, with continued active investigation, the role of tumour markers will become
increasingly important in the management of cancer patients.

REFERENCES

1. Chisholm, G.D. Nephrogenic ridge tumors and their syndromes. *Ann. N.Y. Acad.
    Sci.*, *220*, 403-423 (1974).

2. Silver, H.K.B., Gold, P., Feder, S. and Shuster, J. Radioimmunoassay for
    alpha$_1$-fetoprotein. *Proc. Natl. Acad. Sci. (USA)*, *70*, 526-530 (1973).

3. Shuster, J., Livingston, A., Banjo, C., Silver, H.K.B., Freedman, S.O. and
    Gold, P. Immunologic diagnosis of human cancers, *Am. J. Path.*, *62*, 243-257
    (1974).

4. Herrera, M.A., Chu, M.T., Holyoke, E.D. and Mittelman, A. CEA monitoring of
    palliative treatment for colorectal carcinoma. *Ann. Surg. 185*, 23-20 (1977).

5. Cochran, J.S., Walsh, P.C., Porter, J.C., Nicholson, T.C., Madden, J.D. and
    Peters, P.C. Endocrinology of human chorionic gonadotrophin secreting testi-
    cular tumors: new methods in diagnosis. *J. Urol.*, *114*, 549-554 (1975).

6. Braunstein, G.D., Vaitukaitis, J.L., Carbone, P. and Ross, G. Ectopic produc-
    tion of human chorionic gonadotrophin by neoplasms. *Ann. Int. Med.*, *78*, 39-
    45 (1973).

7. Stone, M., Bagshawe, K.D., Kardana, A., Searle, F. and Dent, J. β-Human
    chorionic gonadotropin and carcino-embryonic antigen in the management of
    ovarian carcinoma. *Br. J. Obstet. Gynaecol.*, *84*, 375-379 (1977).

8. Stolbach, L., Inglis, N., Lin, C., Turksoy, R.N., Fishman, W., Marchant, D.
    and Rule, S. Measurement of Regan isozyme, HCG, CEA and histaminase in the
    serum effusion fluids of patients with carcinoma of the breast, ovary or lung,
    in: *Onco-Developmental Gene Expression*. W.H. Fishman and S. Sell (eds.),
    Academic Press, pp. 433-443 (1976).

9. Lange, P.H., McIntire, K.R., Waldman, T.A., Hakala, J.R. and Fraley, E.E.
    Alpha-fetoprotein and human chorionic gonadotropin in the management of testi-
    cular tumors. *J. Urol. 118*, 593-396 (1977).

0. Broder, L.E., Weintraub, B.D., Rosen, S.W., Cohen, M.H. and Tejada, F.
    Placental proteins and their subunits as tumor markers in prostatic carcinoma.
    Cancer, 40, 211-216 (1977).

11. Scardino, P.T., Cox, D.H., Waldman, T.A., McIntire, R.K., Mittemeyer, B. and
    Javadpour, N. The value of serum tumour markers in the staging and prognosis
    of germ cell tumours of the testis. *J. Urol., 118*, 994-999 (1977).

12. Buckle, R.M., McMillan, M. and Mallinson, C. Ectopic secretion of parathyroid
    hormone by renal adenocarcinoma in a patient with hypercalcemia. *Brit. Med. J.,
    4*, 724-726 (1970).

13. Murphy, G.P., Mirand, E.H. and Staubitz, W.J. The value of erythropoietin
    assay in the follow-up of Wilms tumor patients. *Oncology, 33*, 154-156 (1976)

14. Foti, A.G., Cooper, J.F., Herschman, H. and Malvaez, R.R. Detection of Pros-
    tatic cancer by solid-phase radioimmunoassay of serum prostatic acid phospha-
    tase. *New Engl. J. Med., 297*, 1357-1361 (1977).

15. Lee, C., Wang, M.C., Murphy, G.P. and Chu, T.M. A solid phase fluorescent
    immunoassay for human prostatic acid phosphatase. *Cancer Res., 38*, 2871-
    2878 (1978).

16. Belville, W.D., Cox, H.D., Mahan, D., Olmert, J.P., Mittemeyer, B.T. and Bruce,
    A.W. Bone marrow acid phosphatase by radioimmunoassay. *Cancer, 41*, 2286-
    2291 (1978).

17. Criss, W.E. A review of isozymes in cancer. *Cancer Res., 31*, 1523-1542 (1971).

18. Stolbach, L.L., Krant, M.J. and Fishman, W.H. Ectopic production of an alkal-
    ine phosphatase isoenzyme in patients with cancer. *New Engl. J. Med., 281*,
    757-762 (1969).

19. Fishman, W.H., Nishiyama, R.T., Rule, A., Green, S., Inglis, N.R. and Fishman,
    L. Onco-developmental alkaline phosphatase izosymes, in: *Onco-Developmental
    Gene Expression.* W.H. Fishman and S. Sell (eds.), Academic Press, pp. 433-443
    (1976).

20. Benham, F.J., Povey, M.S. and Harris, H. Placental-like alkaline phosphatase
    in malignant and benign ovarian tumours. *Clinica Chemica Acta 86*, 201-215
    (1978).

21. Silver, H.K.B., Deneault, J., Gold, P., Thompson, W.G., Shuster, J. and
    Freedman, S.O. The detection of α_1-fetoprotein in patients with viral hepa-
    titis. *Cancer Res., 34*, 244-247 (1974).

22. Silver, H.K.B., Gold, P., Shuster, J., Javitt, N., Freedman, S.O. and Finlay-
    son, N.D.C. Alpha$_1$-fetoprotein in chronic liver disease. *New Engl. J. Med.,
    291*, 506-508 (1974).

23. Thompson, W.G., Gillies, R.R., Silver, H.K.B., Shuster, J-, Freedman, S.O. and
    Gold, P. Carcinoembryonic antigen and alpha$_1$-fetoprotein in ulcerative colitis
    and regional enteritis. *Can. Med. Assoc. J., 110*, 775-777 (1974).

24. Talerman, A., Haije, W.G. and Baggerman, L. Serum alphafetoprotein (AFP) in diagnosis and management of endodermal sinus (yolk sac) tumor and mixed germ cell tumor of the ovary. *Cancer, 41,* 272-278 (1978).

25. Bourgeux, C., Martel, N., Sizaret, P. and Guerrin, J. Prognostic value of alpha-fetoprotein radioimmunoassay in surgically treated patients with embryonal cell carcinoma of the testis. *Cancer, 38,* 1658-1660 (1976).

26. Kohn, J., Orr, A.H., McElwain, T.J., Bentall, M. and Peckham, M.J. Serum alpha$_1$-fetoprotein in patients with testicular tumours. *Lancet, ii,* 433-436 (1976).

27. Grigor, K.M., Detre, S.I., Kohn, J. and Neville, A.M. Serum alpha$_1$-fetoprotein levels in 153 male patients with germ cell tumours. *Br. J. Cancer, 35,* 52-5 (1977).

28. Wahren, B., Alpert, E., and Esposti, P. Multiple antigens as marker substances in germinal tumors of the testis. *J. Natl. Cancer Inst., 58,* 489-498 (1977).

29. Merrin, C., Baumgartner, G. and Zew, W. Benign transformation of testicular carcinoma by chemotherapy. *Lancet, i,* 43-44 (1975).

30. Braunstein, G.D., McIntire, K.R. and Waldman, T.A. Discordance of human chorionic gonadotropin and alpha-fetoprotein in testicular teratocarcinomas. *Cancer, 31,* 1065-1068 (1973).

31. Silver, H.K.B., Bright, J.L., Grimm, E. and Chee, D.O. Detection and partial purification of tumor associated antigen in human melanoma cell line supernatants. *Proc. Amer. Assoc. Cancer Res., 17,* 150 (1976).

32. Grimm, E.A., Silver, H.K.B., Roth, J.A., Chee, D.O. and Morton, D.L. Detection of tumor associated antigen in human melanoma cell-line supernatants. *Int. J. Cancer, 17,* 559-564 (1976).

33. Knauf, S. and Urbach, G.I. Purification of human ovarian tumor-associated antigen and demonstration of circulating tumor antigen in patients with advanced ovarian malignancy. *Am. J. Obstet. Gynecol., 127,* 705-712 (1977).

34. Burton, R.M., Hope, N.J. and Lubbers, L.M. A thermostable antigen associated with ovarian carcinoma. *Am. J. Obstet. Gynecol. 125,* 472-277 (1976).

35. Khoo, S.K. and MacKay, E.V. Carcinoembryonic antigen (CEA) in ovarian cancer factors influencing its incidence and changes which occur in response to cytotoxic drugs. *Br. J. Obstet. Gynaecol., 83,* 753-759 (1976).

36. Van Nagell, J.R., Meeker, W.R., Parker, J.C. and Harralson, J.D. Carcinoembryonic antigen in patients with gynecologic malignancy. *Cancer, 35,* 1372-1376 (1975).

37. Seppälä, M., Pihko, H. and Ruoslahti, E. Carcinoembryonic antigens and alpha-fetoprotein in malignant tumours of the female genital tract. *Cancer, 35,* 1357-1381 (1975).

38. Rutanen, E.M., Lundgren, J., Sipponen, P., Stenman, U-H., Saksela, E. and Seppälä, M. Carcinoembryonic antigen in malignant and nonmalignant gynecologic tumors. *Cancer, 42,* 581-590.

39. Koj, A. Acute phase reactants, in: *Structure and Function of Plasma Proteins.* A.C. Allison (ed.), Plenum Press, pp. 72-125 (1974).

40. Hollinshead, A.C., Chuang, C-Y., Cooper, E.H. and Catalona, W.J. Interrelationship of prealbumin and α_1-acid glycoprotein in cancer patient sera. *Cancer, 40,* 2993-2998 (1977).

41. Ward, M.A., Cooper, E.H., Turner, R., Anderson, J.A. and Neville, A.M. Acute phase reactant protein profiles: an aid to monitoring large bowel cancer by CEA and serum enzymes. *Br. J. Cancer, 35,* 170-178 (1977).

42. Ward, M.A., Cooper, E.H. and Houghton, A.L. Acute phase reactant proteins in prostatic cancer. *Br. J. Urol., 49,* 411-418 (1977).

43. Theofilopoulos, A.N., Andrews, B.S., Urist, M.M., Morton, D.L. and Dixon, F.J. The nature of immune complexes in human cancer sera. *J. Immunol., 119,* 657-663 (1977).

44. Rossen, R.D., Reisberg, M.A., Hersh, E.M. and Gutterman, J.U. The Clq binding test for soluble immune complexes: clinical correlations obtained in patients with cancer. *J. Natl. Cancer Inst., 58,* 1205-1215 (1977).

45. Gupta, R.K., Silver, H.K.B., Reisfield, R. and Morton, D.L. Isolation and immunochemical characterization of antibodies from cancer patients' sera reactive against human melanoma cell membranes by affinity chromatography. *Surgery* (in press).

46. Salinas, F.A., Sheikh, K.M. and Chandor, S.B. Serological reactivity in cancer patients to human and mouse fetal liver cells. *Cancer Res., 38,* 401-407 (1978).

47. Salinas, F.A., Wee, K.H., and Silver, H.K.B. Evaluation of fetal liver-cell binding mechanism. *Exp. Hemat. 6* (Suppl. 3), 76 (1978).

48. Salinas, F.A. and Wee, K.H. Circulating immune complexes detected with FLC assay in cancer patients' sera. *Proc. XII Int. Cancer Congress, 1,* 152-153 (1978).

49. Hellström, I., Sjögren, O.S., Warner, G. and Hellström, K.E. Blocking of cell-mediated tumor immunity by sera from patients with growing neoplasms. *Int. J. Cancer, 7,* 226-237 (1971).

50. Cochrane, C.G. and Koffler, D. Immune complex disease in experimental animals and man. *Adv. Immunol. 16,* 185-264 (1973).

51. Morell, A.G., Gregoriadis, G., Scheinberg, I.H., Hickman, J. and Ashwell, G. The role of sialic acid in determining the survival of glycoproteins in the circulation. *J. Biol. Chem., 246,* 146111467 (1971).

52. Mabry, E.W. and Carubelli, R. Sialic acid in human cancer. *Experientia, 28,* 182-183 (1972).

53. Van Beek, W.P., Smets, L.A. and Emmelot, P. Increased sialic acid density in surface glycoprotein of transformed and malignant cells — a general phenomenon? *Cancer Res., 33,* 2913-2922 (1973).

54. Silver, H.K.B., Rangel, D.M. and Morton, D.L. Serum sialic acid elevations in malignant melanoma patients. *Cancer, 41,* 1497-1499 (1978).

55. Silver, H.K.B., Salinas, F.A., Swenerton, K. and Fraser, A. Immune complexes, sialylglycoproteins and CEA as tumour markers in ovarian carcinoma (submitted for publication).

56. Silver, H.K.B., Rangel, D.M. and Morton, D.L. Serum sialic acid elevations in malignant melanoma patients. *Annals of the Royal College of Physicians and Surgeons of Canada, 10,* 73 (1977).

57. Silver, H.K.B., Karin, K.A. and Archibald, E.A. Serum sialic acid and sialyl-transferase as monitors of tumor burden in malignant melanoma patients. *Proc. Amer. Soc. Clin. Oncology, 19,* 403 (1978).

Syndromes Arising from Tumors of the Branchial Cleft

Glenn D. Braunstein

*Departments of Medicine, Cedars-Sinai Medical Center and
UCLA School of Medicine, Los Angeles, California 90048, U.S.A.*

ABSTRACT

Tumors of the thymus and parathyroid glands, the structures derived from the branchial clefts, are associated with several clinical syndromes. Patients with thymomas may develop myasthenia gravis, red cell aplasia, hypogammaglobulinemia, and
mucocutaneous candidasis. These disorders appear to be the result of a defect in
lymphocyte mediated adaptive immunity. An increased incidence of nonthymic neoplasms has also been noted in patients with thymomas. The reasons for this association are unknown. Hyperplastic or neoplastic changes in the parathyroid glands
may result in hyperparathyroidism with clinical symptoms related to the hypercalcemia, hypophosphatemia, and enhanced bone resorption. An association between
primary hyperparathyroidism and development of malignancies of the breasts, gastrointestinal tract, thyroid, genitourinary system and lung has been found by several
investigators. This observation has revised the concept of pseudohyperparathyroidism or ectopic production of parathormone by tumors since the majority of patients
with malignancy, hypercalcemia, and elevated serum parathormone levels harbor hyperplastic parathyroids or a parathyroid adenoma in addition to their nonparathyroid
neoplasm.

Branchial cleft Thymus Parathyroid glands Thymoma Myasthenia gravis Red cell
aplasia Hyperparathyroidism Hypercalcemia Cancer syndromes

INTRODUCTION

The thymus and parathyroid glands are derived embryologically from the branchial
clefts and the third and fourth pair of pharyngeal pouches (Weller, 1933). These
organs commonly give rise to clinically distinct syndromes following hyperplastic
or neoplastic changes. The calcitonin - producing C-cells of the thyroid are felt
to be derived from neural crest tissue that migrates into the area of the ultimo-
branchial bodies and then into the thyroid (Hazard, 1977). The syndromes associated with C-cell hyperplasia and medullary carcinoma of the thyroid will be discussed elsewhere.

SYNDROMES ASSOCIATED WITH NEOPLASMS OF THE THYMUS

During the past decade an explosive growth in our knowledge in the physiologic
function of the thymus has taken place. It is now clear that this organ plays a
pivotal role in the development of lymphocyte mediated adaptive immunity (Playfair,
1975). The thymic or T-lymphocytes are derived from bone marrow precursor cells

239

(prothymocytes) which are then processed in the thymus under the influence of one or more thymic polypeptide hormones, named by different investigators, thymosin, thymic factor, thymic humoral factor, and thymopoietin (Goldstein, 1977). Followi thymic processing, these lymphocytes further differentiate into cells that help the B-cells to produce antibodies ("helper cells"), cells that suppress the activity of clones of lymphocytes that retain or have developed the capacity to react against normal tissue constituents ("suppressor cells"), and cells that are capabl of destroying target cells ("killer cells") (Asherson and Zembala, 1976; Barnes and Willis, 1976; Calder, McLennan, and Irvine, 1973; Cantor and Boyse, 1975; Greenberg, Shen and Riott, 1973; Taylor and Basten, 1976).

Since the thymus is intimately involved in the development and maintance of a functional immune system, it is not unexpected that the syndromes associated with thymic neoplasms are primarily autoimmune in nature. These syndromes include myasthenia gravis, red cell aplasia, hypogammaglobulinemia, mucocutaneous candidasis, and possibly increased oncogenesis.

Myasthenia Gravis (MG)

MG is a disorder of neuromuscular function that affects approximately 1 in 10,000 to 1 in 40,000 individuals (Havard, 1977; Pirskanen, 1977). Clinically it is characterized by weakness primarily of the extraocular, bulbar and neck muscles that worsens with effort and improves after rest and administration of cholinesterrase inhibitors (Drachman, 1978; Havard, 1977). This neuromuscular dysfunction has been clearly defined as postsynaptic with a reduced number of available acetylcholine receptors at the neuromuscular junction (Drachman, 1978; Havard, 1977).

Approximately 75% of patients with MG have gross or microscopic abnormalities of th thymus (Drachman, 1978; Rosai and Levine, 1976). The majority show lymphoid follicles with germinal centers in the medulla ("thymic hyperplasia") while 10-15% have benign or malignant epithelial thymomas (Rosai and Levine, 1976). Conversly close to half of the patients with thymomas do not have local or systemic symptoms while 25% present with or develop local symptoms (cough, dyspnea, chest pain) from the anterior superior mediastinal mass and approximately 30% have associated MG (Rosai and Levine, 1976).

Females less than 40 years of age generally have thymic germinal centers and a high prevelance of HLA-8 antigen while thymomas usually are found in older males who have an increased incidence of HLA-2 (Drachman, 1978; Feltkamp and co-workers, 1974; Fritze and colleagues, 1974; Havard, 1977; Pirskanen, Tiilikainen and Hokkanen, 1972). The HLA antigen dysequilibrium and the 3-7% incidence of familia MG suggests a genetic predisposition towards the development of MG (Namba and Grob 1970; Pirskanen, 1977).

Havard (1977) and Drachman (1978) have recently reviewed the evidence favoring an autoimmune etiology for MG. The evidence includes the high frequency of antibodies present in the sera of MG patients that are directed against the acetylcholine receptor and antibodies that react to both skeletal muscle and the myoid cell that are present in the hyperplastic thymus or thymoma. Other serologic abnormalities such as antinuclear antibodies, LE cells, rheumatoid factor, antithyroid and antigastric parietal cell antibodies, false positive tests for syphilis, and positive Coombs tests are present to a lesser extent. In addition, MG co-exists with a greater than chance frequency with rheumatoid arthritis, agammaglobulinemia prenicious anemia, autoimmune hemolytic anemia, systemic lupus erythematosis and Sjogren's syndrome - - disorders in which an autoimmune derangement has also been implicated. Some of the evidence that a problem with cell mediated immunity is present in these patients include the inhibition of migration of leucocytes from MG patients in the presence of muscle extracts, the demonstration that thymic

lymphocytes from MG patients are cytotoxic for fetal muscle in culture, the ability
of thymic cells from MG patients to stimulate autologus peripheral blood lymphocytes in the mixed leucocyte reaction, and the enhanced responsiveness of MG thymic
lymphocytes in the presence of pokeweed mitogen   (Abdou and colleagues, 1974;
Lisak, 1975).

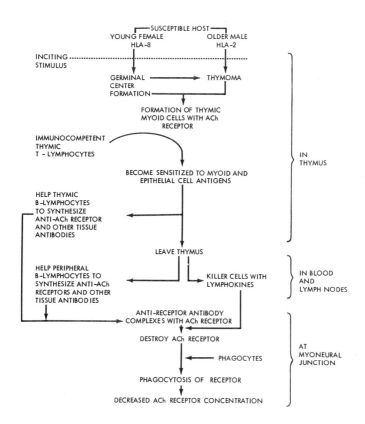

Fig. 1. Hypothesis for the pathogenesis of myasthenia gravis.

Figure 1 is an attempt to summarize the current evidence relating to the pathogenesis of MG in patients with thymic hyperplasia and thymomas (Drachman, 1978; Havard,
1977; Wekerle and Ketelsen, 1977). As noted above there exists a genetic predisposition for the development of MG. In response to an appropriate stimulus, which
may be viral in origin (Datta and Schwartz, 1974), thymic abnormalities develop and
include   the reappearance of the acetylcholine receptor-containing myoid cells
which are normally present in the fetus but are absent in the adult (Kao and
Drachman, 1977). Because of the appearance of an antigen not normally present in
the thymus or because of a defect in immunosurveillance by the competent T-lymphocytes (suppressors cells), a population of T-cells become sensitized to the acetylcholine receptor and other cellular constituents and help intra- and extrathymic
B-cells produce acetylcholine receptor antibodies which attach to acetylcholine

receptors in striated muscle.   The antigen – antibody complex attracts killer T-
cells and phagocytes which destroy the receptors and reduce their concentration
and the ability of the muscle cells to respond to the quanta of acetylcholine released from the nerve endings.

The treatment of MG involves the administration of anticholinesterase drugs and in
selected individuals glucocorticoids or other immunosuppressive agents or measures
(Drachman, 1978; Havard, 1977).   Thymectomy is clearly indicated for patients with
thymomas in order to prevent spread and this procedure may improve or ameliorate
the myastenic symptoms.   Post operative irradiation is generally recommended for
patients with malignant thymomas.   Although controversy exists   concerning the
indication for thymectomy in patients without thymomas, it is clear that a substantial portion of patients have a remission of their symptoms following the procedure
(Drachman, 1978; Havard, 1977; Papatestas and co-workers, 1971a).

Red Cell Aplasia (RCA)

RCA is characterized by an absence or marked diminution of erythropoiesis manifest
by an anemia without reticulocytosis and few or no bone marrow erythoblasts.   Iron
incorporation into hemoglobin is greatly diminished while granulocyte and platlets
remain normal.   Less than 200 cases of RCA have been reported and approximately
half the patients harbor a thymoma (Jacobs and colleagues, 1959; Roland, 1964).
The incidence of RCA in patients with thymomas is 4-5% (Hirst and Roberston, 1967;
Rogers, Manaligod and Blazek, 1968).   The mean age of patients with RCA associated
with thymomas is approximately 60 years with a 2-to-1 female proponderance, in
contradistinction to the 2-to-1 male proponderance in RCA unassociated with thymoma
(Brown and Rubin, 1967; Dameshek, Brown and Rubin, 1967; Hirst and Robertson, 1967;
Rogers, Manaligod and Blazek, 1968).   Histologically, two-thirds of the thymomas
are of the spindle cell variety and less than 10% are malignant (Hirst and Robertson
1967; Rogers, Manaligod and Blazek, 1968).   Germinal centers are generally not seen
in this disorder (Dameshek, Brown and Rubin, 1967).

The presenting symptoms relate   to the anemia or the tumor.   The tumor may be present for months or years before the anemia is discovered and in some incidences the
anemia occurs following removal of the thymoma (Dameshek, Brown and Rubin, 1967;
Hirst and Robertson, 1967; Rogers,Manaligod and Blazek, 1968).   Only two-thirds
of the patients with erythroblastopenic anemia and thymoma have strict "pure" RCA,
while 7% of the patients ahve an associated neutropenia, 12% anemia and thrombocytopenia and 10% have pancytopenia (Rogers, Manaligod and Blazek, 1968).   Approximately 7% of the patients present with pure RCA that progresses to pancytopenia
(Rogers, Manaligod and Blazek, 1968).

The pathogenesis of the disorder is unknown but strong evidence exists that impli-
cates an autoimmune etiology.   This evidence includes the frequent association of
other autoimmune phenomenon including hypo- and hypergammaglobulinemia, antinuclear
antibodies, positive LE-cells, false positive serologic tests for syphilis, and
myasthenia gravis (Hirst and Robertson, 1967; Rogers, Manaligod and Blazek, 1968).
Several investigators have provided evidence that anti-erythroblast antibodies
exist in this disorder (Jepson and Vas, 1974; Krantz, 1974; Krantz and Kao, 1967,
1969; Krantz, Moore and Zaentz, 1973; Safdar, Krantz and Brown, 1970; Zalusky and
colleagues, 1973).   Collectively these workers have demonstrated that many of the
patients with this syndrome have an IgG globulin in their serum which inhibits the
rate of heme synthesis in the marrow of RCA and normal patients cultured in vivo,
binds to erythroblast nuclei, and in conjunction with complements is cytotoxic for
erythroblasts.   Injection of the serum of such patients into mice results in an
anemia, reticulocytopenia, suppression of the incorporation of iron into erythrocytes and a rise in erythropoietin levels in the serum, thus mimicking the human
disease (Zalusky and associates, 1973).   Since the antibodies described appear to
be specifically directed against erythroblasts, it is unknown why some patients

evelop leucopenia, thrombocytopenia or both in association with the anemia. Per-
aps these patients have an autoimmune pluripotent stem cell failure as suggested
y Geary and associates (1975).

pproximately 25 - 30% of the patients with RCA have a remission of their disease
ollowing thymectomy, while patients with associated leucopenia, thrombocytopenia
r pancytopenia do not appear to respond (Hirst and Robertson, 1967; Krants, 1974;
ogers, Manaligod and Blazek, 1968). If the patient does not respond to thymectomy,
steroid or immunosurpressent therapy may be of beneift (Geary and co-workers, 1975;
rantz, 1974; Marmont and associates, 1975). Of interest the remissions following
such therapy are preceeded by disappearance of the anti-erythroblast antibody
(Krantz, 1974; Safdar, Krantz and Brown, 1970), again supporting an autoimmune
etiology of the syndrome.

Iypogammaglobulinemia

immunoglobulin deficiency accompanies many of the congenital dysplastic diseases
of the thymus (Ambrus and Ambrus, 1973) and, therefore, it is not surprising that
acquired hypogammaglobulinemia has been noted in 8 - 9% of the patients with thymomas (Waldmann and co-workers, 1967). Approximately 10% of the patients with
acquired late onset hypogammaglobulinemia have an associated thymoma, usually of
the spindle cell variety (Peterson, Cooper and Good, 1965). Although all the
patients have been found to have depressed IgG levels, the IgA and IgM concentrations have been variable with 60% demonstrating panhypoimmunoglobulinemia and 20%
showing depressed IgA and increased IgM levels (Waldmann and associates, 1967).

The disorder presents after the age of 30 and two-thirds of the patients are women
(Peterson, Cooper and Good, 1965). Repeated infections and diarrhea are the common
clinical manifestations (Mallinson, 1971; Peterons, Cooper and Good, 1965). The
gammaglobulin abnormalities may be discovered concominately with the thymoma or may
appear following it's removal (Jacox and co-workers, 1964). Co-existent aplastic
anemia or pure red cell aplasia have been noted in 30 - 40% of the patients
(Peterson, Cooper and Good, 1965; Waldmann and associates, 1967). Removal of the
thymoma is not associated with amelioration of the disorder (Peterson, Cooper and
Good, 1965).

The pathogenesis of this disorder is poorly understood. Clearly a B-cell defect
exists but it is unclear whether this is secondary to a primary T-cell problem.
Decreased synthesis of immunoglobulins and suppression of in vitro differentiation
of lymphocytes into normal B-cells have noted (DeLaConcha and associates, 1977;
Litwin and Zangani, 1977; Siegal, Siegal and Good, 1976; Waldmann and co-workers,
1967). In addition, circulating lymphocytes from a patient with a thymoma and
immunodeficiency suppressed the ability of pokeweed mitogen to cause normal donor
B-cells to differentiate into plasma cells (Siegal, Siegal and Good, 1976). Litwin
and Zanjani (1977) have provided evidence that T-lymphocytes from patients with the
thymoma-hypogammaglobulinemia syndrome may suppress the maturation of both B-lymph-
ocytes and erythroid precursors in culture, suggesting that this syndrome may result
from overproduction or overactivity of suppressor T-cells.

Chronic Mucocutaneous Candidasis

Less than 20 patients with the combination of thymoma and mucocutaneous candidasis,
with or without associated myasthenia gravis have been reported (Mobaken, Lindholm
and Olling, 1977). The syndrome is characterized by persistent candida infections
of the mucous membranes, skin, hair, and nails (Edwards and associates, 1978).
These patients have normal humoral immunity but lack adequate cellular immunity to
candida and antigenically similar fungi, although immunity to bacteria, viruses and
other fungi remains intact (Edwards and co-workers, 1978). This syndrome is clearly
due to a problem in T-cell function but the precise defect has not been defined.

Thymectomy does not appear to bring about a resolution of the candidal infections (Mobacken, Windholm and Olling, 1977).

Associated Nonthymic Neoplasms

Sovadjian, Siberstein and Titus (1968) found that 21% of 146 patients with a thymoma who were followed for at least 20 years developed a malignant lesion of a nonthymic tissue. Papatestas, Osserman and Kark (1971b) retrospectively reviewed the records of 1243 patients with myasthenia gravis and found that 8.9% of the patient with thymomas had extrathymic neoplasms while 7.4% of myasthenia gravis patients without thymomas had second neoplasms. The greatest increase in frequency of nonthymic malignancy was found after the onset of myasthenia gravis and in those who did not undergo thymectomy, while the incidence was found to decrease following thymectomy. These observations suggest that the presence of thymoma predisposes to the development of an extrathymic malignancy, possible through defective immunologic surveillance.

SYNDROMES ASSOCIATED WITH NEOPLASMS OF THE PARATHYROID GLANDS

The parathyroid glands are primarily responsible for maintenance of normal calcium homeostasis through the secretion of parathormone. Parathormone is an 84 aminoacid protein that is synthesized in the parathyroids initially in precursor forms (preproparathormone, proparathormone) (Keutmann, 1974). Concomenent with or following secretion, parathormone is cleaved into a biologically active aminoterminal fragment and a biologically inactive carboxyterminal fragment (Keutmann, 1974). The biologically active portion of the molecule either directly or indirectly increases the intestinal absorbtion of calcium, phosphate and magnesium, increases bone reabsorption with release of calcium, phosphorus and magnesium into the blood, increases the tubular reabsorption of calcium and magnesium and decreases the tubular reabsorption of phosphate and bicarbonate (Lockwood, Bruun and Transobol, 1975) The primary stimulus for the secretion of parathormone is a decrease in the ionized level of serum calcium while increases in the ionized calcium reduce parathormone secretion (Rasmussen, 1971). In addition the serum magnesium concentration as well as the concentration of vitamin D and its' metabolites modulate parathormone secretion (Rasmussen and co-workers, 1974).

Hyperparathyroidism

Hyperparathyroidism occurs with a frequency of 1-4 cases per 1000 individuals (Boonstra and Jackson, 1971; Christensson and co-workers, 1976). The vast majority of patients with hyperparathyroidism develop the disorder on a sporadic basis. Hyperparathyroidism also occurs in a familial setting with an autosomal dominant transmission with or without associated tumors of the endocrine pancreas, pituitary, thyroid and/or adrenals (multiple endocrine neoplasia syndrome, type I) or medullary carcinoma of the thyroid and pheochromocytomas (multiple endocrine neoplasia syndrome, type II) (Ballard, Frame and Hartsock, 1964; Goldsmith and colleagues, 1964; Steiner, Goodman and Powers, 1968). Although there is a considerable amount of controversy regarding the current relative frequencies of parathyroid adenomas and hyperplasia, most series note that approximately 80% of the patients have a solitary adenoma, 3-5% have a parathyroid carcinoma and parathyroid hyperplasia is present in the remaining patients (Garman, Myers and Marshall, 1978; Schantz and Castleman, 1973; Williams, 1974).

The etiology of the sporadic form of pimary hyperparathyroidism is unknown. Failkow and associates (1977) examined the glucose-6-phosphate dehydrogenase isoenzymes in parathyroid tumors and noted the presence of both A and B isoenzymes in porportions similar to those observed in normal tissues, providing evidence for a multicellular origin of parathyroid adenomas. This is in contrast to the clonal origin of some neoplasms and rise the possiblity that presently unknown stimuli lead to parathyroid hyperplasia, followed by the development of autonomus

secretion of parathormone by one or more glands which ultimately suppresses the
activities of the other glnads. Recently several investigators have noted an increased incidence of parathyroid adenomas or hyperplasia following x-ray therapy
to the head and neck for benign diseases in infancy, childhood and adolescence or
young adulthood (Christensson, 1978; Prinz and colleagues, 1977; Tisell and others,
1977). The mechanisms responsible for the development of parathyroid neoplasms
following irradiation are not clear but may relate to chromosomal or tissue injury,
damage to the immunosurveillance mechanism, or activation of latent viruses (Mole,
1974, Prinz and co-workers, 1977).

The clinical features of hyperparathyroidism may be divided into those that are
manifestations of hypercalcemia and those that which are specific for hyperparathyroidism. Thus hypercalcemia may lead to polyuria, polydipsia, fatigue, depres-
sion, psychosis, personality changes, lethargy, coma, muscle weakness, corneal and
conjunctival calcium deposits, abdominal pain, peptic ulcer disease, pancreatitis,
constipation, anorexia, vomiting, weight loss and hypertension. Renal stones,
arthralgias, pseudogout, bone pain and tenderness with or without cystic bone
changes and diffuse bony demineralization are more specific for hyperparathyroidism
(Bone, Snyder and Pak, 1977; Lockwood, Bruun and Transbol, 1975; Watson, 1974).

The biochemical abnormalities are generally those that would be anticipated from
the overproduction of parathormone and include hypercalcemia, hypophosphatemia,
hypomagnesmia, hyperchloremia with a mild acidosis, decreased tubular reabsorption
of phosphate and an inconsistent elevation of uric acid and alkaline phosphatase
of bone origin (Lockwood, Bruun and Transbol, 1975). These abnormalities are
associated with an increase concentration of immunoreactive parathormone while in
the other causes of hypercalcemia (with the exception of ectopic production of
parathormone by tumors) the parathormone levels are low due to suppression of the
parathyroid glands by the elevated calcium.

The therapy for hypercalcemia includes restoration of normal hydration, promotion
of calcium loss via the urine, inhibition of bone resorption and correction of
electrolyte problems. The various therapies have been recently reviewed by Myers
(1977). In patients with primary hyperparathyroidism; removal of the parathyroid
adenoma or adenomas is curative while in patients with diffuse hyperplasia resection of the three and one-half glands may restore normocalcemia. A number of
authors have reviewed the surgical managment of hyperparathyroidism and the therapy
of the post-operative complications (Lockwood, Bruun and Transbol, 1975; Purnell
and associates, 1974; Purnell, Scholz and Beahrs, 1977; Seyfer, Sigdestad and
Hirata, 1976).

Association of Hyperparathyroidism and Non-parathyroid Malignancies

As previously noted, hyperparathyroidism is a frequent manifestation of the multiple
endocrine neoplasia syndromes. The frequency of co-existing endocrine tumors in
patients with hyperparathyroidism varies from 2-17.5% (Boey and co-workers, 1975).
In addition, numerous investagators have noticed an increase incidence of malignant
breast, gastrointestinal, thyroid, genitourinary, and pulmonary neoplasms in patients
with hyperparathyroidism (Drezner and Lebovitz, 1978; Farr, 1976; Kaplan and co-
workers, 1971; Katz and associates, 1970; Newman and Plucinski, 1977; Petro and
Hardy, 1975; Samaan and others, 1974). These authors have noted that between 34
and 42% of patients with parathyroid adenomas or hyperplasia have an associated
malignant neoplasm,raising the possiblity that hyperparathyroidism or hypercalcemia
may predispose a patient to neoplasia, or conversely,malignancies may produce a
parathyrothropic substance that leads to the development of parathyroid hyperplasia
or adenoma. Since x-ray therapy to the head and neck appears to be an inciting
factor for the subsequent development of parathyroid adenomas and well differentiated thyroid carcinomas (DeGroot and colleagues, 1977; Prinz and colleagues, 1977;
Tisell and others, 1977), the 5.4 - 16% incidence of co-existence of these two

diseases may represent patients who received childhood or adolescent head and neck irradiation (Farr, 1976; Kaplan and associates, 1971; Newman and Plucinski, 1977; Petro and Hardy, 1975; Samaan and co-workers, 1976).

The most frequent etiology of hypercalcemia and cancer is the dissolution of bone secondary to osseous metastesis (Besarb and Caro, 1978; Buckle, 1974; Myers, 1977) A variety of neoplasms have also been shown to eleborate various humoral factors that may enhance bone resorption. Thus, secrction of prostaglandins by solid tumc (Robertson and associates, 1976; Seyberth and co-workers, 1975), osteoclast stimula ing factor in patients with myeloma and lymphoma (Mundy and others, 1974 a, b) an parathormone by a variety of tumors, especially squamous cell carcinomas of the lung and hypernephromas (Buckle, 1974; Hamilton and co-workers, 1977; Lafferty, 1976) has been demonstrated. Although many of the early reports suggested that th ectopic production of parathormone was a relatively common cause of non-metastatic hypercalcemia, the more recent studies indicate that co-existent primary hyperpara thyroidism accounts for the majority of patients with cancer, hypercalcemia and elevated serum parathormone concentrations (Samaan and associates, 1976).

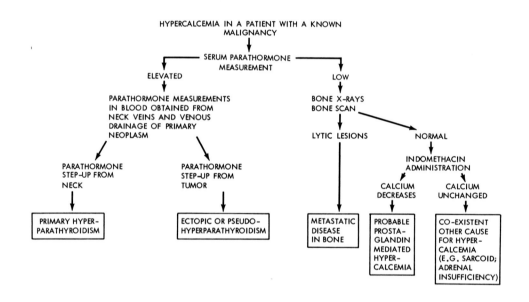

Fig. 2.   Scheme for evaluation of hypercalcemia associated with cancer.

In order to define the etiology of hypercalcemia in a patient with cancer we follow the procedures outline in Fig. 2.   The serum parathormone level is used to differ- entiate between patients with hypercalcemia due to metastatic disease, prosta- glandin or other non-parathormone mediated causes of hypercalcemia and those patients with co-existing primary hyperparathyroidism or ectopic production of parathormone.   The later two possiblities are differentiated by a venous sampling procedure in which blood is obtained from the neck and mediastinal veins as well as from the vessels draining the non-parathyroid neoplasm (Doppman, 1976; Samaan and others, 1976).   Analysis of the parathormone concentrations in these samples is then performed and if the highest levels are found in the neck, the diagnosis of primary hyperparathyroidism is made. Conversly if the step-up in parathormone levels is found in the blood from the tumor bed, pseudohyperparathyroidism is assumed to be present. We consider this differentiation to be important since successful removal of the hyperplastic parathyroids or a parathyroid adenoma is accompanied by the return of the calcium to normal which usually improves the quality of life for the patient and allows the discontinuation of potentially toxic agents, such as mithramycin or phosphates, used to treat the hypercalcemia.

REFERENCES

1. Abdou, N.I., R.P. Lisak, B. Zweiman, I. Abrahamsohn and A.S. Penn (1974). The thymus in myasthenia gravis. Evidence for altered cell populations. N. Engl. J. Med., 291, 1271-1275.
2. Ambrus, J.L. and C.M. Ambrus (1973). Disorders of the thymus gland and thymus transplantation in man. In T.D. Luckey (Ed.), Thymic Hormones, Baltimore Univ. Park Press, Baltimore. pp. 19-38.
3. Asherson, G.L. and M. Zembala (1976). Suppressor T-cells in cell-mediated immunity. Br. Med. Bull., 32, 158-164.
4. Ballard, H.S., B. Frame and R.J. Hartsock (1964). Familial multiple endocrine-peptic ulcer complex. Medicine, 43, 481-516.
5. Barnes, R.D. and E.J. Willis (1976). "Normal" elimination of aberrant auto-immune clones. Lancet, 2, 20-22.
6. Besarb, A. and J.F. Caro (1978). Mechanisms of hypercalcemia in malignancy. Cancer, 41, 2276-2285.
7. Boey, J.H., T.J.C. Cooke, J.M. Gilbert, E.C. and S. Taylor (1975). Occurrence of other endocrine tumors in primary hyperparathyroidism. Lancet, 2, 781-784.
8. Bone, H.G. III, W.H. Snyder III and C.Y.C. Pak (1977). Diagnosis of hyperpara-thyroidism. Ann. Rev. Med., 28, 111-117.
9. Boonstra, C.E. and C.E. Jackson (1971). Serum calcium survey for hyperpara-thyroidism. Results in 50000 clinic patients. Am. J. Clin. Path., 55, 523-526.
10. Buckle, R. (1974). Ectopic PTH syndrome, pseudohyperparathyroidism, hypercal-cemia of malignancy. Clin. Endocrinol. Metab., 3, 237-251.
11. Calder, E.A., D. McLennan and W.S. Irvine (1973). Lymphocyte cytotoxicity induced by preincubation with serum from patients with Hashimotos thyroiditis. Clin. Exp. Immunol., 15, 467-470.
12. Cantor, H. and E.A. Boyse (1975). Functional subclasses of T lymphocytes bear-ing differnet Ly antigens. I. The generation of functionally distinct T-cell subclasses in a differentiative process independent of antigen. J. Exp. Med., 141, 1376-1389.
13. Christensson, T., K. Hellström, B. Wengle, A. Alveryd and B. Wikland (1976). Prevalence of hypercalcaemia in a health screening in Stockholm. Acta Med. Scand., 200, 131-137.
14. Christensson, T. (1978). Hyperparathyroidism and radiation therapy. Ann. Int. Med., 89, 216-217.
15. Dameshek, W., S. Brown and A.D. Rubin (1967). "Pure" red cell anemia (erythro-blastic hypoplasia) and thymoma. Semin. Hemat., 4, 222-232.
16. Datta, S.K. and R.S. Schwartz (1974). Infectious (?) myasthenia. N. Engl. J. Med., 291, 1304-1305.
17. DeGroot, L.J., L.A. Frohman, E.L. Kaplan and S. Referoff (1977). Radiation-Associated Thyroid Carcinoma. Grune and Stratton, New York.
18. DeLaConcha, E.G., G. Oldham, A.D.B. Webster, G.L. Asherson and T.A.E. Platts-Mills (1977). Quantitative measurements of T and B-cell function in "variable" primary hypogammaglobulinemia: Evidence for a consistent B-cell defect. Clin. Exp. Immunol., 27, 208-215.
19. Doppman, J.L. (1976). Parathyroid localization. Arteriography and venous sampling. Rad. Clin. N. Amer., 14, 163-188.
20. Drachman, D.B. (1978). Myasthenia gravis. N. Eng. J. Med., 298, 136-142, 186-193.

21. Drezner, M.K. and H.E. Lebovitz (1978). Primary hyperparathyroidism in para-
    neoplastic hypercalcemia. Lancet, 1, 1004-1006.
22. Edwards, J.E., R.I. Lehrer, E.R. Stiehm, T.J. Fischer and L.S. Young (1978).
    Severe candidal infections. Clinical perspective, immune defense mechanisms
    and current concepts of therapy. Ann. Int. Med., 89, 91-106.
23. Farr, H.W. (1976). Hyperparathyroidism and cancer. CA, 26, 66-73.
24. Feltkamp, T.E.W., P.M. Van den Berg-Looner, L.E. Nijenhuis, C.P. Engelfriet,
    A.L. Van Rossum, J.J. Van Loghem and H.J.G.H. Oosterhuis (1974). Myasthenia
    gravis, autoantibodies and HL-A antigens. Brit. Med. J., 1, 131-133.
25. Fialkow, P.J., C.E. Jackson, M.A. Block and K.A. Greenawald (1977). Multi-
    cellular origin of parathyroid "adenomas". N. Engl. J. Med., 297, 696-698.
26. Fritze, D., C. Herman Jr., F. Naeim, G.S. Smith and R.L. Walford (1974).
    HL-A antigens in myasthenia gravis. Lancet, 1, 240, 242.
27. Geary, C.G., P.R. Byron, G.Taylor, J.E. MacIver and J. Zervas (1975). Thymoma
    associated with pure red cell aplasia, immunoglobulin deficiency and an inhib-
    itor of antigen-induced lymphocyte transformation. Brit. J. Hem., 29, 479-485.
28. Goldsmith, R.E., G.W. Sizemore, I.W. Chen, E. Zalme and W.A. Altemeir (1976).
    Familial hyperparathyroidism. Description of a large kindred with physiologic
    observations and a review of the literature. Ann. Int. Med., 84, 36-43.
29. Goldstein, G. (1977). The thymus as an endocrine gland. In V.H.T. James (Ed.)
    Proceedings of the V International Congress of Endocrinology, Excepta Medica,
    Amsterdam-Oxford. pp. 500-503.
30. Greenberg, A.H., L. Shen and C.M. Riott (1973). Characteristics of the effecto-
    cells mediating anti-dependent cytotoxicity. Cur. Titles Immun. Transp. Aller-
    gy, 1, 33-35.
31. Hamilton, J.W., C.R. Hartman, D.H. McGregor and D.V. Cohn (1977). Synthesis of
    parathyroid hormone-like peptides by a human squamous cell carcinoma. J. Clin.
    Endocrinol. Metab., 45, 1023-1030.
32. Havard, C.W.H. (1977). Progress in myasthenia gravis. Brit. Med. J., 11, 1008-
    1011.
33 Hazard, J.B. (1977). The C-cell (parafollicular cells) of the thyroid gland
    and medullary thyroid carcinoma. Am. J. Path., 88, 214-249.
34. Hirst, E. and R.I. Robertson (1967). The syndrome of thymoma and erythroblasto-
    penic anemia. A review of 56 cases including 3 case reports. Medicine, 46,
    225-264.
35. Jacobs, E.M., R.V.P. Hutter, J.L. Pool and A.B. Ley (1959). Benign thymoma
    and selective erythroid aplasia of the bone marrow. Cancer, 12, 47-57.
36. Jacox, R.F., E.S. Mongan, J.B. Hanshaw and J.P. Leddy (1964). Hypogammaglobul-
    inemia with thymoma and probable pulmonary infection with cytomegalovirus.
    N. Engl. J. Med., 271, 1091-1096.
37. Jarman, W.T., R.T. Myers and R.B. Marshall (1978). Carcinoma of the parathyroid
    Arch. Surg., 113, 123-125.
38. Jepson, J.H. and M. Vas (1974). Decreased in vivo and in vitro erythropoiesis
    induced by plasma of ten patients with thymoma, lymphosarcoma, or idiopathic
    erythroblastopenia. Cancer Res., 34, 1325-1334.
39. Kao, I. and D.B. Drachman (1977). Thymic muscle cells bear acetylcholine re-
    ceptors. Possible relation to myasthenia gravis. Science, 195, 74-75.
40. Kaplan, L., A.D. Katz, C. Ben-Isaac and S.G. Massry (1971). Malignant neoplasms
    and parathyroid adenoma. Cancer, 28, 401-407.
41. Katz, A., L. Kaplan, S.G., R. Heller, D. Plotkin and I. Knight (1970). Primary
    hyperparathyroidism in patients with breast carcinoma. Arch. Surg., 101, 582-
    585.
42. Keutmann, H.T. (1974). The chemistry of parathyroid hormone. Clin. Endocrinol.
    Metab., 3, 173-197.
43. Krantz, S.B. and V. Kao (1967). Studies on red cell aplasia. I. Demonstration
    of a plasma inhibitor to heme synthesis and an antbody to erythroblast nuclei.
    Proc. Natl. Acad. Sci. (USA), 58, 493-500.
44. Krantz, S.B. and V. Kao (1969). Studies on red cell aplasia. II. Report of a

second patient with an antibody to erythroblast nuclei and a remission after immunosuppressive therapy. J. Hematol., 34, 1-13.

5. Krantz, S.B., W. H. Moore and S.D. Zaentz (1973). Studies on red cell aplasia. V. Presence of erythroblast cytotoxicity in γG-globulin fraction of plasma. J. Clin. Invest., 52, 324-336.

6. Krantz, S.B. (1974). Pure red cell aplasia. N. Engl. J. Med., 291, 345-350.

7. Lafferty, F.W. (1966). Pseudohyperparathyroidism. Medicine, 45, 247-260.

8. Lisak, R.P. (1975). Immunologic aspects of myasthenia gravis. Ann. Clin. Lab. Sci., 5, 288-293.

9. Litwin, S.D. and E.D. Zanjani (1977). Lymphocytes suppressing both immunoglobulin production and erythroid differentiation in hypogammaglobulinemia. Nature, 266, 57-58.

0. Lockwood, K., E. Bruun and I.B. Transbol (1975). Diseases of the parathyroid glands. Adv. Surg., 9, 177-209.

1. Mallinson, W.J.W. (1971). Hypogammaglobulinaemia with thymoma. Proc. Roy. Soc. Med., 64, 53-54.

2. Marmont, A., C. Peschle, M. Sanguineti and M. Condorelli (1975). Pure red cell aplasia (PRCA): Response of three patients to cyclophosphamide and/or anti-lymphocyte globulin (ALG) and demonstration of two types of serum IgG inhibitors to erythropoiesis. Blood, 45, 247-261.

3. Mobacken, H., L. Lindholm and S. Olling (1977). Deficient neutrophil function in a patient with chronic mucocutaneous candidiasis, thymoma and myasthenia gravis. ACTA Dermat. (Stock), 57, 335-339.

4. Mole, R.H. (1974). Late effects of radiation: Carcinogenesis. Br. Med. Bull., 29, 78-83.

55. Mundy, G.R., R.A. Luben, L.G. Raisz, J.J. Oppenheim and D.N. Buell (1974a). Bone-resorbing activity in supernatants from lymphoid cell lives. N. Engl. J. Med., 290, 867-871.

56. Mundy, G.R., L.G. Raisz, R.A. Cooper, G.P. Schechter and S.E. Salmon (1974b). Evidence for the secretion of an osteoclast stimulating factor in myeloma. N. Engl. J. Med., 291, 1041-1046.

57. Myers, W.P.L. (1960). Hypercalcemia in neoplastic disease. Arch. Surg., 80, 308-318.

58. Myers, W.P.L. (1977). Differential diagnosis of hypercalcemia and cancer. CA., 27, 258-272.

59. Namba, T. and D. Grob (1970). Familial concurrence of myasthenia gravis and rheumatoid arthritis. Arch. Int. Med., 125, 1056-1058.

60. Newman, H.K. and T.E. Plucinski (1977). Unsuspected nonmedullary carcinoma of the thyroid in patients with hyperparathyroidism. Am. J. Surg., 134, 799-802.

61. Papatestas, A.E., L.I. Alpert, K.E. Osserman, R.S. Osserman and A.E. Kark (1971a). Studies in myasthenia gravis: Effects of thymectomy. Results in 185 patients with nonthymomatous and thymomatous myasthenia gravis, 1941-1969. Am. J. Med., 50, 465-474.

62. Papatestas, A.E., K.E. Osserman and A.E. Kark (1971b). The relationship between thymus and oncogenesis. A study of the incidence of non thymic malignancy in myasthenia gravis. Brit. J. Cancer, 25, 635-645.

63. Peterson, R.D., M.D. Cooper and R.A. Good (1965). The pathogenesis of immunologic deficiency diseases. Am. J. Med., 38, 579-607.

64. Petro, A.B. and J.D. Hardy (1975). The association of parathyroid adenoma and non-medullary carcinoma of the thyroid. Ann. Surg., 181, 118-119.

65. Pirskanen, R., A. Tiilikainen and E. Hokkanen (1972). Histocompatibility (HL-A) antigens associated with myasthenia gravis. A preliminary report. Ann. Clin. Res., 4, 304-306.

66. Pirskanen, R. (1977). Genetic aspects in myasthenia gravis. A family study of 264 Finnish patients. Acta Neurol. Scand., 56, 365-388.

67. Playfair, J.H. (1975). Introduction to autoimmunity in endocrine diseases. Clin. Endocrinol. Metab., 4, 229-239.

68. Prinz, R.A., E. Paloyan, A.M. Lawrence, J.R. Pickleman, S. Braithwaite and M.H. Brooks (1977). Radiation-associated hyperparathyroidism. A new syndrome?

Surgery, 82, 296-302.

69. Purnell, D.C., D.A. Scholz, L.H. Smith, G.W. Sizemore, B.M. Black, R.S. Goldsmith and C.D. Arnaud (1974). Treatment of primary hyperparathyroidism. Am. J. Med., 56, 800-809.

70. Purnell, D.C., D.A. Scholz and O.H. Beahrs (1977). Hyperparathyroidism due to single gland enlargement. Prospective postoperative study. Arch. Surg., 112, 369-372.

71. Rasmussen, H. (1971). Ionic and hormonc control of calcium homeostasis. Am. J. Med,, 50, 567-588.

72. Rasmussen, H., R. Bordier, K. Kurokawa, N. Nagata and E. Ogata (1974). Hormonal control of skeletal and mineral homeostasis. Am. J. Med., 56, 751-758.

73. Robertson, R.P., D.J. Baylink, S.A. Metz and K.B. Cummings (1976). Plasma prostaglandin E in patients with cancer with and without hypercalcemia. J. Clin. Endocrinol. Metab., 43, 1330-1335.

74. Rogers, B.H., J.R. Manaligod and W.V. Blazek (1968). Thymoma association with pancytopenia and hypogammaglobulinemia. Report of a case and review of the literature. Am. J. Med., 44, 154-164.

75. Roland, A.S. (1964). The syndrome of benign thymoma and primary aregenative anemia: An analysis of forty-three cases. Am. J. Med. Sci., 247, 719-731.

76. Rosai, J. and G.D. Levine (1976). Tumors of the thymus in ATLAS of Tumor Pathology, Second Series, Fascicle 13, Armed Forces Institute of Pathology, Washington, D.C.

77. Safdar, S.H., S.B. Krantz and E.B. Brown (1970). Successful immunosuppressive treatment of erythroid aplasia appearing after thymectomy. Brit. J. Hematol., 19, 435-443.

78. Samaan, N.A., R.C. Hickey, C.S. Hill Jr., H. Medellin and R.B. Gates (1974). Parathyroid tumors: Preoperative localization and association with other tumors Cancer, 33, 933-939.

79. Samaan, N.A., R.C. Hickey, M.R. Sethi, K.P. Yang and S. Wallace (1976). Hypercalcemia in patients with known malignant disease. Surgery, 80, 382-389.

80. Schantz, A. and B. Castleman (1973). Parathyroid carcinoma. A study of 70 cases. Cancer, 31, 600-605.

81. Seyberth, H.W., G.V. Segre, J.L. Morgan, J.B. Sweetman, J.T. Potts Jr. and J.A. Oates (1975). Prostaglandins as mediators of hypercalcemia associated with certain types of cancer. N. Engl. J. Med., 293, 1278-1283.

82. Seyfer, A.E., J.B. Sigdestad and R.M. Hirata (1976). Surgical considerations in hyperparathyroidism. Reappraisal of the need for multigland biopsy. Am. J. Surg., 132, 338-340.

83. Siegal, F.P., M. Siegal and R.A. Good (1976). Suppression of B-cell differentiation by leukocytes from hypogammaglobulinemic patients. J. Clin. Invest., 58, 109-122.

84. Souadjian, J.V., M.N. Silverstein and J.L. Titus (1968). Thymoma and cancer. Cancer, 22, 1221-1225.

85. Steiner, A.L., A.D. Goodman and S.R. Powers (1968). Study of a kindred with pheochrome tumor, medullary thyroid carcinoma, hyperparathyroidism and Cushing's syndrome: MEN type 2. Medicine, 47, 371-409.

86. Taylor, R.B. and A. Basten (1976). Suppressor cells in humoral immunity and tolerance. Br. Med. Bull., 32, 152-157.

87. Tisell, L.E., G. Hansson, S. Lindberg and I. Ragnhult (1977). Hyperparathyroidism in persons treated with x-rays for tuberculous cervical adenitis. Cancer, 40, 846-854.

88. Vichayanrat, A., A. Auramides, B. Gardner, S. Wallach and A.C. Canter (1976). Primary hyperparathyroidism and breast cancer. Am. J. Med., 61, 136-139.

89. Waldmann, T.A., W. Strober, R.M. Blaese and A.J.L. Strauss (1967). Thymoma hypoglobulinemia, and absence of eosinophils. J. Clin. Invest., 46, 1127-1128.

90. Waldmann, T.A., S. Broder, M. Durm, M. Blackman, R. Krakauer and B. Meade (1975). Suppressor T cells in the pathogenesis of hypogammaglobulinemia associated with a thymoma. Trans. Assn. Amer. Phys., 88, 120-134.

1. Watson, L. (1974). Primary hyperparathyroidism. Clin. Endocrinol. Metab., 3, 215-235.
2. Wekerle, H. and V.P. Ketelsen (1977). Intrathymic pathogenesis and dual genetic control of myasthenia gravis. Lancet, 1, 678-680.
3. Weller, G.L. Jr. (1933). Development of the thyroid parathyroid and thymus glands. Man. Contrib. Embryol. Carnegie Inst., (No. 141) 24, 93-140.
4. Williams, E.D. (1974). Pathology of the parathyroid glands. Clin. Endocrinol. Metab., 3, 285-303.
5. Zalusky, R., E.D. Zanjani, A.S. Gidari and J. Ross (1973). Site of action of a serum inhibitor of erythropoiesis. J. Lab. Clin. Med., 81, 867-875.

"APUD" Cell Syndromes

Judith L. Vaitukaitis

Section of Endocrinology and Metabolism, Thorndike Memorial Laboratory,
Boston City Hospital, Boston University School of Medicine,
Boston, Massachusetts, U.S.A.

In 1966, Pearse described a collection of endocrine cells with common cytochemical and functional characteristics and further suggested a common origin of those cells from the neuroectoderm of the neural crest (1966a,b). Their common cytochemical and histologic characteristics gave rise to the acronym, "APUD," which refers to Amine content, amine Precursor Uptake and amino acid Decarboxylase activity within those cells. APUD cells are thought to be diffusely located in both endocrine and non-endocrine tissues. Specifically, APUD cells have been localized in normal thyroid, pancreas, gastrointestinal tract, adrenal and lung. APUD cells share with neural tissue the capacity to synthesize and release the biogenic amines, histamine, 5-hydroxytryptamine and dopamine; in some cells, norepinephrine and epinephrine may be derived from dopamine. In addition to the variety of biogenic amines associated with APUD cells, several secrete polypeptide hormones, including insulin, glucagon, ACTH, gastrin, secretin, gastric inhibitory peptide (GIP), enteroglucagon, motilin, vasoactive intestinal peptide (VIP) and parathormone.

Under experimental conditions, Pearse and Polak (1971) observed APUD cells migrate from the ectodermal neural crest through the mesoderm to the foregut entoderm. Other cells with APUD characteristics, but not all, have similarly been observed to migrate considerable distances, in some cases to the adrenal and thyroid enlage, respectively (Pearse, 1975; Weston, 1970).

APUDOMAS

Theoretically, a tumor of the APUD cell, termed "apudoma," may arise in any anatomic site in which those cells are located. There are a variety of criteria by which these tumors may be identified and these are listed in Table 1. Those criteria are sent forth by Pearse and Polak (1971).

Paraneoplastic Syndromes

Secretion of hormones, as well as biologically active amines by apudomas may result in a variety of paraneoplastic syndromes, providing clinical clues to an otherwise occult tumor. In some cases, monitoring serial hormone levels may provide a useful basis for monitoring therapy and recurrence of the tumor. Secretion of hormones by apudomas may be "eutopic," i.e., the substances are normally produced by the cell of origin of the tumor, or the secretion may be "ectopic." In

TABLE 1   Identification of Apudomas

Histologic techniques	Masked metachromasia Argyrophilia Lead haematoxylin
Non-specific cytochemistry	α-glycerophosphate dehydrogenase Esterases Cholinesterases
Specific chemistry	Uptake and decarboxylation of amine precursors (formaldehyde- induced fluorescence)

the latter case, the hormone secreted is not usually associated with the cell of origin of the tumor. However, the distinction between eutopic and ectopic secretion may be semantic, since growing evidence suggests that any cell type can produce a given hormone, but in markedly varying amounts and its detection is somewhat limited by the available assay techniques. Table 2 lists the more common apudomas and their associated biogenic amines or polypeptides.

TABLE 2   Apudomas

Tumor	Hormones	
	Eutopic	Ectopic
Islet cell adenoma	insulin, glucagon	ACTH, ADH, VIP, hCG and its subunits, parathormone
GI carcinoid	gastrin, VIP, glucagon, GIP, secretin, CCK, motilin	ACTH, ADH, hCG and its subunits, insulin, VIP
Bronchial carcinoid		growth hormone, ADH, calcitonin, insulin, glucagon, prolactin
Small cell lung carcinoma		ADH, ACTH, calcitonin, VIP glucagon, oxytocin, prolactin, neurophysin, parathormone
Thymoma		ACTH, calcitonin
Medullary thyroid carcinoma	calcitonin	ACTH, VIP
Pheochromocytoma	epinephrine, norepinenephrine	ACTH, VIP, ?calcitonin

Humoral substances characteristically secreted by apudomas include several biogenic amines: histamine, 5-hydroxytryptamine (serotonin, 5-HT), and dopamine, and in some cases, catecholamines derived from dopamine. Table 3 lists the variety of biogenic amines and the clinical syndromes associated with them. The physiologic effect of the biogenic amines is exerted locally, usually at the site of synthesis of those substances. However, with some tumors, considerably larger quantities of substance are released into the peripheral blood, inducing a variety of vascular symptoms and diarrheal syndromes, which provide clinical clues to the presence of an otherwise occult tumor.

TABLE 3   Clinical Syndromes Associated with Apudomas

Syndrome	Putative Substance
Diarrhea of carcinoid syndrome	Serotonin
Hypertensive paroxysms associated with pheochromocytoma	Catecholamines
Peptic ulceration associated with gastric carcinoids	Histamine
Verner-Morrison syndrome (watery diarrhea, hypokalemia, achlorhydria)	Vasoactive Intestinal Peptide

The variety of apudomas may be associated with a rather characteristic collection of signs and symptoms. At this point, I will describe several of the more common paraneoplastic syndromes associated with apudomas.

Medullary Thyroid Carcinoma

Medullary carcinoma of the thyroid is perhaps the prototype of the neuroendocrine tumors. The term "apudoma" was first used in association with a C cell tumor (medullary carcinoma of the thyroid) which ectopically secreted ACTH (Sziff et al., 1969). Subsequently, that term has become engrained within the literature. Table 4 lists the several features of this syndrome.

TABLE 4   Medullary Carcinoma of the Thyroid

1. Sporadic or familial; may be inherited as an autosomal dominant

2. Constitutes 5-10% of all thyroid carcinomas of the medullary type

3. Clinical manifestations

   Marfanoid habitus
   Watery diarrhea
   Flushing
   Peptic ulcer disease
   Hypertension
   Hypercalcemia
   Intestinal motility disorders (serotonin, calcitonin, vasoactive intestinal peptide, prostaglandin)
   May be associated with an ectopic ACTH syndrome

4. Secretes calcitonin

5. Increased tissue histaminase usually with increased serum histamine activity in some

6. May be associated with multiple endocrine adenomatosis, type IIa

Carcinoids

Carcinoid tumors may arise in the foregut, midgut, hindgut and, in some cases, the

lung. Characteristically, carcinoid tumors arising in the foregut are more likely
to secrete the variety of peptides characteristic of neuroendocrine tumors. Those
tumors which produce biologically active substances may be associated with diarrhea
and flushing. Flushing is thought to be mediated by bradykinin and the diarrhea
usually by serotonin. Extensive discussion of tumors of the various portions of the
gut has been discussed elsewhere in this symposium.

Small Cell Carcinomas of the Lung

Small cell carcinomas of the lung are frequently associated with paraneoplastic syndromes associated with the APUD cell type. A variety of polypeptides, including
ACTH, ADH, glucagon, insulin, vasoactive intestinal peptide, growth hormone, pro-
lactin and calcitonin, have been identified in small cell carcinomas of the lung.
In addition, histaminase and L-Dopa decarboxylase activities have been identified
histochemically in some of those tumors, further suggesting a relationship to the
APUD neuroendocrine system (Baylin et al., 1978). In addition to having APUD
characteristics, the small cell carcinomas of the lung have a wide range of biochemical variation between patients, as well as within the same patient (Baylin et al.,
1978). If the tumors predominantly secrete calcitonin, there are rarely any associated signs and symptoms with ectopic production of calcitonin. On the other hand
ectopic production of parathormone, ACTH and ADH is frequently associated with
marked metabolic aberrations of electrolytes which may constitute a more immediate
threat to the patient's well being than the underlying tumor itself. Consequently,
recognition of those syndromes is important so that appropriate therapy may be initiated to correct the metabolic aberrations so that the patient can then better
tolerate specific anti-tumor therapy, be it surgery, radiotherapy or chemotherapy
which, in turn, should significantly decrease production of substances responsible
for inducing marked metabolic aberrations. The metabolic aberrations induced by
PTH, ADH and ACTH are briefly summarized in Table 5.

TABLE 5   Small Cell Lung Carcinoma

Hormone	Syndrome	Presentation
ACTH	Cushing's	hypokalemic alkalosis, edema, hyperten-sion, hyperglycemia, pigmentation, mus-cle weakness and wasting
ADH	Inappropriate antidiuresis	hyponatremia, symptoms of water intoxi-cation (lethargy → convulsions, coma)
Parathormone	Hypercalcemia	polyuria, thirst, nausea, abdominal pain, headache, psychosis, coma, normal or low serum phosphate

Multiple Endocrine Adenopathies (MEA) are associated with tumors derived from APUD
cells. Table 6 lists the variety of organs affected along with the classification
of MEA syndromes.

Multiple endocrine adenomatosis, Type I and IIa, is transmitted as an autosomal dominant with a high degree of penetrance. The mode of inheritance for Type IIb, however, is unknown. The relatively common occurrence of hyperplasia, accompanied by
adenomas in some cases, affecting several different endocrine glands in the same
family, is perplexing and suggests a basic regulatory defect of the several "APUD"
cells derived from neuroectoderm. The signs and symptoms of affected patients reflect the various biologically active hormones secreted by the tumors.

Most of the substances secreted by tumors associated with MEA Types I and II are
eutopic and, consequently, respond to physiologic stimuli. Calcium, glucagon and

TABLE 6 <u>Multiple Endocrine Adenopathies</u>

Type I (Wermer Syndrome)
  Pituitary Tumors (ACTH, GH)
  Pancreatic islet tumors
    Zollinger-Ellison syndrome (gastrin)
    Insulinoma
    Glucagonoma
    Secretin
  Parathyroid tumors

Type II
  IIa (Sipple Syndrome)
    Medullary thyroid carcinoma
    Pheochromocytoma
    Hyperparathyroidism
  IIb
    Medullary thyroid carcinoma
    Pheochromocytoma
    Hyperparathyroidism (rare)
    Multiple mucosal neuromas
    Hyperplastic corneal nerves

alcohol infusions have served as provocative stimuli for release of biogenic amines and polypeptide hormones by those neuroendocrine tumors. Both glucagon and calcium infusions stimulate the secretion of calcitonin from medullary carcinomas of the thyroid, insulin from insulinomas, glucagon from glucagonomas and gastrin from gastrinomas. Obviously, if basal hormonal levels are increased, there is no need to further manipulate the patient. In addition, glucagon may stimulate catecholamines from pheochromocytomas. A variety of provocative tests may be needed to evaluate members of a kindred suspected of harboring otherwise occult neuroendocrine tumors.

The APUD cell concept has evolved for more than 15 years. Experimental evidence strongly suggests a common clonal origin for most, but not all, APUD cells sharing common cytochemical and functional characteristics. The classification of cells of that type is clinically functional and assists the clinician in systematic evaluation and therapy of affected patients.

<u>REFERENCES</u>

Baylin, S. B., Weisburger, W. R., Eggleston, J. C., Mendelsohn, G., Beaven, M. A., Abeloff, M. D., and Ettinger, D. S. (1978). Variable content of histaminase, L-Dopa, decarboxylase and calcitonin in small-cell carcinoma of the lung. <u>New Engl. J. Med.</u>,<u>299</u>, 105.
Pearse, A. G. E. (1966a). Common cytochemical properties of cells producing polypeptide hormones, with particular reference to calcitonin and the thyroid C cells. <u>Vet. Rec.</u>, <u>79</u>, 587-590.
Pearse, A. G. E. (1966b). 5-Hydroxytryptophan uptake by dog thyroid C cells and its possible significance in polypeptide hormone production. <u>Nature (Lond)</u>, <u>211</u>, 598-600.
Pearse, A. G. E. (1975). Neurocristopathy, neuroendocrine pathology and the APUD concept. <u>Z. Krebsforsch.</u>,<u>84</u>, 1-8.
Pearse, A. G. E. and Polak, J. M. (1971). Neural crest origin of the endocrine polypeptide (APUD) cells of the gastrointestinal tract and pancreas. <u>Gut</u>, <u>12</u>, 783.
Pearse, A. G. E. and Polak, J. M. (1974). Endocrine tumors of neural crest origin:

neurolophomas, apudomas and the APUD concept. Med. Biology, 52, 3-18.

Sziff, T., Csapo, Z., Lasslo, F. A., and Kovacs, K. (1969). Medullary cancer of
the thyroid gland associated with hypercorticism. Cancer, 24, 167-173.

Watson, J. A. (1970). The migration and differentiation of neural crest cells.
Adv. Morpholol., 8, 41-114.

Sub-Clinical Coagulopathy in Cancer

R. Bugat and A. Boneu

*Centre Claudius Regaud and University Paul Sabatier,
School of Medicine, Toulouse, France*

ABSTRACT

Intravascular coagulation is frequently observed in cancerous patients. Laboratory findings are much more frequent than clinical symptoms. There is general
agreement that intravascular coagulation should be considered as a pathophysio-
logic state which is common to clinical and laboratory abnormalities. When present, fibrinolysis appears to be secondary to intravascular coagulation, even if
localized , rather than being a primary event. Recognition and active treatment
of hematologic problems in cancer patients may allow specific therapy to become
more effective. However , a great deal of further research is required in this
field before it can be translated into clinical management.

KEY WORDS

Intravascular coagulation, cancer, fibrinogen kinetics, heparin.

INTRODUCTION

Neoplastic processes are known to induce a remarkable variety of disturbances
in physiological mechanisms including blood coagulation. Thromboembolic phenomena and disseminated intravascular coagulation (DIC) are recognized complications of neoplastic disease. Clinically evident DIC, however, remains a relatively unusual finding. The occurence of a number of abnormal coagulation parameters
in patients with cancer without clinically obvious DIC have suggested that a subclinical coagulopathy might exist.

The purpose of this review is to explore coagulopathy in cancer as it occurs
without clinical symptoms, corresponding to low grade form of intravascular coagulation.

COAGULATION AND FIBRINOLYSIS

Before discussing the abnormal situation of intravascular coagulation, a brief
restatement of normal coagulation and fibrinolysis is in order.

Figure 1 gives a well accepted overview of coagulation.

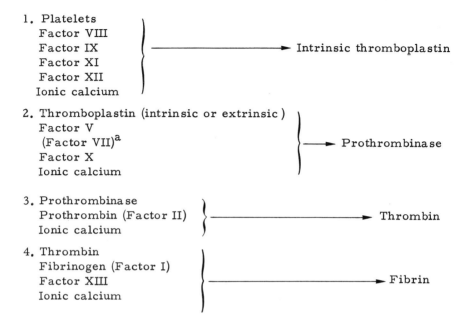

1. Platelets
   Factor VIII
   Factor IX   Intrinsic thromboplastin
   Factor XI
   Factor XII
   Ionic calcium

2. Thromboplastin (intrinsic or extrinsic)
   Factor V
   (Factor VII)[a]   Prothrombinase
   Factor X
   Ionic calcium

3. Prothrombinase
   Prothrombin (Factor II)   Thrombin
   Ionic calcium

4. Thrombin
   Fibrinogen (Factor I)
   Factor XIII   Fibrin
   Ionic calcium

Fig. 1 - Blood clotting factors.

According to the waterfall scheme, blood coagulation can actually be subdivided into three phases (6).

I - The intrinsic factor X̶ activating system, the mechanism by which factor X is activated following the contact of blood with a foreign surface.

II- The extrinsic factor X̶ activating system which is initiated when the blood is exposed to damaged tissues.

III- The common pathway which is the sequence of events following the activation of factor X to the formation of a fibrin clot.

Figure 2 depicts suggested alternative of the entire sequence of in vivo clotting. Once the coagulation system has been activated , the fibrinolytic system is brought into action and exerts a large influence on the products of coagulation (fig. 3).

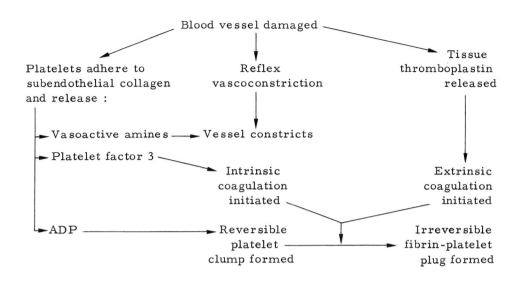

Fig. 2 - Schema of coagulation (from C.A. OWEN Jr.)

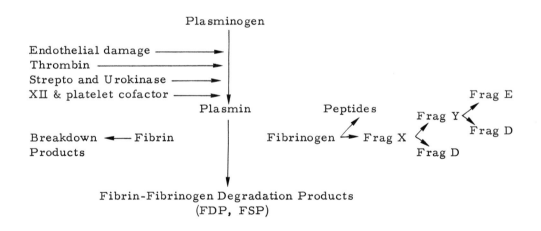

Fig. 3 - The fibrinolytic pathway (from ref. 4).

A strong proteolytic enzyme -plasmin- has the ability to digest both fibrinogen and fibrin, resulting in fibrin-fibrinogen degradation products (FDP) or fibrinogen-fibrin-related antigen (10). These products may then render blood incoagulable by their action on thrombin, fibrin monomer and platelets. Fibrinogen is composed of three pairs of polypeptides chains, respectively called, alpha

beta and gamma. The alpha and beta chains contain fibrinopeptides A and B at
the amino terminal end groups (1). (fig. 4).

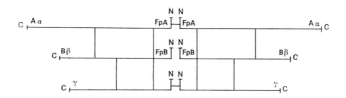

Fig. 4- The fibrinogen molecule

Thrombin splits fibrinopeptides A and B from the parent fibrinogen molecule,
after which the remaining so-called fibrin monomer spontaneously polymerizes
to form a fibrin clot. Clots are normally stabilized by covalent bonds between
fibrin molecules with cross-linking seen between lysine and glutamine residues
(8). Cross-linking results in a compound rendered insoluble in urea 5 M. Then,
both fibrinogen and fibrin are cleaved by plasmin. Fragment X, the first to be
formed, has a molecular weight of 240,000, it is clottable by thrombin. Neither
of fragments Y or D is clottable; fragment D is responsible for the disordered
fibrin polymerization frequently seen in intravascular coagulation. During intravascular clotting, some fibrin monomer molecules may remain in solution by
complexing with fibrinogen or with FDP. Soluble fibrin monomer complexes
will precipitate as cryofibrinogen when plasma is chilled, they will also clump
suspension of staphylococci (7). A variety of agents called paracoagulants, will
convert soluble fibrin monomer complexes into insoluble fibrin. The demonstration of a positive plasma para-coagulation test means that the circulating blood
contains fibrin monomers which are symptomatic of in vivo clotting, whereas
fibrinolytic split products only represent evidence of fibrinolysis.

INTRAVASCULAR COAGULATION

Figure 5 illustrates the pathogenesis of intravascular coagulation. Coagulation
may be activated in three essential circumstances:

       - endothelial injury
       - tissue injury
       - cytolysis.

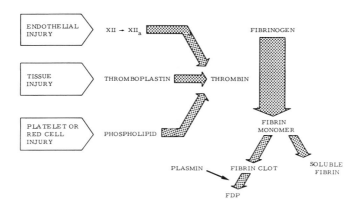

Fig. 5 - Pathogenesis of intravascular coagulation

Malaria offers an example of cytolysis induced coagulopathy . Infectious diseases activate coagulation by injuring endothelium,whereas cancer acts by injuring tissues In fact, no single mechanism that causes the chronic intravascular
coagulopathy in cancer has been identified (9). Cell products-secretion and en-
zymes- and the cells themselves have been proposed as the procoagulant res-
ponsable for the syndrome. The vascular structure and the caracteristics of the
interstitial fluid of tumor masses may also play a great role. Several studies
have revealed for a long time defective and often dilated vessels with areas of
inadequate blood supply in tumors. Muscular and nervous elements appear to be
lacking and contraction is defective. Deformation and varicosities are frequently found. Stasis and consequent hypoxia increase permeability of the vasculature which results in release of thromboplastic agents. Although there is as yet
no identified thromboplastic material common to all neoplastic states which
can be assigned the role of causing the syndrome, there is agreement that the
presence of thrombin in the circulation leads to fibrin formation, aggregation
and subsequent loss of platelets, consumption of plasmatic coagulation factors,
activation of the fibrinolytic system and transient hypocoagulability. The intensity of the problem may vary from undetectable to catastrophic bleeding . Figure
6 reprinted from S. I. RAPAPORT (11) shows mechanisms by which diffuse intravascular coagulation produces clinical disease.

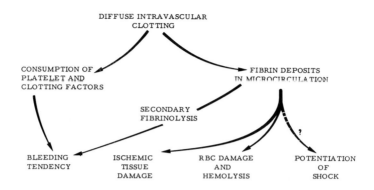

Fig. 6 - Intravascular coagulation produces clinical disease (from ref. 11).

When fibrin is laid down in loose strands in small blood vessels, blood will still flow through the vessels but the red cells are damaged. A striking hemolytic anemia may be produced with a characteristic morphologic abnormality of the red blood cells which appear fragmented , and twisted , they are called schizocytes.

There is no single diagnostic test for intravascular coagulation. Both screening and confirmatory tests have been described .As shown on the following table, examples of the former include prothrombin time, platelet counts, fibrinogen determinations. They are simple tests available at any hospital. In case of negative tests, it seems that subtle changes in the dynamic of coagulation process might better be monitored by dynamic tests, for example , studying fibrinogen or platelets kinetics.

Clinically evident DIC	Sub-clinical IC
◆ Screening tests 　　Platelet counts 　　Prothrombin time 　　Partial thromboplastin time 　　Fibrinogen determinations	◆ Immunologic measurements 　　Beta thromboglobulin 　　Platelet factor 4 　　Fibrinopeptide A 　　Thrombin-anti-thrombin III 　　complexes
◆ Confirmatory tests 　　Paracoagulation tests 　　Euglobulin clot lysis time 　　FDP determinations 　　Specific assays (Factors V, VIII, 　　　　　　II).	◆ Dynamic studies 　　Fibrinogen and platelets 　　kinetics

Fig. 7 -Diagnostic tests for intravascular coagulation

FIBRINOGEN KINETICS IN CANCEROUS PATIENTS -PERSONAL DATA.

One hundred patients, not recently operated on, free of clinical bleeding, thrombosis or infection, suffering from malignant tumors at different stage of their development underwent in the department of Nuclear Medicine of our Institution a fibrinogenkinetics study (including, when possible, external countings over the tumors) by monitoring survival of administred 131 I- labeled autologous fibrinogen. A concomitant study of haemostasis whith F D P measurement and para-coagulation test determination was also performed in each case.

Sixty to one hundred microcuries of sterile isotope were injected intravenously. Serial plasma samples were collected for one week. Iodine uptake by the thyroid was supressed by daily potassium iodide administration. The isotope data was resolved into logarithmic equations using a two compartment model. The half disappearance time (T 1/2) of the late component was chosen as parameter for expressing results. In case of palpable malignant bulk , the tumoral uptake was evaluated by studying daily change in the ratio: tumoral radioactivity over cardiac radioactivity. An increase of this ratio above twenty per cent at day 4 was considered pathologic. Results of this study which have been published elsewhere (2) showed that :

◆ T 1/2 is significantly shortened in 90% of cancerous patients (Fig. 8)

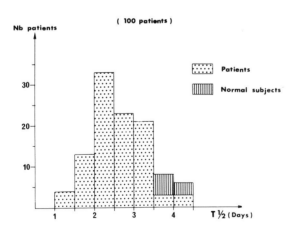

Fig. 8 - Fibrinogen kinetics = distribution of patients according to T 1/2

◆ The abnormality is correlated with serum FDP level
◆ Tumoral uptake is significantly high
◆ Calcium heparinate * (15, 000 IU/SC/24h given from day 5 to day 8) restores T 1/2 up to normal range in 95.% of cases (fig. 9).

*CALCIPARINE® : Laboratoire CHOAY. Paris. France.

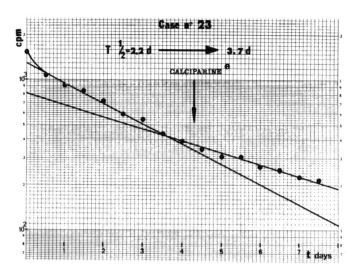

Fig. 9 - Fibrinogen kinetics : Pharmacological test.

These results confirm the high incidence of altered fibrinogen kinetics in patients with malignant disease and suggest the existence of a compensated (sub-clinical) localized intravascular coagulation (LIC), dependent on active tumoral process. However, there is no evidence that associated non malignant conditions do not account for these findings. In order to approach the mechanism which induces altered fibrinogen kinetics in patients bearing malignant tumor, some additional pharmacological tests were performed using drugs of different types (3). Results, as compared to those observed with calcium heparinate, are summarized on the following table.

Drug.	Dose /24h.	Pharmacological effects			Improvement in fibrinogen kinetics.
		Anticoag.	Antiagg.	Anti infl.	
Calcium Heparinate	15,000 IU	+/-	-	+	23/24
Prednisone	40 mg/m^2	-	-	+++	7/8
Indomethacin	100 mg	-	+	++	2/9
Aspirin	1g	-	+++	+/-	7/15
Aspirin	2g	-	+++	+	3/6
Ticlopidin	1g	-	+++	?	7/12

PREDNISONE appears as potent as calcium HEPARINATE , whereas ASPIRIN , whatever the daily dose (1 or 2 grams) and TICLOPIDIN , which is a true platelet antiaggregating agent, improve   fibrinogen kinetics in about 50% of cases.

The signification of these results remains dubious and not clear. All drugs share
out TICLOPIDIN ?) an antiinflammatory effect which suggest that these drugs
could counteract with the early stages of coagulation (kinin forming system and
factor XII) since some data (12) indicate that complement , hemostatic factors
and kinin constitute three complex systems which have numerous inter-relations
leading to reciprocal activations. In an attempt to evaluate what is either due to a
non specific inflammatory process or to truly impaired coagulation, further studies should be aimed at exploring on the one hand contact factors and on the other
hand, specific products of the release reaction, namely beta thromboglobulin and
platelet factor 4.

PERSPECTIVE IN TREATMENT

Deposition of fibrin and platelets within tumour vasculature probably accounts for
most findings in LIC . Fibrin has been detected within and around solid tumors
and is was assumed that this would favour the invasive growth of malignant tissue
and hamper free access of cytotoxic drugs into tumours. In other respects, fibrin
formation around intravascular tumour cell emboli is considered to play a role
in metastasis formation. Although no conclusive study has yet been published in
humans, antifibrinolytic drugs seem to decrease the growth rate of some experimental tumours. Nevertheless , if one considers evidence that the pathologic
process in the intravascular or localized coagulation syndrome is that of thrombosis more than of fibrinolysis , this approach remains open to criticism.
According to our experience using the subcutaneous route, it is possible to improve impaired fibrinogen kinetics with low doses of heparin, without recording
any gross disturbance in blood coagulation (normal thrombin time). This could
be in keeping with action that low dose of heparin has on its cofactor, antithrom-
bin III and which explains the efficient effect of this prescription in preventing
post-surgical thrombosis.

Recognition and effective treatment of hematologic problems in cancer patients
may prolong their life and allow specific therapy to become more effective. However , the lack of sufficient information currently available calls for further
experimental research.

REFERENCES

1- Blömback, B. Johnson, A. J. (1971). Joint report of the subcommittees
    on nomenclature and fibrinolysis , thrombolysis, and intravascular coa-
    gulation. Thromb. Diath. Haemorrh. (suppl) 51, 251-156.

2- Boneu, A. , Armand, J. P. , Blasco, A. , Bugat, R. , Boneu, B. , Lucot, H.
    Pris, F. , Combes, P. F. (1976). Demie-vie du fibrinogène marqué à
    l'iode 131 chez les cancéreux. Effets de l'héparine. Nouv. Presse Med.,
    5 , 415-418.

3 - Boneu, A. , Bugat, R. , David, J. F. , Combes, P. F. (1977). Cinétique du
    fibrinogène marqué à l'iode 131 chez les cancéreux. Approche pharmaco-
    logique. C. R. Soc. Biol. , 171, 1293-1296.

1- Dixon , R.E. (1973). Intravascular coagulation : a paradox of thrombosis and hemorrage. Obstet. Gynecol. Surg. , 28, 385-395.

5- Hilgard, P., Thornes , R.D. (1976). Anticoagulants in the treatment of cancer. Europ. J. Cancer, 12, 755-762.

6- Esnouf , M.P. (1976). Biochemestry of blood coagulation. Br. Med. Bull. 33, 213-218.

7- Marder, V.J., Matchett, M.O., Sherry, S. (1971). Detection of serum fibrinogen and fibrin degradation products : comparison of six technics using purified products and application in clinical studies. Am. J. Med. , 51, 71-82.

8- Marder , V.J., Budzynski, A. Z. (1974). Degradation products of fibrinogen and cross-linked fibrin-projected clinical application. Throm. Diath. Haemorrh. , 32, 49-56

9- McKay, D.G. (1965). Disseminated intravascular coagulation. An intermediary mechanism of disease. Harper and Row. New-York.

10- Merskey , C., Johnson, A.J. (1971). The clinical significance of fibrinogen -fibrin-related antigen in serum. Scand. J. Haematol. (suppl.) , 51, 313-315.

11- Rapaport, S.I. (1972). Defibrination syndromes in hematology . In W.J. Williams, E. Beutler, A.J., Erslev, R.W. Rundles (Ed.). Hematology. Mc. Graw-Hill Book Company, 1234-1255.

12- Sobel, A., Marcel, G.A., Lagrue, G. (1974). Complement hemostase et kinines. Sem. Hop. Paris. 50, 549-556.

Address reprint requests to Roland Bugat, M.D., Centre Claudius Regaud 11, rue Piquemil, 31052 Toulouse. Cedex. France.

Subclinical Cancer—Concepts and Management

LaSalle D. Leffall, Jr.

*Professor and Chairman, Department of Surgery,
Howard University College of Medicine, Washington, D.C., U.S.A.*

ABSTRACT

To place the concept of subclinical cancer in proper perspective, some definitions and guidelines are important. Subclinical cancer is cancer that produces no symptoms and that is not detected on standard physical examination. For our discussion, standard physical examination does not include Papanicolaou smears or stools for occult blood. Although many phsycians perform these procedures as part of standard physical examination in adults, some physicians do not include them. Thus, there is the need to emphasize their use in the detection of subclinical cancer. With these guidelines, we can bring more sharply into focus the principles underlying the concepts and management of subclinical cancer. Our discussion will deal with newly occurring primary subclinical cancers. Some subclinical cancers, like breast or cervix, when diagnosed early can lead to high survival rates while subclinical cancer of the pancreas, ovary or prostate when first diagnosed may be advanced and show poor survival rates. The major emphasis will be on the common worldwide cancers-breast, uterus, lung, prostate, oral cavity, esophagus, stomach, colon and rectum. Some comments will be made about the less common cancers.

Screening programs, which have as their primary aim the detection of cancer in the subclinical stage, must be cost effective. It is often difficult to determine the effectiveness of screening due to the following factors: 1) changes in disease patterns over time; 2) self selection of screenees; 3) chance variation; 4) small numbers of patients in most clinical trials; 5) lead time and length bias and 6) certain intrinsic theoretical difficulties in ascertaining a complex process from limited data. One of the most reliable methods for overcoming these problems is the comparison of total mortality in the entire screened population with that in a randomly selected control population.[1]

Certainly subclinical cancers must be looked for in high risk patients. All data, including retrospective analysis, must be used to determine high risk groups whether by age, race, sex, personal

habits (smoking), or geography. A careful search for synchronous
and metachronous subclinical cancers is mandatory especially when a
predisposing factor, as heavy smoking, is known to be associated
with cancers of the respiratory and upper gastrointestinal tracts.

BREASTS

Minimal breast cancer, which is usually subclinical, has been
defined as cancer which is either non-infiltrating or infiltrating
but smaller than 5 mm.[2,3] McDivitt has reported that if non-
infiltrating breast cancer was not treated adequately eight per
cent would develop into infiltrating cancer at 5 years and 15 per
cent at 10 years.[4] If breast cancer can be detected and treated
while still in a non-infiltrating or minimally infiltrating stage,
the overall prognosis and survival is predictably good. Gallager
and Martin classified minimal breast cancer to include lobular
carcinoma in situ, intraductal carcinoma in situ, and minimally
invasive carcinoma, either lobular or ductal, less than 5 mm. They
predicted that such patients have a ten year survival rate in
excess of 90 per cent.[5,6]

Studies which compared cancerous with non-cancerous removed breasts,
as well as comparisons with autopsy specimens, indicated that the
ductal proliferation in cancerous breasts was greater than in non-
cancerous breasts, and both had more proliferation than the autopsy
specimens. Animal models and human data suggest a continuum from
hyperplasia to atypical hyperplasia, to in situ carcinoma to
infiltrating carcinoma with metastases. The finding of significant
atypia may indicate an initiator mechanism. Whether one or several
promotors are required for progression through the continuum is
unknown. However, more and better understanding of the latency,
expressivity or promoting activity has become important with more
frequent identification of these minimal lesions.[7,8]

Gallager and Martin studied breast cancer by correlating mammography
and subserial whole organ sectioning and came to these conclusions:
1) human breast cancer is not a focal process but a disease which
affects breast epithelial diffusely; 2) the supporting connective
tissue of breast is also affected by the carcinogenic agent; 3) the
earliest histologically recognizable change in the sequence which
eventuates in invasive breast cancer is epithelial hyperplasia, a
nonobligate, preneoplastic lesion meaning that, although hyperplasia
is a stage through which epithelium must pass en route to neoplasia,
there are other possible outcomes of hyperplasia including reversion
to normal; 4) a stage of "intraepithelial" noninvasive carcinoma
precedes infiltrating mammary cancer; 5) concurrent invasion at
multiple sites from pre-existing carcinoma in situ is a common
phenomenon; 6) breast cancer may spread within the breast either by
the formation of new invasive nodules from intraductal carcinoma or
by local lymphatic spread, or both and 7) the configuration of an
invasive breast cancer may be a reflection of its rate of growth.[5,6]

Mammography has had a major influence on both the recognition of
minimal lesions and the understanding of the evolution of clinical
breast cancer. Wolfe has developed a classification system for
xeromammographic images that he believes encompasses a high-risk
group of women. In younger and perimenopausal women the P2 pattern,

or prominent duct pattern, does seem to suggest that any radio-
graphically demonstrable localized abnormality in these women
deserves biopsy. In addition, it appears that the DY pattern,
severe dysplasia often obscuring an underlying prominent duct
pattern, is associated with the highest rate of carcinoma and
hyperplastic conditions. Further definition as well as clarification
and verification by diverse groups studying this problem is needed
before definitive statements regarding patient management, based
on these patterns, can be made.[9]

Most clinicians believe that these minimal, often subclinical
cancers, should be disassociated from the ordinary clinical cancer
for management purposes. For in situ carcinoma, there is general
agreement that less than radical mastectomy is acceptable. Many
surgeons prefer to do a total (simple) mastectomy with an
incontinuity, low axillary lymph node dissection. The same
procedure or a true Patey-type modified radical mastectomy is
considered acceptable for the small invasive cancers.[10] For certain
minimal cancers, an alternative to total mastectomy has been
bilateral subcutaneous mastectomy with immediate prosthetic
replacement. Although there is no general agreement among surgeons,
the possible indications for this procedure are: 1) lobular
carcinoma in situ; 2) a single microscopic focus of intraductal
carcinoma; 3) a microscopic focus of invasive carcinoma in one
high-power field and 4) a combination of two or more of the
following: a) borderline histology; b) high-risk epidemiologic
factors and c) patient's anxiety about future development of
cancer.[11]

UTERUS

Carcinoma in situ of the cervix is not the inevitably progressive
disease that it was once considered to be. Unequivocal invasive
cancer develops in only a small percentage of cases and can be
controlled, if not cured, by current standard therapy. Most
oncologists agree that cancer of the cervix is the end stage of a
steady, although not necessarily orderly, progression of
abnormalities. The progression from dysplasia to carcinoma-in-situ,
to invasive carcinoma when it occurs, varies greatly from one
patient to another. Not all patients with abnormal cervices
develop cancer, or even a severe form of cervical intra-epithelial
dysplasia. Therefore in those lesions which may undergo spontaneous
regression or may turn into overt cancer in 10-15 years, there is
much to be gained by adopting a conservative approach especially
when most of these patients are young and have not completed their
family. Furthermore, the complications of conization cannot be
ignored. In recent years, the use of colposcopy guided biopsy has
been of increasing value. Electrocautery and cryosurgery are used
to treat non-malignant cervical lesions with cytocolposcopic follow-
up.[12,13,14]

Christopherson and his associates one hundred and eleven patients
with microinvasive carcinoma of the cervix over a 21-year period.
The sole pathologic criterion for inclusion was unequivocal
invasion to a depth of no more than 5.0 mm. Ninety-one patients
were followed for 5 years or until death, and 80 patients for 19
years or until death. From these data, simple hysterectomy
would seem to be the maximal treatment required. Since the

prognosis of microinvasive carcinoma is similar   to that of
carcinoma in situ, it is suggested that such cases not be included
when considering the end results of Stage I cervix cancer.[15]

One of the best studies of cancer of the cervix was done by a
task force that produced the "Walton Report", which outlined the
value of cervical screening, of Canadian women preventing death
from cervical cancer. The conclusions of the task force were as
follows: 1) squamous carcinoma of the cervix lends itself to
control by means of a cytologic screening program because: a)
invasive squamous carcinoma of the cervix is preceded by a spectrum
of disease extending over many years, which may be recognized at
the stages of dysplasia and carcinoma in situ; b) in a significant
proportion of patients with evidence of dysplasia or carcinoma in
situ the disease, if untreated, will develop into invasive squamous
carcinoma; c) cytologic evidence of the existence of dysplasia and
carcinoma in situ can be easily, safely and economically obtained
by the preparation and examination of smears and d) once dysplasia
or carcinoma in situ has been identified, further progress of the
disease can be prevented by simple therapeutic procedures and
continuing surveillance. On the basis of the conclusions, the
task force recommended the following: 1) health authorities
encourage and support the development of cytologic screening
programs designed to detect the precursors of clinical invasive
carcinoma of the cervix; 2) appropriate means should be employed:
a) to inform women of their degree of risk of developing carcinoma
of the cervix; b) to persuade all women at risk to participate in
the screening program; 3) an effective and sufficient frequency of
examination is as follows: a) initial smears should be obtained
from all women over the age of 18 who have had sexual intercourse;
b) if the initial smear is satisfactory and without significant
atypia, a second smear should be taken within one year; c)
provided the initial two and all subsequent smears are satisfactory
and without significant atypia, further smears should be taken at
approximately, a 3-year interval until the age of 35, and thereafter at 5-year intervals until the age of 60; d) women over the
age of 60 who have had repeated satisfactory smears without
significant atypia may be dropped from a screening program for
squamous carcinoma of the cervix; e) women who are not at high
risk should be discouraged from having smears more frequently than
is recommended above and f) women at continuing high risk should
be screened annually.[16]

Women at higher risk for later carcinoma of the endometrium are
those who have: 1) obesity; 2) diabetes mellitus; 3) infertility;
4) irregular menses and failure of ovulation; 5) adenomatous
hyperplasia and 6) long term estrogen therapy (risk increased with
dosage and duration). To identify high risk patients, we must pay
more attention to menopausal women and devise a method of screening
them by histologic sampling. Gusberg also believes it may be
necessary to screen all menopausal women with special attention to
those at higher risk by introducing methods of histologic sampling
which will be as complete as   curettage under anesthesia
but which can be done with a local anesthetic or no anesthetic at
all. A method that can be performed with minimal discomfort as an
outpatient has now become technically feasible. Aspiration

techniques may enable us to obtain histologic samples which are
virtually the equivalent of those produced by a diagnostic curettage
under anesthesia.[17] Cohen et al studied the correlation between
the histology obtained by suction curettage and subsequent formal
sharp curettage under anesthesia. An absolute correlation of over
95% was demonstrated and no cancers or precursors of cancer were
missed. The technique is considered useful and accurate for
screening patients at increased risk for developing endometrial
cancer.[18] Gusberg believes that some of the essential factors in
the control of endometrial cancer are: 1) recognition of
adenomatous hyperplasia and carcinoma in situ of the endometrium
as true precursors of invasive endometrial cancer; 2) recognition
of the high risk menopausal patient, through a histological sampling
of patients at the menopause with or without dysfunctional bleeding;
3) further research into the technology of obtaining histologic
samples in all menopausal women on an ambulatory basis without
anesthesia as a means of screening for the precursors of endometrial
cancer and 4) adoption of a staging formula that will allow
rendering the best treatment.[19]

LUNG

Cigarette smoking is the most important cause of lung cancer. In
Auerbach's studies, precancerous lesions of the bronchial epithelium
have always been found in patients who died of lung cancer. All
patients gave a history of having smoked cigarettes. Also, precancerous lesions were always found in patients without lung cancer
who smoked cigarettes heavily. Air pollutants other than cigarette
smoke seem to play a minor role in the production of such precancerous lesions. The question of reversibility of carcinoma in
situ awaits further study. Auerbach applied the term carcinoma in
situ to all bronchial epithelial, lesions composed entirely of
atypical cells and lacking cilia. He does not imply that, given
sufficient time, all in situ cancer would become invasive.[20,21]

Screening programs have been designed to detect lung cancer at a
more curable stage. Chest X-rays, sputum cytology and lung-health
questionnaires have been applied regularly to a study population
of out-patient men over 45 years old who are heavy smokers and
therefore have a higher probability of developing lung cancer.
Small asymptomatic lung cancers have been detected by both X-ray
and cytology. Both of these tests tend to complement each other.
Those tumors detected by cytology only appear to have a better
prognosis. Chest X-ray and sputum cytology testing are the only
procedures which have value in screening for early lung cancer.
Screening programs can detect and localize small asymptomatic lung
cancers. Almost 30 per cent of lung cancers are centrally situated
near the hilum. This location emphasizes the importance of cytology
and the limited value of chest X-ray.

Occult lung cancers not found by X-ray have been identified by the
Mayo Clinic and Memorial Hospital Lung Projects. Localization
procedures, especially fiberoptic bronchoscopy, have been successful
in every case of lung cancer in which they have been applied. The
average time between detection of sputum abnormalities and definitive
treatment has been only four months. Such excellent results could
not have been achieved without the flexible fiberoptic bronchoscope.

Its small diameter permits visualization of distal bronchi and
subdivisions of the upper lobes beyond the range of rigid
bronchoscopes and endobronchial telescopes. Radiologically, occult
cancers tend to arise in the upper lobes, either in subsegmental
bronchi or in more proximal bronchi. Unfortunately, even with the
fiberoptic bronchoscope, techniques for localizing occult lung
cancer are arduous, complex, and cumbersome, requiring carefully
planned sequential endobronchial inspection, biopsy, curettage
and brushing. The tumor may not be visible endoscopically--or
even grossly after pulmonary resection. Precise localization
may require repeated bronchoscopies, during which time the search
is narrowed until the tumor site is identified, visually, by
biopsy or by repeated brushing. Localization is expedited by
reexaminations on a continuing basis rather than at arbitrarily
specified intervals. Occult lung cancer is usually an in situ
or minimally invasive squamous cell carcinoma. Most in situ
or minimally invasive lung cancers are resectable and can be
treated by lobectomy. The five-year survival rates have been
quite good-about 70 per cent. These data and the ability to
localize occult tumors indicate that a five-year survival rate or
20 per cent is theoretically possible by aggressive cytologic
screening alone.[22,23]

Melamed and his associates reported that detailed histologic
examinations of the bronchial tree is resected specimens through
sixth generation subsegmental bronchi revealed that: 1) invasive
epidermoid carcinoma arises from carcinoma in situ of bronchial
surface epithelium or an extension of that neoplastic epithelium
in bronchial glands; 2) the site of origin is a segmental bronchus
in most instances and 3) each carcinoma should be considered as
unifocal in origin even though there is a continuing risk of
another primary lung cancer. It seems unlikely that squamous
metaplasia or basal hyperplasia is an essential step toward cancer.
Patients who have had malignant cells in sputum and have not had
a cancer identified in the lung after thorough rigid and fiberoptic
bronchoscopy with brushing of all segmental bronchi, have consistently
been found to have upper airway cancer.[23]

PROSTATE

By definition Stage A prostatic cancer is subclinical and its
incidence increases beyond the age of 50 years. Its recognition is
usually coincidental with pathologic examination of prostatic tissue
removed for the relief of benign prostatic hypertrophy and its
incidence in this setting is about half of the anticipated autopsy
incidence of Stage A lesions in corresponding age groups. The
prevalence of Stage A cancer far exceeds the morbidity and mortality
from prostatic cancer. Although it is reasonable to assume that the
Stage A prostatic cancer is the source of all clinically evident
prostatic cancers, most Stage A tumors never become clinically
manifest. Whether the transition from Stage A to a clinically
evident   cancer is a function of time alone or whether some additional
change in the phenotype of the cancer cell is necessary for the
transition is unknown. In any event, that Stage A cancer has a
long course is evidenced by the normal or close to normal five-year
expectancy of patients with Stage A lesions receiving either no
therapy or conservative therapy. However, there are enough exceptions

to this general rule to demonstrate the malignant potential of at least some Stage A tumors, particularly those of high grade. Patients may remain well following detection of Stage A cancer because the very operation that produces the tissue for diagnosis may also accomplish total excisions. Perhaps the natural history of the tumor predetermines a long survival. Prostatectomy for benign prostatic hypertrophy does not prevent the development of cancer. Autopsy studies show pathologic evidence that not all Stage A cancers are "early". Stage A cancer is far more common than clinical prostatic cancer, indicating that not all Stage A tumors become clinically manifest cancers within the lifetime of the host. High-grade Stage A cancers behave more aggressively than the low-grade Stage A tumor. Clinical identification of Stage A cancer in an indeterminate way, may influence the subsequent behavior of the disease and thus may impair, as yet undetermined, the validity of conclusions regarding the natural history of the disease in that setting. Stage A cancer may progress to a Stage B but may also: a) remain a Stage A tumor throughout the natural history of the host; or b) bypass the Stage B phase completely and progress directly to a Stage C or D lesion before the cancer becomes evident.[24] Whitmore says that decisions regarding the therapy of prostatic cancer are made difficult by: 1) the occurrence of the disease at a time of life when life expectancy is rapidly diminishing; 2) the relative multiplicity of useful treatments available-- irradiation, surgery and endocrine therapy and 3) the natural history of the tumor. Clinical judgment must rest on individualizing appropriate treatment for the particular cancer and patient. More information is needed about prostatic cancer to make the best judgement.[24]

Foti and his associates compared their radioimmunoassay with the standard enzyme assay for prostatic acid phosphatase in the diagnosis of prostatic cancer. In constrast to the enzyme assay, the radioimmunoassay for prostatic acid phosphatase has the potential to detect well over half the cases of intracapsular (some subclinical), and thus surgically curable, Stages A and B prostatic cancer. Statistical analyses show no advantage to the use of the enzyme assay along with the radioimmunoassay for the measurement of serum prostatic acid phosphatase concentration to improve the rate of correct diagnosis.[25]

A national study of the new specific assays for prostatic acid phosphatase was conducted by the National Prostatic Cancer Project (USA). The results of the study have confirmed that the counter- immunoelectrophorectic method is easily reproducible, semi-specific and sufficiently sensitive. Based on tests as performed by different institutions, the counterimmunoelectrophoretic method was also shown to have high reproducibility and was found to be of much greater sensitivity than the conventional biochemical methods for the detection of earlier stages of prostatic cancer. The national study of the radioimmunoassay has shown that although being a highly sensitive method, it could not be readily distributed at this time from one specialized center. It requires highly specific, expensive technical assistance and is not yet available nationwide. Counter- immunoelectrophoresis is recommended at this time to be used as the preferred method in the evaluation and diagnosis of prostatic cancer. The value of counterimmunoelectrophoresis in detecting early

prostatic cancer as a screening method is promising, but still
under study.[26]

Mass screening for Stage A disease might make it difficult for the
clinicians who are responsible for the care of patients with a
microscopic focus of prostatic cancer. Prostatic cancer is found
at autopsy in half of all men over 70 years of age. In most
instances such foci appear and persist in such old men but do not
progress to a clinically dangerous stage. Why they remain dormant
is unknown. There is general agreement that Stage A cancer, occult
cancer of the prostate, should not be considered a "benign"cancer.
Another biopsy should be recommended. If further cancer is
identified in the specimen, radical prostatectomy or radiation
therapy is advised. The organ-specific enzyme that is being sought
by a sensitive radioimmunoassay or by counterimmunoelectrophoresis
as a marker for cancer is not an abnormal molecule made by the
tumor cells. It is not a tumor-specific antigen but rather a
normal organ-specific component of the exocrine secretion of the
prostate.[27]

ORAL CAVITY

Although erythroplastic lesions are found on intraoral examination
and therefore cannot be called truly subclinical by our definition,
we must emphasize that such lesions may be asymptomatic cancers.
Most reports stress the relationship between leukoplakia and cancer
but not between erythroplakia and cancer. Leukoplakia, or white
lesion, has been indicated as the most common precancerous lesion
of the oral cavity. It has therefore been assumed that early cancer
is frequently a white lesion. Mashberg's studies, however, show
that no more than 2 per cent of white lesions are either invasive
carcinoma or carcinoma-in-situ.[28,29] A recent study in India, where
leukoplakia abounds, indicated that of more than 11,000 leukoplakias,
only 0.1 per cent became malignant in two years-a low rate of
transformation.[30] In spite of noting too much emphasis on the
malignant potential of leukoplakia, the concept that white lesions
of the oral mucosa are precancerous or early cancer persists in the
literature and in teaching institutions. Mashberg found, that the
asymptomatic, red, erythroplastic lesion is really the most common
sign of early asymptomatic oral cancer. Shedd confirmed this.[31]
Ninety-seven per cent of intraoral cancers are found in these sites:
1) floor or the mouth; 2) ventrolateral tongue and 3) soft palate-
anterior pillar complex.[28]

Two types of erythroplasia suggest the presence of cancer. One is
granular, red, and velvety with stippled or patchy areas of
keratin (white) in or peripheral to the lesion. The other is smooth,
nongranular, red, with minimal or no keratin (white). These
changes in the mucosa may not have well defined boundaries. Many
are irregular, with a blending of inflammation and normal mucosa.
Palpation is not helpful because only 20 per cent are elevated
above 1 mm. Asymptomatic erythroplastic lesions that persist in
high risk patients, (heavy smokers and drinkers) for more than 2
weeks may be precancerous, carcinoma in situ or invasive carcinoma.
Biopsy is essential.[28,29]

ESOPHAGUS

The incidence and mortality rates of esophageal cancer, including
cancer of the gastric cardia, are high in parts of North China,
where in some counties it is ranked first as the cause of all
deaths. In 1959 a series of epidemiological surveys were started.
The most recent one covered the period 1969 to 1971 and included
181 counties and cities with a population of nearly 50 million.
Preliminary clinical and experimental studies were also done on
geography, etiology, associated conditions, pathogenesis and mode
of evolution from earliest subclinical to clinical stages. Trials
of prophylactic measures, consisting of vitamins and herbal
medicines, were conducted in experimental animals and in selected
groups of high risk persons discovered during mass screening by
cytological examination. Patients found to have epithelial
hyperplasia on cytology were noted to be in the high risk group.
Cytology specimens were obtained by using a friction balloon in
the esophagus. The geographic distribution showed that the
incidence of esophageal cancer was highest in counties and cities
in the southern part of the Taihang Mountain Range, especially
in Linhsien county. Trace elements in the soil and drinking water,
nitrosamines, secondary amines, nitrites and nitrates in food as
well as fungus contimation were analysed to evaluate the high and
low incidence areas. There was a correlation between the high and
low incidence of pharyngeal and esophageal cancer in domestic fowl
and the human high and low incidence areas. A large scale
cytological examination of esophageal mucosa in the high risk
areas revealed a high frequency of epithelial hyperplasia in the
adult population of these same areas. Apart from the finding of
precancerous lesions many very early subclinical esophageal cancers
were also identified. This study, which established the geographic
distribution of esophageal cancer in North China and analyzed some
of the presumed etiological factors, has helped the Chinese obtain
a better understanding of subclinical and clinical esophageal
cancer.[32]

STOMACH

In Japan, Kaneko and his associates studied the outcome of gastric
cancer in six selected mass survey groups. One hundred and thirty
seven cases of gastric cancer were detected and followed post-
operatively for up to 16. The five-year survival rate of 83
patients in the survey, who were followed for more than five years,
was higher than that of the outpatients who were symptomatic and
seeking medical advice. The better prognosis is explained by the
fact, that many early gastric cancers were detected in the survey.[33]
In screening, the gastrocamera markedly increased the detection rate
of gastric cancer. Mass survey was performed once a year on
volunteers of each group. Photofluorography, a photographic recording of fluoroscopic images on small films of the stomach, was done
after 250 ml barium meal. Six exposures were taken in a proscribed
sequence of positions.[34] Gastrocamera examination was performed,
without local anesthesia, by using a small calibre instrument
specially devised for gastric mass survey. This was done just
before photofluorography.[33] Survival rates for mass survey groups
are higher than for outpatient groups, thus demonstrating the

importance of gastric mass survey. In mass survey cases, the
percentage of early carcinoma is extremely high in contrast with
outpatient cases. Even for advanced cancer the prognosis is better
in mass survey than in symptomatic outpatients, perhaps related to
less extensive muscle invasion.

For a proper evaluation of the role of gastric mass survey, a
study must be made in a population in which all the cases of
gastric cancer are registered. Therefore, the workplace mass
surveys are most suitable since the subjects' work is stable and
their medical status is well investigated. The main problem of the
survey is the possibility of overlooking cancer in the patients
examined. To overcome, this Kaneko and his associates have
emphasized the importance of repeated annual surveys. Many cases of
early cancers were actually detected through subsequent examinations.
The detection rate of gastric cancer was highest when photofluorography and gastrocamera investigation were combined. Endoscopy
must be included in gastric mass survey because its value is great
in high risk populations.[33]

COLO-RECTUM

In the U.S. screening programs for colorectal cancer using guaiac
stool testing, almost 10,000 patients have been examined. Twenty-
two cases of early colorectal cancer were found. The prevalence of
colorectal cancer in the United States is 45 per 100,000 population.
Accordingly, one would have expected to find three to four cases of
colorectal cancer in these 10,000 patients. The actual detection
rate was approximately five times the expected rate. The guaiac
testing method has been valuable in identifying patients with
colorectal cancer. Proctosigmoidoscopy and stool testing for occult
blood have detected colorectal cancer at an earlier stage. The
guaiac stool test, is inexpensive and can be used routinely, is
easy for patients to do and is esthetically satisfactory to both
patients and medical personnel. Proctosigmoidoscopy and guaiac
testing stools for occult blood are complementary. Both should be
done annually in patients over 40.[35]

At Memorial Sloan-Kettering Cancer Center, a screening program for
colorectal cancer and adenomas has been applied to 6500 asymptomatic
patients, age 40 and older, using occult-blood testing followed by
investigation of patients with positive slides by air-contrast barium
enema and colonoscopy. A control population of more than 7,000
patients had sigmoidoscopy only and no occult blood testing.
Approximately 1% of the patients had positive slides. Most patients
had only one or two positive slides. About half of patients with
positive slides had neoplasms including 23 patients with large
adenomas and 7 patients with cancers. Pathological staging of cancers
was more favorable (less invasion of the muscle wall) in the screened
asymptomatic group compared with the controls. Neoplasms seen on
sigmoidoscopy in screened patients who had negative occult-blood
tests included 12 cancers and 15 large adenomas. Reason for false
negatives is the possible conversion of initially positive slides
to negative perhaps related to the drying effect on the specimen
when not tested within 3-4 days. Screening for colorectal cancer
and adenomas by occult-blood testing is feasible, and has good

patient compliance with detection of early cancers. False positives
are uncommon. False negatives need further study.[36]

BLADDER

Cytologic study of urine and bladder washings for exfoliated cells
is receiving widespread attention in the early detection of bladder
carcinoma. At the Mayo Clinic, more than 46,000 cytologic procedures
have been performed on 35,000 patients. Among them, 106 had
findings indicative of cancer in the absence of cystoscopic or other
evidence of a urothelial neoplasm; and subsequently, of these, 69
had in situ carcinoma. Clinical observation revealed the prolonged
course of some in situ lesions.[37] The study suggested that cytology
detected the anaplastic cancers most commonly. The earliest
recognizable manifestations of bladder cancer are morphological.
Their recognition depends on examining exfoliated cells or biopsy
material. Biochemical, immunological, or other markers may be
useful in the future, but for the time being cytology and tissue
from the bladder is the only means of establishing a presumptive
or positive diagnosis of bladder cancer.[38] Cytology can detect
recurrent and persistent transitional cell carcinoma following
chemotherapy, radiation, or surgery. In such cases the abnormal
area of epithelium in the bladder may be extremely difficult for
the urologist to find by biopsy. He should not be lulled into
believing that the cytology report is incorrect by abnormal
appearing bladder and negative biopsies.[39]

MELANOMA

Melanoma is included in this report to discuss the role of elective
or prophylactic node dissections for patients with clinically
negative lymph nodes (subclinical disease may be present). There
are divergent views about this procedure. From September 1967, to
January 1974, a clinical trial was done by the WHO Melanoma Group
to evaluate the efficacy of elective lymph node dissection in the
treatment of malignant melanoma of the extremities with no evidence
of involved regional lymph nodes. Treatment was prospectively
randomized: 267 patients had excision of the melanoma and
immediate regional lymph node dissection and 286 had excision of
the melanoma and regional lymph node dissection when metastases
appeared. Statistical analysis showed no difference in survival
between the two groups, regardless of how the data were analyzed
(sex, site of origin, maximum diameter of primary tumor, Clark's
level or Breslow's thickness). It was concluded that elective
lymph node dissection in malignant melanoma of the extremities
does not improve prognosis and is not recommended when patients can
be examined at three month intervals.[40] Southwick believes that
elective discontinuous node dissection offers no different prognosis
than a therapeutic dissection and is therefore not indicated in the
primary treatment of malignant melanoma.[41] However, additional
prospective randomized studies are needed.

BOWEN'S DISEASE

Clinicians must be alert to certain diseases that may be associated
with subclinical cancers. An example is Bowen's disease, a specific
variant of cutaneous intraepidermal squamous cell carcinoma. Although
this disease has overt clinical manifestations, it may be associated

with other cancers, often subclinical, in the respiratory, gastrointestinal and genitourinary tracts. At least five per cent of
patients with Bowen's disease have multiple extracutaneous cancers
involving more than one anatomic site. It is noteworthy that five
per cent of patients harbor occult (subclinical) cancers.
Approximately one-third of patients with Bowen's disease develop
extracutaneous cancers about six to ten years after initial
diagnosis.[42]

TUMOR MARKERS

Tumor markers can identify subclinical cancer and provide a means
of detecting localized and possibly curable cancer. These markers
also determine the effectiveness of treating nonmeasurable cancer.
Hepatocellular cancer produces alpha fetoprotein. Choriocarcinoma
and testicular cancer produce human chorionic gonadotropin.
Elevated serum thyrocalcitonin may be the only clue to a diagnosis
of medullary carcinoma of the thyroid. Tumor markers remain a
fruitful area for further investigation.

SUMMARY

This discussion reviewed the concepts and management of subclinical
cancers. Emphasis has been placed on commonly occurring worldwide
cancers. Even now, clinicians should be able to detect and
diagnose many subclinical cancers. Earlier diagnosis will afford
patients a better chance for cure, less functional impairment, and
an improved quality of life. As physicians, it is our responsibility
to be vigilant in finding subclinical cancer.

BIBLIOGRAPHY

1. Feinleib, M. and Zelen, M.: Some Pitfalls in the Evaluation of Screening Programs. Arch. Environ. Health, Vol. 19, pp. 412-415, 1969.

2. Ackerman, L.V. and Katzenskin, A.L.: The Concept of Minimal Breast Cancer and the Pathologist's Role in the Diagnosis of Early Carcinoma. Cancer, 39:2755-2763, 1977.

3. Ashikari, R., Huvos, A.G., Snyder, R.E., Lucas, J.C., Hutter, R.V.P. et al: A Clinicopathologic Study of Atypical Lesions of the Breast. Cancer, Vol. 33, No. 2, 1974.

4. McDivitt, R.W., Hutter, R.V.P., Foote, Jr., F.W. and Stewart, F.W.: In Situ Lobular Carcinoma. JAMA, 201:82-86, 1967.

5. Gallager, H.S. and Martin, J.E.: Early Phases in the Development of Breast Cancer. Cancer, 28:1505, 1971.

6. Gallager, H.S. and Martin, J.E.: An Orientation of the Concept of Minimal Breast Cancer. Cancer, Cancer, Vol. 6, 1170-1178, 1967.

7. Gallager, H.D.: View from the Giant's Shoulder. Cancer, Vol. 40, 185-191, 1977.

8. Gullino, P.M.: Natural History of Breast Cancer. Cancer, 39:2697-2703, 1977.

9. Wolfe, N.J.: Breast Patterns as an Index of Risk for Developing Breast Cancer. Am. J. Roentgenol. 126:1130-1139, 1976.

10. Wanebo, H.J., Huvos, A.G. and Urban, J.A.: Treatment of Minimal Breast Cancer. Cancer, 33:349-357, 1974.

11. Hutter, R.V.P. and Rickert, R.R.: Pathological Basis for Therapeutic Considerations in Minimal Lesions of the Breast. Diseases of the Breast, Vol. 2, No. 1, 26-30, 1976.

12. Burrowes, J.T., Sengupta, B.S. and Persaud, V.: Carcinoma In-Situ of the Cervix Treated with Colposcopy Guided Epithelial Conization (Report of a 4-7 year Follow-Up Study). Int. J. Gynecol. Obstet., 14:273-279, 1976.

13. Creasman, W.T. and Parker, R.T.: Management of Early Cervical Neoplasia. Clin. Obstet Gynecol. 18:233-245, 1975.

14. Murphy, W.M. and Coleman, S.A.: The Long Term Course of Carcinoma In-Situ of the Uterine Cervix. Cancer 38:957-963, 1976.

15. Christopherson, W.M., Gray, L.A. and Parker, J.E.: Micro-invasive Carcinoma of the Uterine Cervix. Cancer 38:629-632, 1976.

16. Cervical Cancer Screening Program: The Canadian Med. Assn.
     Journal, pp. 1003-1033, June 5, 1976.

17. Gusberg, S.B.: Opinions. Ca-A Cancer Journal for Clinicians.
     Vol. 27, No. 1, pp. 47-49, 1977.

18. Cohen, C.J., Gusberg, S.B. and Koffler, D.: Histologic
     Screening for Endometrial Cancer. Gynec. Oncol., 2, 279-286,
     1974.

19. Gusberg, S.B.: An Approach to the Control of Carcinoma of
     the Endometrium. Ca-A Cancer Journal for Clinicians, 23:99-
     105, 1973.

20. Auerbach, O., Gere, L.B., Ravlowski, J.M., Muchsan, G.E.,
     Smolin, H.J., and Stout, A.P.: Carcinoma In Situ and Early
     Invasive Carcinoma Occurring in the Tracheobronchial Trees
     in Cases of Bronchial Carcinoma. J. Thor. Sur., 34:298-309,
     1957.

21. Auerbach, O., Stout, A.P., Hammond, E.C. and Garfinkel, L.:
     Changes in Bronchial Epithelium in Relation to Cigarette
     Smoking and in Relation to Lung Cancer. The New Eng. J.
     Med. 265:253-267, 1961.

22. Fontana, R.S., Sanderson, D.R., Woolner, L.B., Miller, W.E.:
     Benatz, P.E., and Taylor, W.E.: The Mayo Lung Project for
     Early Detection and Localization of Bronchogenic Carcinoma:
     A Status Report. Chest, 67:511-522, 1975.

23. Melamed, M.: Glehinger, B.: Miller, D.: Osborne, R.: Zaman,
     M.: McGinnis, G., and Martini, N.: Preliminary Report of the
     Lung Cancer Detection Program in New York. Cancer, Vol. 39,
     No. 2, 369-382, 1977.

24. Whitmore, R.: The Natural History of Prostatic Cancer. Cancer,
     Vol. 32, 1104-1112, 1973.

25. Foti, A.G.: Cooper, J.F.: Herschman, H. and Malvae, R.R.:
     Detection of Prostatic Cancer by Solid-Phase Radioimmunoassay
     of Serum Prostatic Acid Phosphatase. The New Eng. J. of Med.
     Vol. 297, No. 25, 1357-1361, 1977.

26. Chu, T.M.: Wang, M.D.: Scott, W.W.: Gibbons, R.P.: John-
     son, D.E.: Schmidt, J.D.: Loening, S.A.: Prout, G.R. and
     Murphy, G.P.: Immunochemical Detection of Serum Prostatic
     Acid Phosphatase Methodology and Clinical Evaluation. In-
     vest. Urol., 15:319, 1978.

27. Gittes, R.: Acid Phosphatase Reappraised. The New Eng. J.
     Med., Vol. 297, No. 25, 1398-1399, 1977.

28. Mashberg, A., and Meyers, H: Anatomical Site and Size of
     222 Early Asymptomatic Oral Squamous Cell Carcinomas: A
     Continuing Prospective Study of Oral Cancer. II. Cancer
     37:2149-2157, 1976.

29. Mashberg, A., Morrissey, J.B. and Garfinkel, L.: A Study of
     the Appearance of Early Asymptomatic Squamous Cenn Carcinoma.
     Cancer 32:1436-1445, 1973.

30. Malawalla, A.M.: Silverman, Jr., S.: Mani, M.J. et al: Oral
     Cancer in 57, 518 Industrial Workers of Gujarat India: A
     Prevalence and Follow-up Study. Cancer 37:1882-1886, 1976.

31. Shedd, D.P.: Clinical Characteristics of Early Oral Cancer.
     JAMA, 215:955-956, 1971.

32. The Coordinating Group for Research on the Etiology of Eso-
     phageal Cancer of North China, The People's Republic of China,
     Peking: The Epidemiology of Esophageal Cancer in North China
     and Preliminary Results in the Investigation of its
     Etiological Factors, 1974.

33. Kaneko, E., Nakamura, T., Umeda, M. and Fujino, N.H.: Outcome
     of Gastric Carcinoma Detected by Gastric Mass Surgery in
     Japan. Gut., 18:626-630, 1977.

34. Ichikawa, H., Yamada, T., Horikoshi, H., Doi, H., Matsue,
     H., Tobayashi, K., Sasagawa, M. and Higa, A.: X-ray diagnosis
     of early gastric cancer. Jap. J. Clin. Oncol. 1(1), 1-8
     1971.

35. Miller, S.F.: Colorectal Cancer: Are the Goals of Early
     Detection Achieved? Ca-A Cancer Journal for Clinicians.
     Vol. 27, No. 6, pp. 338-343, 1977.

36. Winawer, S.J., Miller, D.G., Schottenfeld, D.M., Leidner,
     S.D., Sherlock, P. and Befler, B.S. Jr.: Feasibility of
     Fecal Occult Blood Testing for Detection of Colorectal
     Neoplasia. Cancer, 40:2616-2619, 1977.

37. Farrow, G.W., Utz, D.C. Rife, C.C. and Greene, L.F.: Clinical
     Observations on Sixty-Nine Cases of In Situ Carcinoma of the
     Urinary Bladder. Cancer Research, 37, 2749-2789, 1977.

38. Friedell, G.H.: Recognition of Early Bladder Cancer and
     Premalignant Epithelial Changes. Current Practice of Urinary
     Cytology. Cancer Research 37, 2792-2793, 1977.

39. Frable, W.J., Parson, L., Barksdale, J.A. and Koontz, W.W.:
     Current Practice of Urinary Bladder Cytology. Cancer Research,
     37, 2800-2805, 1977.

40. Veronesi, A., Adamus, J., Bandiera, D.C, Brennhovd, J.E.,
     Caceres, E., et al. Inefficacy of Immediate Node Dissection
     in Stage I Melanoma of the Limbs. N. Engl. J. Med. 297:
     627-630, 1977.

41. Southwick, H.W.: Malignant Melanoma-Role of Node Dissection
     Reappraised. Cancer, 37:202-205, 1976.

42. Rickert, R.R., Brodkin, R.H. and Hutter, R.V.P.: Bowen's
     Disease, Ca-A Cancer Journal for Clinicians, Vol. 27, No. 3,
                       160-169,1977.

Diagnosis and Treatment of Primary Hepatocellular Carcinoma in Early Stage

A Preliminary Report on 134 Cases Detected in Mass Survey

The Shanghai Coordinating Group for Research on Liver Cancer,
The People's Republic of China

ABSTRACT

During 1971-1976, 1,967,511 natural population were screened by alpha-fetoprotein (AFP) in Shanghai, and 300 cases of primary hepatocellular carcinoma (PHC) (mass survey group) detected. This paper represents the diagnosis and treatment of 134 early cases (early stage group) without symptoms and signs of PHC. When the mass survey group is compared with the clinical group (1,200 cases), a marked increase (from 0.4% to 44.7%) in the proportion of early cases is observed. In the early stage group, operations revealed that 81.6% of cases had small hepatomas with nodules $\leq$ 5 cm. The results of extirpation of tumors are superior to that of other modalities in the long run, the 1-year, 2-year and 3-year survival rates being 86.7%, 75.0% and 57.1%. It is concluded that AFP screening is of significant diagnostic value in the early detection of PHC. The long-term survival rate has increased after early treatment of mass survey cases, especially when surgical resection has been performed. Some unsolved problems are discussed.

KEYWORDS

Hepatocellular carcinoma, early detection, early treatment, alpha-fetoprotein screening, mass survey, small hepatomas, preclinical diagnosis.

INTRODUCTION

In the past, early cases of primary hepatocellular carcinoma (PHC) were rarely discovered in clinical practice. Since the advent of mass survey with alpha-fetoprotein (AFP) in this country in 1971, not only the diagnostic accuracy has been greatly increased, but detection of preclinical cases has become possible. This paper described the diagnosis and treatment of 134 cases of asymptomatic PHC detected by AFP during the mass survey (early stage group) carried out by 15 hospitals in Shanghai from 1971 to 1976.

MATERIALS AND METHODS

1. Number of people screened. 1,967,511 people (natural population aged 16 to 60 were screened. Among these, 300 persons were found to bo cases of PHC (mass survey group), a discovery-rate of 15.25/ 100,000.

2. Methods of screening. AFP detection was carried out by double agar gel diffusion (AGD) and countercurrent immunoelectrophoresis (CIEP) in 1971-1973 and by passive reverse hemagglutination (PHA) test in 1974-1976. Rechecking was done in positive cases by CIEP, radio-rocket-electrophoresis autography (RREA) or radioimmunoassay (RIA).

3. Criteria for diagnosis. Diagnosis was established when positive CIEP or AFP level $\geq$ 500 ng/ml persisted over 1 month, with pregnancy, active liver disease (other than PHC) or teratoma of gonads excluded.

Of the 134 cases, 59 (44.0%) were confirmed by operation and/or histological examination, 55 patients (41.1%) died of PHC afterwards (50 within two years), and the remaining 20 patients (14.9%) had positive AFP (CIEP) persisting over 6 months with no evidence of active liver disease. In the majority of cases clinical features of PHC eventually appeared.

RESULTS

In order to facilitate the analysis of results, a comparative study was made between 1,200 clinical patients (clinical group, analysed in 1973) and the early stage group of the present series.

1. Early detection in mass screening. The proportion of early stage cases in the mass survey group and clinical group was 44.7% (134/300) and 0.4% respectively, and of late stage cases 15.7% (47/300) and 41.6%.

2. Distribution of positive rates for various objective examinations. Of the early stage group, liver scintiscan was positive in 26.7% (31/116), ultrasonography detection was positive in 20.6% (21/ 102), and enzymology (including alkaline phosphatase, gamma-glutamyl transpeptidase or the ALP and LDH isoenzyme was positive in 25.0% (20/80). The corresponding figures for the clinical group were 88.7%, 83.7% and 70.3-89.0%.

3. Treatment and results. Of the 134-cases, resection was performed on 31 cases (23.1%) without death, the resectability rate being 58.5% (31/53). This included left lateral hepatolobectomy, 11 cases; left hemihepatectomy, 8 cases; right hemihepatectomy, 7 cases; local or wedge-shaped resection, 3 cases; right posterior hepatolobectomy, 1 case; and middle lobe hepatolobectomy, 1 case. Seven cases underwent cryosurgery; 2 hepatic artery catheterization, and 9 irradiation (including 6 unresectable cases in which markers were placed at laparotomy to guide post-operative irradiation). 68 cases were treated by traditional Chinese medicine alone, 7 with medicinal herbs in combination with chemotherapy, and 10, in which PHC was not diagnosed because of lack of experience in the early days or the patients refused any definite treatment because of being asymptomatic, underwent symptomatic therapy.

The results of resection were better than those for other treatments,

the 1-year, 2-year and 3-year survival rates for the former were
86.7% (26/30), 75.0% (18/24) and 57.1% (4/7) as against 70.4% (50/71), 26.8% (15/56) and 10.0% (2/20) for the cases conservatively
treated with Chinese medicinal herbs alone or in combination with
chemotherapy. The difference in 2- and 3-year survival rates between
these 2 groups was significant (χ^2 = 7.910, P< 0.05 and χ^2 = 4.219,
P < 0.05), and in 1-year survival rate insignificant (χ^2 = 2.991,
P > 0.05).

4. Survival rates. The 1-year, 2-year and 3-year survival rates
(calculated by direct method) in the entire series were 73.4%, 38.5%
and 18.9% respectively. On the other hand, only 10.7% of cases in
the clinical group survived 1 year.

DISCUSSION

1. Reliability of AFP in the diagnosis of PHC. All the 134 cases in
our series were diagnosed on the basis of positive AFP alone. Our
routine method was to monitor serially, at intervals of 1-2 weeks,
the dynamic status of AGD, CIEP, PHA, RREA or RIA. In some patients
the establishment of diagnosis was delayed until AFP rose gradually
from a low level (PHA 1:10 positive or $\sim$50 ng/ml), in a period of
several months, to a height diagnostic of PHC. During the past 6
years, we encountered only 1 case presenting false positive AFP, in
which operation revealed intrahepatic cholelithiasis. Judged by our
PHC criteria, the diagnostic accuracy was 98.2% (53/54) for cases
operated on. However, the possibility of a false positive reaction
caused by various factors should be kept in mind. It is rather
difficult to differentiate it from active liver diseases. Our experience showed that in differential diagnosis the following are of
value: (1) The appearance of a synchronous curve of AFP and SGPT
in serial monitoring suggests active liver diseases, whereas the
appearance of divergence of the two curves suggests PHC. (2) When
the value of SGPT is several times higher than normal active liver
disease should be considered; when the value is about twice the
normal, the possibility of PHC should not be excluded. (3) When
AFP is $\geqslant$ 500 ng/ml, PHC should be considered.

2. Value of AFP in the early diagnosis of PHC. Although AFP has
been clinically applied in the diagnosis of PHC for more than 10
years, its value in early diagnosis of the disease has not yet been
extensively accepted. At the 11th International Cancer Congress,
the Chinese delegation reported on a mass survey of 494,304 population and affirmed the value of AFP in early detection of PHC. In
this survey early cases detected accounted for 44.7% as against 0.4%
found at clinics. Furthermore, of the operative cases in this
series, 81.6% (40/49) of the tumor nodules measured less than 5 cm,
the smallest being 0.8 cm. In the past, such "small hepatomas" were
found only when a PHC ruptured or at laparotomy for other illnesses.
This also points to the value of AFP. In 1977, Okuda and others reported 20 small hepatomas, of which only 4 were found clinically by
AFP in patients with liver diseases, whereas the rest were diagnosed
postmortem.

An additional evidence of the superiority of AFP over other conventional procedures in early diagnosis of PHC is that of the clinical
cases with positive findings, only 20% were early stage cases.

Survival in the definitively treated group is longer than that for those receiving merely symptomatic treatment, the 1-year survival rate being 76.5% (91/119) and 33.3% (3/9) (χ^2 = 5.924, P< 0.05) and the 2-year survival rates 39.8% (39/98) and 16.7% (1/6) (P > 0.05) respectively. This shows that definite therapeutic intervention prolongs survival of the patient and that mass survey by AFP is an ideal approach to early detection of PHC.

3. Modalities of choice and the position of resection in the treatment of early PHC. Based on our experience resection with post-operative composite adjunctive treatment should be the method of choice for PHC unless surgery is contraindicated. Generally the resectability rate is higher, the operative mortality rate lower, and survival longer in early stage cases.(Table 1).

TABLE 1 Comparison of Results of Resection Between
the Early Stage Group and Clinical Groups
(Shanghai)

	Early Stage Group 1971-1976	Clinical Group	
		1958-1973	1973-1976
Cases resected	31	258	112
Resectability rate (%)	58.5	28.2	37.3
Operative mortality rate (%)	0	14.7	5.4
1-year survival (%)	86.7	34.1	46.8
2-year survival (%)	75.0	22.4	26.4
3-year survival (%)	57.1	15.5	25.0

The following are certain problems observed in early stage cases undergoing surgery: (1) Failure to find the tumor. This happened in 7.5% of our cases undergoing laparotomies (4/53), all proved to have PHC on follow-up. The failure is probably because operation was performed too early and the tumor being too small to be identified. (2) Multicentric origin of PHC. In our series, 14.3% (7/49) of the early stage cases had 2 to more grossly identifiable nodules. Furthermore, the fact that AFP did not revert to normal post-operatively in 22.6% (7/31) of the resected cases possibly also indicates a multicentric pattern. (3) The presence of associated liver cirrhosis and a hilar located tumor make resection of PHC more difficult. In spite of these difficulties, early detection by mass survey and removal of the tumor is still an effective way of prolonging survival. The proportion of resectable cases in the present series was 23.1%, while that encountered clinically was only 8%.

REFERENCES

Coordinating Group for Research on Liver Cancer, People's Republic of China (1974). Alpha-fetoprotein assay in primary hepato-cellular carcinoma, mass survey and follow-up studies. Presented at the 11th International Cancer Congress. Oct., 1974, Florence, Italy.
Okuda, K., T. Nakashima, H. Obata, and Y. Kubo (1977). Clinico-pathological studies of minute hepatocellular carcinoma, analy-

sis of 20 cases, including 4 with resection. <u>Gastroenterol.</u>, <u>73</u>,
109-115.

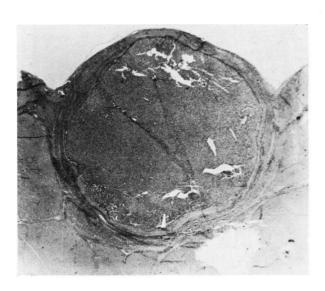

Small hepatocellular carcinoma,
showing well formed fibrous
capsule x 10

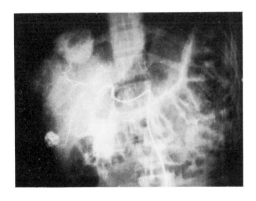

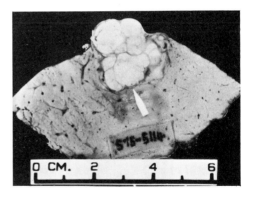

Angiogram of   Surgical specimen
early stage PHC   of early stage PHC

Studies on Alpha-Fetoprotein IV.
Further Studies on Alpha-Fetoprotein in Mass Surveys and Follow-up Studies on Primary Hepatocellular Carcinoma

Coordinating Group for Research on Liver Cancer,
The People's Republic of China

c/o Institute of Biochemistry, Academia Sinica, 320 Yo Yang Road, Shanghai

ABSTRACT

1. The adoption of sensitive methods of AFP assay in mass surveys significantly increases the rate of early diagnosis of liver cell cancer (LCC). Periodic screening at fixed intervals increases the diagnostic rate of stage I LCC from 4.7 per cent to 60 per cent, while the rate of failure in detection is lowered to 15 per cent. 2. Patients with persistently elevated levels of AFP of 50 to 300 ng per ml come out with an incidence of LCC as high as 10.3 to 29.4 per cent during long-term follow-up studies. It is proposed to have them serve as objects of investigation on the interruption of neoplastic transformation at the precancerous stage. 3. Kinetic studies on both serum AFP concentration and SGPT activity in those patients with simultaneously elevated AFP and SGPT may help in the differential diagnosis of malignant from benign diseases. 4. Preliminary results suggest that surgical operations on stage I liver cancer and traditional (Chinese) medical treatment for patients with slightly elevated AFP levels of long duration may prove to be quite promising.

Keywords: Alpha-fetoprotein, hepatoma, mass survey, early diagnosis, slightly elevated AFP levels.

Alpha-fetoprotein (AFP), being an onco-fetal protein (Abelev, 1971) is usually present at a level below 25 ng per ml serum in normal adults (Coordinating Group, 1974). AFP appears at higher levels in most patients with primary liver cell cancer (LCC), in some with terratomas, and also in some cases of hepatitis and liver cirrhosis. In China, AFP levels above 300 ng per ml, with the exception of terratoma cases, are generally considered to be highly indicative of liver cell cancer. In previous papers (Coordinating Group, 1973, 1974), the results of mass surveys and follow-up studies have been reported. Nothing was then known of the prognosis of cases with AFP levels below 300 ng per ml. This paper presents results obtained in further studies of such cases dtected in mass surveys.

1. Relationship between the Sensitivity of the Screening Test Employed and the Early Diagnosis of Liver Cell Cancers in Mass Surveys

The results obtained by different methods of various sensitivity are given in Tables 1a and 1b. As the hemagglutination test (Division Cancer Research, 1976) can be carried out with simple equipment in 30 minutes with only one drop of blood, it has been used as a screening test for mass surveys in the countryside. Radio-rocket-electrophoresis autography (Coordinating Group, 1974), being simple, sensitive, highly specific, easily reproducible, and not requiring a gamma counter, has become the method of choice for quantitative follow-up studies. These two methods combined have been proven to be quite efficacious in conducting mass surveys. The data presented in this paper were all obtained by these methods.

TABLE 1a Relationship between Sensitivity of the Screening Methods and their Diagnostic Rate for Stage I LCC

Year	Method	Sensitivity (ng per ml)	Number of People Examined*	Patients with LCC** Total	Stage I No.	Stage I %
1971	Double diffusion	3,000	13,881	43	2	4.7
1972	Countercurrent electrophoresis	500	66,832	105	31	29.5
1975–1976	Hemagglutination & radio-rocket-electrophoresis	50	31,231	28	17	60.1

* Including the natural population and people with liver disease or history of liver disease.
** "Stage I" liver cell cancer is here defined as that stage of the disease showing no signs and symptoms of hepatoma.

TABLE 1b Relationship between Sensitivity of Different Screening Methods and their Failure in Detecting Stage I LCC

Sensitivity (ng/ml)	Number of People Examined	Number of People with Stage I LCC	1-3	4-6	7-8	Per cent Failure in Detection
3,000	13,881	2	8	4	2	87.5
500	66,832	31	8	7	9	43.6
50	31,231	17	0	1	2	15.0

TABLE 2 Results of Serial Mass Survey for One Population

Survey	Date	Number of People Examined	LCC Cases Prestage I*	Stage I	Stage II-III	Failure in Detection of Stage I LCC
1	Sept.,1975	13,224	10	3	4	2
2	March,1976	6,825	2	1	2	1
3	Sept.,1976	11,182	1	0	0	0

*For cases with persistent slightly elevated levels of AFP and later shown to have cancer in follow-up studies, see Section 3.

2. The Importance of Serial Screening

One population has been screened repeatedly at intervals of six months. The results are shown in Table 2. From Table 2 it can be seen that repeated AFP screening at a fixed interval may greatly decrease the rate of failure in detecting stage I liver cell cancer.

3. Cases Showing Persistent Slightly Elevated Levels of AFP

The term "persistent slightly elevated AFP level" applies only to those cases found in mass surveys with AFP levels between 50 and 300 nanograms per ml and presenting no obvious sign or symptoms of hepatoma, maintained at such levels for at least two months when reexamined at intervals of 3 weeks, but excluding "SGPT correlated positive" cases and other AFP positive tumours or diseases.

Follow-up cases selected randomly according to these criteria are shown in Table 3. It is worth noting that the incidence of liver cancer in this group is very high.

TABLE 3 One-to-Two Year Follow-up Studies of Cases showing
Persistent Slightly Elevated AFP Levels

Group	Number of cases	Follow-up period	Liver cancer proven No.	Liver cancer proven %	Normal No.	Normal %	Under observation No.	Under observation %
1	116	1 year	12	10.3	nd		104	89.7
2	136	1 year	37	27.4	59	43.7	39	28.8
3	51	2 years	15	29.4	24	47.1	12	23.5

4. Treatment of Stage I Liver Cancers and of Cases with Slightly Elevated AFP

Patients were selected randomly showing persistent slightly elevated AFP levels and treated by traditional Chinese medicine. Results from a 1-year period treatment are given in Table 4. The incidence of clinical LCC cases in the treated group is lower than in the control group. Work along these lines are still in progress.

TABLE 4 Results of a One-year Treatment for Cases showing
Persistent Slightly Elevated AFP Levels

	Group	Number of Patients Treated	Clinical LCC Number	Clinical LCC Per cent	Relative Incidence of LCC
I	Control	116	12	10.3	$\frac{4}{1}$ (P<0.05)
	Treated	270	7	2.6	
II	Control	136	37	27.3	$\frac{2.5}{1}$ (P<0.05)
	Treated	63	7	11.1	

Some of the stage I liver cell cancer patients discovered in mass surveys were given surgical treatment. The effectiveness of such measures is shown in Table 5.

TABLE 5 The Effectiveness of Surgical Treatment
on Stage I LCC Patients

Group	One-year Follow-up		Two-year Follow-up	
	Number	Per cent Survival	Number	Per cent Survival
I	30	86.7(26/30)	24	75.0(18/24)
II	24	83.3(20/24)	13	77.0(10/13)

5. SGPT Correlated AFP Positive Cases and the Separation of AFP and SGPT Dynamic Curves

Due to the presence of elevated AFP levels in liver diseases other
than hepatoma, differential diagnosis is often difficult. 29 patients
with persistent elevated levels of AFP were consequently selected at
random for quantitative follow-up in SGPT activity as well as AFP concentration. Two types have been observed during a two-year period
(Fig. 1). 13 of the 29 appeared to be SGPT correlated AFP positive.
In follow-up observations for more than two years both AFP and SGPT
returned to normal. None of them showed any symptoms of liver cancer
(Fig. 1a). In 6 out of the 29, all of whom were clinically deteriora-
ting, a separation of the AFP and SGPT dynamic curves was manifest
(Fig. 1b). The other 10 cases are still under observation.

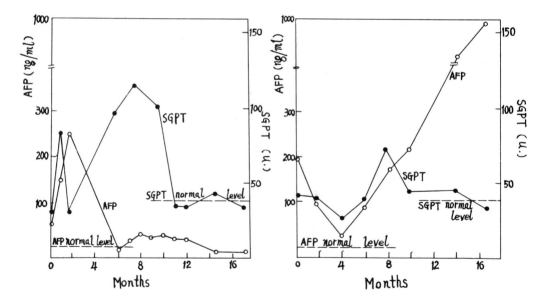

Fig. 1a SGPT correlated AFP   Fig. 1b Separation of the SGPT
dynamic curve (case Chang)   and AFP dynamic curves (case Kou)

DISCUSSION

From Tables 1a and 1b it may be surmised that more sensitive methods are necessary in order for the AFP assay for primary liver cancer in mass surveys to assume greater significance. It is now possible to realize the early detection and early treatment of liver cancer by a combination of simple, sensitive and specific methods with serial mass surveying at fixed periods on a large scale. In cases showing persistent slight elevation of AFP, treatment by traditional Chinese medicine seems to have better effects, while stage I cancer patients fare better with surgical treatment.

It has always been difficult to distinguish between hepatoma and other liver diseases, particularly when the AFP concentration falls within the range of 50 to 300 ng per ml. However, most slightly elevated AFP would become normal within two months. Among people whose serum AFP concentrations persist at slightly elevated levels, some are at the same time SGPT elevated. Cases showing diverging AFP-SGPT dynamic curves should be closely followed. As the percentage of patients who ultimately turn out to have liver cancer is always very high among those showing persistent slight elevation of AFP, this group should form the main object of study with a view to interrupting the course of carcinogenesis and preventing the onset of liver cancer.

REFERENCES

Abelev, G. I. (1971). Alpha-fetoprotein in ontogenesis and its association with malignant tumors. Adv. Cancer Res., 14, 295-358.

Coordinating Group for the Research on Liver Cancer, the People's Republic of China. (1973). Application of serum alpha-fetoprotein assay in mass survey of primary carcinoma of liver. In 2nd International Symposium on Cancer Detection and Prevention. April, 1973, Bologna, Italy.

Coordinating Group for the Research on Liver Cancer, the People's Republic of China. (1974). Studies of human alpha-fetoprotein. Presented at the 11th International Cancer Congress. Oct., 1974, Florence, Italy.

Division of Cancer Research, National Vaccine and Serum Institute, Peking. (1976). Hemagglutination test for alpha-fetoprotein in the diagnosis of primary liver carcinoma. Scientia Sinica XIX, 641-646.

Studies on Alpha-Fetoprotein V.
Influence of Alpha-Fetoprotein on
Immunological Function

Coordinating Group for Research on Liver Cancer,
The People's Republic of China

c/o Institute of Biochemistry, Academia Sinica, 320 Yo Yang Road, Shanghai

ABSTRACT

1. Purified AFP displays suppression of phagocytosis of macrophages.
2. AFP positive serum shows the same type of suppression which is
relieved after removing AFP from the serum. 3. AFP attaches to macrophages. It is possible that receptors for AFP are present on the
surface of these cells.

Keywords: Alpha-fetoprotein, immunosuppression, macrophages, peritoneal cells, receptor.

During the fetal development of human beings and animals, AFP, a main
component in fetal serum, was shown to be of great importance for
normal pregnancy (Mizejewski & Grimley, 1976). In patients with primary liver cell cancer, more than 90% have AFP concentrations higher
than normal controls, in some it may reach a level as high as a few
mg per ml. Thus, the search for the biological function of AFP
during development or carcinogenesis has become a subject of great
interest.

It has been observed clinically that macrophages, which otherwise
play an important role in immunological reactions, do not appear to
function properly in cancer patients. Studies on the effect of AFP
on immunological function would therefore be of importance in expli-
cating the physiology of AFP. This paper is a report on the influence of human AFP on the immunological functions of macrophages.

MATERIALS AND METHODS

Human AFP

Fetal AFP and hepatoma AFP were purified by immunoadsorbent columns
of sepharose 4B conjugated with monospecific anti-AFP antibody. The
purified sample showed a single band in immunoelectrophoresis and
polyacrylamide gel electrophoresis (AFP content greater than 95%).

The Preparation of Macrophages and the Examination of Phagocytosis

Macrophages were obtained from exudates of human blisters and rat peritoneal cavity. Chicken red blood cells served as markers for phagocytosis in observations on the influence of AFP on macrophage function.

RESULTS

1. Suppression of Phagocytosis by AFP Positive Sera before and after Removal of AFP by means of Immunoadsorption

Suppression of phagocytosis was shown for AFP positive sera. The degree of suppression depended on the AFP concentration in the sera used (Table 1). Those sera, in which AFP had been removed by an immunoadsorbent column of sepharose 4B coupled with monospecific anti-AFP antibody, showed reduced suppression. The higher the original AFP concentration, the less was the suppression on phagocytosis after removing AFP.

TABLE 1 Suppression of Phagocytosis by AFP Positive
Sera before and after Removal of AFP

Sera	1	2	3	4	5	6	7	8	9	10
AFP (μg/ml)	12	12	21	29	40	41	45	68	97	99
Per cent suppression of phagocytosis in presence of AFP	15	18	23	25	18	16.5	17	28	28	38
Per cent suppression of phagocytosis in absence of AFP	6.7	6.9	4.4	23.9	10.1	6.5	7	0	-3	2
Per cent recovery of phagocytosis after removal of AFP	8.3	11.1	18.6	1.1	7.9	10	10	28	31	36

2. Suppression of the Phagocytosis and the Electrophoretic Mobility of Human Macrophages by Human Fetal AFP (HAFP) and Human Serum Albumin (HSA)

HAFP showed suppression of phagocytosis and electrophoretic mobility of macrophages with HSA as control (Fig. 1).

3. Suppression of Phagocytosis of Rat Macrophages by HAFP and HSA

Fig. 2 shows that fetal AFP and liver cancer AFP are both capable of suppressing the phagocytosis of rat macrophages. HSA showed much lower suppression than HAFP.

4. Comparison of the Binding Capacity of HAFP and HSA with Rat Peritoneal Exudate Cells

^{131}I-HAFP and ^{131}I-HSA were separately incubated with rat peritoneal exudate cells, the excess free ^{131}I-labeled proteins were removed by

electrophoresis and the cells subjected to radioautography and radioactivity measurement (Table 2). It may be seen that the binding capacity of HAFP for such cells were in all cases greater than HSA. To
obtain the same amount of binding, one has to employ an HSA concentration one order of magnitude higher than HAFP (Fig. 3).

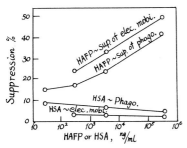

Fig. 1 Suppression of phagocytosis and electrophoretic mobility
by HAFP and HSA

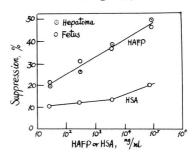

Fig. 2 Suppression of phagocytosis of rat macrophages by HAFP
and HSA

TABLE 2 Percentage of Binding of HAFP and HSA to Rat
Peritoneal Exudate Cells

	Peritoneal Cells	Chicken Red Blood Cells
^{131}I-HAFP	2.85 ± 0.15	0
^{131}I-HSA	0.55 ± 0.35	0

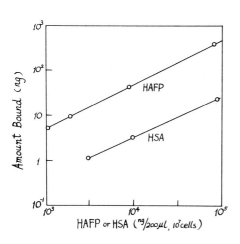

Fig. 3 Comparison of the binding
capacity of HAFP and HSA for rat
peritoneal cells

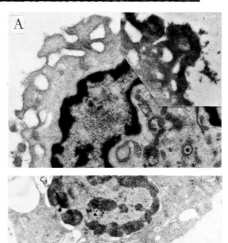

Fig. 4a The electron micrograph
of HAFP bound to the macrophage,
24,000 x;   Insert: 60,000 x;
Fig. 4b Control.

5. Binding of HAFP to the Rat Peritoneal Macrophage Surface

Fig. 4 shows the localization of HAFP on the macrophage surface by the electron microscope using the immunoperoxidase technique.

6. Binding of HAFP to Rat Peritoneal Exudate Cells

The relationship between binding capacity of HAFP and HAFP concentration is shown in Fig. 5. Binding capacity is defined as cpm retained on macrophage/cpm total x 100. Fig. 6 shows the relationship between amount of HAFP bound and HAFP concentration.

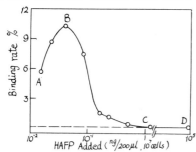

Fig. 5 Relationship between concentration of HAFP and binding capacity

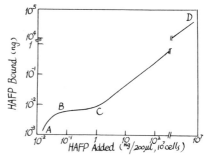

Fig. 6 Relationship between concentration of HAFP and amount of HAFP bound by rat peritoneal cells

It may be noted that at HAFP concentrations less than 0.25 ng/ml, both the amount of HAFP bound and binding capacity increases with HAFP concentration. At concentrations ranging from 0.25 ng to 1 ng per ml, the amount of HAFP bound remained constant (at 5.3×10^{-3}ng) but the binding capacity decreased (Fig. 5 $\overline{BC}$). One peritoneal cell binds approximately 8 molecules of HAFP. Taking peritoneal cells as roughly 80% macrophages, 1 macrophage cell binds approximately 10 molecules HAFP. At concentrations greater than 1 ng/ml, the amount bound increases again with AFP concentration (Fig. 6 $\overline{CD}$), but there is no change in binding capacity (Fig. 5 $\overline{CD}$).

When treated according to Boeynaems and Dumont (1975), ABC in Fig. 6 gives a dissociation constant of 2.5×10^{-12}M for HAFP to macrophage binding (Fig. 7). This value is obtained when log HAFP is plotted against f, where f equals number of receptor bound/maximum number of receptors bound or, more specifically, amount of HAFP bound/saturation value for amount HAFP bound. When f/HAFP is plotted against f, a concave curve like that shown in Fig. 8 is obtained.

7. Comparison of Binding Capacity of HAFP of Human Blister Cells and Rat Peritoneal Exudate Cells

The binding capacity of HAFP with human blister cells is found to be one order of magnitude stronger than that with rat peritoneal cells.

DISCUSSION

Human AFP is able to suppress phagocytosis by macrophages (Fig.1 & 2), the extent of suppression being proportional to its concentration.

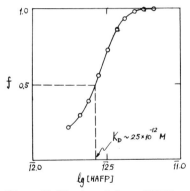
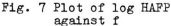

Fig. 7 Plot of log HAFP
against f

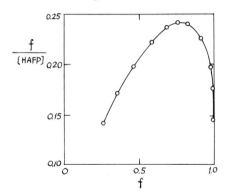

Fig. 8 Plot of f/HAFP
against f

Such an effect is not shared by HSA. AFP positive sera, however, also suppress macrophage phagocytosis, suggesting that AFP may be instrumental in weakening the immunological state of the patient.

With rat peritoneal exudate cells containing 70-80% macrophages as material, it has been possible to demonstrate the same type of effect (Table 2, Fig. 3). It has also been possible to demonstrate the attachment of HAFP to the surface of macrophages, suggesting the existence of receptors on macrophage membranes (Fig. 4). As shown in Fig. 5 & 6, the binding capacity of such cells increases with AFP concentration. However, on increasing AFP concentration above the saturation plateau, a second rise in binding capacity of a looser nature is indicated (CD portion of Fig. 6). From replacement experiments, it can be shown that such a looser binding is still much stronger than that of HSA. As shown in Fig. 7 & 8, the binding complex at low AFP concentrations has a K_D value of 2.5×10^{-12}M and shows a positive cooperative effect. The nature of the constituents on the macrophage cell as well as the exact domains on the AFP molecule responsible for the binding are targets of current investigation in our laboratory.

It has been shown that macrophage phagocytosis decreases in the cancerous state. The above experimental findings suggest the possibility for cancer cells to operate by liberating AFP molecules which in binding with specific receptors on the surface of macrophages render these cells insensitive to the presence of cancer cells (loss of cognitive capacity).

REFERENCES

Boeynaems, J.-M. & J.E. Dumont (1975). Hormone receptor interaction a theoretical approach to the experimental data. In Vokaer & De Bock (Eds), Reproductive Endocrinology, pp. 71-85. Pergamon Press, London.
Mizejewski, G.J. & P.M. Grimley (1976). Abortogenic activity of antiserum to alpha-fetoprotein. Nature 259,222-224.

Establishment of an Epithelioid Cell Line and a Fusiform Cell Line from a Patient with Nasopharyngeal Carcinoma

Laboratory of Tumor Viruses of Cancer Institute, Laboratory of Tumor Viruses of Institute of Virology, Department of Radiotherapy of Cancer Institute and Laboratory of Cell Biology of Cancer Institute, Chinese Academy of Medical Sciences, China

Laboratory of Electron Microscopy, Department of Microbiology and Laboratory of Pathogenesis, Chung Shan Medical College, China

ABSTRACT

An epithelioid cell line and a fusiform cell line were established from a tumor biopsy from a patient with nasopharyngeal carcinoma which was histologically diagnosed as a well differentiated squamous cell carcinoma. Based on studies of the cell growth pattern, chromosome analysis, heterotransplantation, and electron microscopy, these two cell lines were considered to be squamous carcinoma cells, and the fusiform cells might have originated from the epithelioid cells. There were many round cells on top of the epithelioid and fusiform cell sheets, many of which became continuously detached into the medium. No EB virus particle, early antigen or EBNA could be detected in this two cell lines.

INTRODUCTION

Extensive attempts have been made in establishing a permanent epithelial cell line from NPC patients in order to investigate further the relationship between EBV and NPC but no successful results have been reported (de-Thé and others, 1970, de-Thé, 1972, Trumper, Epstein and Giovanella, 1976). In our laboratory, we have succeeded in establishing an epithelioid cell line and a fusiform cell line from a patient with NPC. These cell lines have been maintained in culture for 3 years and subcultured for more than 100 times. This paper describes the establishment and the characteristics of these cell lines.

MATERIALS AND METHODS

The tissue used for cultures was obtained from a tumor biopsy from a 58-year-old woman with NPC on August 13, 1975. The patient had severe headache, tinnitus, and epistaxis. Clinical examination show-

ed the presence of a tumor in the nasopharynx which had invaded the
base of the skull, with compression signs of cranial nerves (III, IV,
IX, XII), and with metastases to the lymph nodes on both sides of the
neck. The soft tissue tumor mass on the posterior wall of nasopharynx was also confirmed on roentgenography. X-ray film of the
base of the skull showed suspected bony destruction of the left side
of the external plate of pterygoidal process of sphenoid. Tumor
biopsy revealed a well-differentiated squamous cell carcinoma.

The tumor specimen was cut into approximately 0.5-1.0 mm pieces.
Minced tumor fragments were placed on the surface of flasks which
had been pretreated with rat tail collagen to aid the attachment of
explants. RPMI 1640 medium supplemented with 40% of calf serum, 100
units of penicillin, and 100 μg of streptomycin per ml were added to
the flasks at the opposite side of the explants. The cultures were
incubated at 37°C for 3 hr in an incubator with 5% CO_2 in air, and
the flasks were turned over to allow the medium to cover the explants. The medium was changed twice a week. Subcultures were made
by dispersing the cells with 0.25% trypsin : 0.2% versene solution.

COURSE OF ESTABLISHMENT OF PERMANENT CELL LINES

Epithelioid cells began to outgrow around the tissue fragments in two
of the five flasks on the 10th day of cultivation, after which the
cell sheet increased in size gradually. Attempts to transfer the
epithelioid cells by dispersing part of the cell sheet with trypsin:
versene (0.25%:0.02%) or by scraping cells with capillary pipette
failed. The first successful subculture was made by trypsin: versene
11 weeks after cultivation. Thereafter the cells were successively
transferred once every week. Thus an epithelioid cell line designated as CNE was established. The epithelioid cells were polygonal
is shape with the nuclei varying in size. Some multinucleated giant
cells and cytoplasmic vacuoles were present. In old cultures some
cells frequently had part of the cytoplasm protruded and finally detached from the cell sheet as dead cells. At the 12th passage a few
fusiform cells appeared among the epithelioid cells and gradually
increased in number. The fusiform cells were isolated as an independent line and designated as CNF. There were many round cells on
the top of both cell sheets, especially on the fusiform ones. Many
of them became continuously detached into the medium. Cultures
initiated from the floating round cells recovered their original
epithelioid or fusiform cell morphology. No fibroblast cells appeared during the course of establishment of cell lines.

The CNE and CNF cells were dispersed by trypsin: versene (0.25%:0.2%)
and inoculated into separated dishes with 5 ml of medium containing
40, 20, and 10 cells respectively. Ten days after cultivation at
37°C in 5% CO_2, the typical clones of the epithelioid and fusiform
cells were isolated from dishes at terminal dilutions. This procedure was repeated twice. The clonal epithelioid and fusiform cell
lines thus obtained were designated as CNEC and CNFC respectively.
The epithelioid cell sheet was not as readily dispersed by trypsin:
versene (0.25%:0.02%) as fusiform cell sheet unless the concentration of versene was increased to 0.2%.

GROWTH CURVE, SATURATION DENSITY, AND PLATING EFFICIENCY

Monolayer cells of CNE and CNF cell lines were dispersed with trypsin and versene (0.25%:0.2%). 30 ml flasks were plated with 1×10^5 cells in 3.5 ml of complete RPMI 1640 medium. Cell cultures were kept at $37^{\circ}C$. The medium was changed and the cell counting from 2 flasks was performed every 3 days for 12 days. The effect of different concentrations of calf serum on the growth of both cell lines was studied. The growth curves of CNE and CNF cell lines were similar in media with 20% of calf serum. The cell number increased logarithmically on the 6th-9th day, reaching more than 20 times of that originally seeded. The growth rate of both cell lines in medium containing 5% of calf serum was slower. The cell number on the 12th day was 14-15 times of that originally seeded.

The value where two successive harvests showed no increase in cell number was taken as saturation density. The saturation densities of CNE and CNF cell lines were $2.13 \times 10^5/cm^2$ and $2.26 \times 10^5/cm^2$ respectively. The plating efficiencies of CNE and CNF cell lines were 22% and 52% respectively. The colonies of CNE cell consisting of epithelioid cells were uniform in size with regular margin, whereas the colonies of CNF consisting of fusiform cells showed variable size with irregular margin.

ASSAY OF AGGLUTINATION BY CONCANAVALIN-A

2×10^5 cells of CNE, CNF, CNEC, and CNFC cell lines in 3 ml of complete RPMI 1640 medium were plated into separate flasks and incubated at $37^{\circ}C$ for 24 hours. After washing twice with PBS lacking calcium and magnesium, the cells were dispersed with versene (0.02%), washed again with PBS, and then suspensed in PBS containing calcium and magnesium at a concentration of 4×10^5 cells per ml. 0.1 ml of concanavalin-A at different concentrations in PBS was mixed with 0.1 ml of the cell suspension in 100 x 12 mm tubes at room temperature for 30 minutes. The aggregates were scored under inverse microscope in a scale from – to ++++. Cells of all four lines could be agglutinated by 4 μg of concanavalin-A, and the size of the aggregates increased with the increasing concentrations of concanavalin-A.

CHROMOSOME ANALYSIS

Cell lines of the CNE (51st passage), CNEC (20th passage), CNF (34th & 38th passages), and CNFC (16th passage) were treated with colchicine (final concentration 0.02 μg/ml) for 2 4 hours during the logarithmic growing phase. The chromosome preparation was made according to an air-dried technique. 100-200 metaphase plates of each line were counted and chromosome aberrations also recorded.

Chromosome numbers of these cell lines showed a wide distribution with a mode between hypotriploid and hypotetraploid. Although the stemline of the CNEC and CNF cell lines was not formed, yet cells with chromosomes numbering over 100 appeared frequently. In the CNE cell line the mode accumulated between hypertriploid and hypotetraploid with a stemline of 80 chromosomes. For the CNFC cell line, a stemline of 70 chromosomes was noted at the 16th passage.

Various types of chromosome aberration, such as the dicentric, multicentric, fragmental, minute, and superfragmental, were observed in different cell lines. About 2-5% of chromosome aberrations occurred

in the CNE and CNFC cell lines. Besides other types of chromosome
aberration, dicentric chromosome was most frequently encountered in
the CNF cell line, accounting for 22% of all types. The dicentric,
fragmental, and minute types of chromosome aberration were frequently
observed in the CNFC cell line, 54% of them were classified as the
dicentric type.

HETEROTRANSPLANTATION

0.1 ml each of the CNE (33rd passage) and CNF (19th passage) cell
suspension were transplanted subcutaneously into newborn rats. Antithymocyte serum (0.4 ml) was given on the day of transplantation and
subsequently on the 3rd, 5th, and 8th days. 11 days after implantation the animals were sacrificed. The tumors measured 0.5-0.7 cm in
diameter and were examined histologically. The transplantability of
CNE and CNF was 77% and 100% respectively. Histologically, these
tumors were poorly differentiated squamous carcinoma.

ELECTRON MICROSCOPIC EXAMINATION

CNE and CNF cells were scraped off with a rubber policeman and centrifuged at 1000 rpm for 1-2 minutes. Cell pellets were fixed in 5%
gluteraldehyde followed by osmic acid, then embedded in butyl metha-
crylate. Thin-section specimens were stained with uranyl acetate
and lead citrate, and examined under electron microscope.

Electron microscopy showed that the CNE cells maintained typical
features of epithelial cells, including desmosomes, tonofibrils,
keratohyalin granules and membrane coating granules. The CNF cells
were polymorphic; some of them contained minute desmosomes and tono-
filaments, but not as typical as those seen in CNE cells. The ratio
of nucleus to cytoplasm of CNF cells was larger, and more endoplasmic
reticula, free ribosomes, and mitochondria were seen in the cytoplasm. It is rather difficult to identify the nature of some fusiform cells, so CNF cells are temporarily classified as poorly differentiated carcinoma cells.

No EB viral capsid antigen (VCA), early antigen (EA) or nuclear
antigen (EBNA) could be demonstrated in these cell lines by means of
complement fixation test, indirect immunofluorescence test and anti-
complement immunofluorescence test.

DISCUSSION

Based on studies of the cell growth pattern, chromosome analysis,
heterotransplantation, and electron microscopy, the CNE cell line
had the characteristics of epithelial cells and was confirmed to be
squamous carcinoma cells. The fusiform cells could not be seen in
cultures of the epithelioid cell line until the 12th passage. The
CNF cell line also had some characteristics of epithelial cells and
formed poorly differentiated squamous cell carcinoma in animals
treated with antithymocyte serum. Therefore, the fusiform cells
probably originated from the epithelioid cell line. Contamination
by other malignant epithelial cell line could be ruled out, because
no other epithelial cell line was present in our laboratory.

Many round cells were observed on the top of monolayer or multilayers

of the both cell lines, and became continuously detached into the
medium.   These floating cells, after seeding into another flask,
could grow into their original epithelioid cell or fusiform forms.
Since many patients with nasopharyngeal carcinoma had lymph node metastases in the neck region in the absence of notable tumor in the
nasopharynx when they first came to the outpatient clinic, the easy
detachment of cancer cells from the original tumor might be similar
to the phenomenon as observed in tissue culture. No EB virus particle or early antigen could be detected in these two cell lines
either treated or untreated with IUDR. These cell lines were established from an NPC patient with well differentiated squamous cell
carcinoma. This might be similar to the results as reported by
Klein and others (1974) who could not demonstrate EBV DNA, and EBNA
in the well-differentiated squamous carcinoma cells of NPC transplanted in nude mice. But Liang and others (1962) reported that
nasopharyngeal carcinomas showed, during their course of development,
a definite tendency to change their histological pattern, and did so
in a definite sequence, i.e. from highly differentiated type toward
poorly differentiated type and from poorly differentiated type toward
undifferentiated type. Even in the same biopsy specimen of the primary growth, different parts of the tumor revealed different histologic patterns. Our two cell lines formed poorly differentiated
squamous cell carcinoma in immunosuppressive animals. Whether there
are viral genome and its expression in these two cell lines or not
needs further study by other methods.

REFERENCES

de-Thé, G., H. C. Ho, H. C. Kwan, C. Desgranges and H. C. Favre
    (1970). Nasopharyngeal carcinoma (NPC). 1. Type of cultures
    derived from tumor biopsies and non-tumorous tissues of Chinese
    patients with special reference to lymphoblastoid transforma-
    tion. Int. J. Cancer, 6, 189-206.
de-Thé, G. (1972). Virology and immunology of nasopharyngeal carci-
    noma: Present situation and outlook - a Review. In Biggs, P.
    M., G. de-Thé and L. N. Payne (Eds), Oncogenesis and Herpes
    Virus, IARC, Lyon, pp 275-284.
Klein, G., B. C. Gioranella, T. Lindahl, P. J. Fialkow, S. Singh,
    and J. S. Stehlin (1974). Direct evidence for the presence of
    Epstein-Barr Virus DNA and nuclear antigen in malignant epi-
    thelial cell from patient, with poorly differentiated carcinoma
    of the nasopharynx. Proc. Nat. Acad. Sci. (USA). 71, 4737-4741.
Liang, P. C., C. C. Chen, C. C. Chu, Y. F. Hu, H. M. Chu, and Y. S.
    Tsung (1962). The histopathologic classification, biologic
    characteristics and histogenesis of nasopharyngeal carcinoma.
    Chinese M. J., 81, 629-658.
Trumper, P. A., M. A. Epstein, and B. C. Giovanella (1976). Acti-
    vation in vitro by BUdR of a productive EB virus infection in the
    epithelial cells of nasopharyngeal carcinoma. Int. J. Cancer,
    17, 578-587.

Index

The page numbers refer to the first page of the article in which the index term appears.